The Cult of Youth

In this major new study, James F. Stark provides the first historical account of the most dominant ideas, practices and material cultures associated with anti-ageing and rejuvenation in modern Britain. With a focus on the interwar period, his study uncovers the role of the commercial world in influencing attitudes towards ageing and youth. Stark argues that the technologies of anti-ageing, their commercialisation and their consumption made rejuvenation a possible and desirable aim in a period of sociopolitical instability, mechanised conflict and extending lifespans. Ultimately, Stark offers an innovative historical account which draws together bodies, gender, science, medicine, advertising and ageing, and shows how the quest for youth was transformed by social anxieties about an ageing population and economic crisis.

JAMES F. STARK is an historian of modern medicine and science and is Associate Professor of Medical Humanities at the University of Leeds.

The Cult of Youth

Anti-Ageing in Modern Britain

James F. Stark

University of Leeds

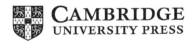

CAMBRIDGE
UNIVERSITY PRESS

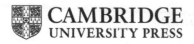

CAMBRIDGE
UNIVERSITY PRESS

Shaftesbury Road, Cambridge CB2 8EA, United Kingdom

One Liberty Plaza, 20th Floor, New York, NY 10006, USA

477 Williamstown Road, Port Melbourne, VIC 3207, Australia

314–321, 3rd Floor, Plot 3, Splendor Forum, Jasola District Centre, New Delhi – 110025, India

103 Penang Road, #05–06/07, Visioncrest Commercial, Singapore 238467

Cambridge University Press is part of Cambridge University Press & Assessment, a department of the University of Cambridge.

We share the University's mission to contribute to society through the pursuit of education, learning and research at the highest international levels of excellence.

www.cambridge.org
Information on this title: www.cambridge.org/9781108705974

DOI: 10.1017/9781108695428

First published 2020
First paperback edition 2022

A catalogue record for this publication is available from the British Library

Library of Congress Cataloging-in-Publication data
Names: Stark, James F., author.
Title: The cult of youth : anti-ageing in modern Britain / James F. Stark.
Description: Cambridge ; New York, NY : Cambridge University Press, 2020. |
    Includes bibliographical references and index.
Identifiers: LCCN 2019038306 (print) | LCCN 2019038307 (ebook) |
    ISBN 9781108484152 (hardback) | ISBN 9781108705974 (paperback) |
    ISBN 9781108695428 (epub)
Subjects: LCSH: Aging–Prevention–History. | Aging–Great Britain–History. |
    Youthfulness–Great Britain–History. | Medical innovations–Great Britain–History.
Classification: LCC RA776.75 .S773 2020 (print) | LCC RA776.75 (ebook) |
    DDC 612.6/70941–dc23
LC record available at https://lccn.loc.gov/2019038306
LC ebook record available at https://lccn.loc.gov/2019038307

ISBN   978-1-108-48415-2   Hardback
ISBN   978-1-108-70597-4   Paperback

Contents

List of Figures   *page* vi
Acknowledgements   viii

1   Introduction   1

2   Hormones, 1918–1929   24

3   Diet, 1918–1929   68

4   Electrotherapy, 1925–1932   106

5   Exercise, 1930–1939   138

6   Skin Care, 1930 and Beyond   170

7   Conclusion   205

8   Postscript   214

Bibliography   218
Index   248

Figures

1.1 'The Rejuvenator', as presented in the 1937 Blackpool
Illuminations. (Bolton Council Records, 1993.83.04.35.)   *page* 3
1.2 Elderly, infirm and disabled figures awaiting rejuvenation in
the 1937 Blackpool Illuminations. (Bolton Council Records,
1993.83.04.36.)   4
2.1 Before-and-after images of two patients featured in the Steinach Film.
(Peter Schmidt, *The Conquest of Old Age*, 1931, plate XXXV.)   43
2.2 Before-and-after images of a thirty-four-year-old technician,
one of Peter Schmidt's patients. (Peter Schmidt, *The Conquest
of Old Age*, 1931, plate XXXVII.)   44
2.3 An imagination of the social consequence of rejuvenation in
a number of contexts, from the pen of the illustrator Will Owen
(1869–1957). ('When All the World Is Young', *The Sketch*,
15 October 1919, 75.)   46
2.4 A rejuvenated old man, bearing a striking resemblance to an
aged Charles Darwin, dances with a young flapper on the cover
illustration of the satirical song, 'Be Rejuvenated'. (Annie Salter
and W. R. Barwick, *Be Rejuvenated*. Sydney: W. M. Nash, 1925,
front cover.)   52
2.5 A sketch printed as one of the 'Prize Jokes' in the *Ballymena
Weekly Telegraph*. ('Prize Jokes' *Ballymena Weekly Telegraph*,
2 February 1929, 5.)   56
3.1 An advertisement for Yeast-Vite demonstrating its supposed effects,
promoting models of both male and female health, happiness and,
crucially, productivity. ('Yeast-Vite and YOUR health register',
Aberdeen Press and Journal, 19 October 1929, 5.)   96
4.1 Patent images showing Otto Overbeck's US patent for an electric
body comb. (Otto Overbeck, 'Electric Body Comb', US Patent
1,638, 407, 9 August 1927.)   116
4.2 An outline of a large-scale, clinical electrotherapy device.
(Chisholm Williams, *High-Frequency Currents in the Treatment
of Some Diseases*. New York: Rebman Company, 1903, 130.)   121

4.3 Violet Ray was also the stage name of a popular singer during
the 1920s. ('An old lady asking her doctor about "Violet Ray"
referring to high-frequency rays. Reproduction of a drawing
after H.M. Brock, 1925', reproduced by permission of the
Wellcome Collection CC BY.)   125
4.4 Peter Schmidt included images of various rejuvenation devices,
including the Vienna Youth Mask, which deployed similar techniques
to those used in the female Steinach Operation. (Peter Schmidt,
*The Conquest of Old Age: Methods to Effect Rejuvenation and to
Increase Functional Activity.* London: George Routledge &
Son, 1931, plate XXXIX.)   130
5.1 Muller's family were typically included as demonstrators of the
stretches, in a manner later mirrored by mother and daughter,
Mary and Prunella Bagot Stack, in the context of the Women's
League of Health and Beauty. (J. P. Muller, *My System: 15 Minutes'
Exercise a Day for Health's Sake.* London: Athletic Publications
Ltd., c.1925, 67.)   143
5.2 Abplanalp's devices were marketed as a way of extending his
exercise regimen rather than an essential component. (Arthur
Abplanalp, 'Exercising Apparatus for use in a Lying Position',
US Patent 1,144,085, 22 June 1915, 1.)   147
5.3 Brochures outlining beauty regimes often contextualised these
within a broader sweep of lifestyle habits which were also
said to influence the complexion. ('Beauty', 1935, 1,
WBA/BT/11/40/4/1/1, Boots Company Archive.)   163
6.1 Advertisement for Aspinall's Neigeline highlighting its
beneficial action on the complexion and rejuvenating effects.
('Aspinall's "Neigeline"', (March 1895), Beauty Parlour 3 (33) –
Cosmetics, John Johnson Collection, available online at:
http://gateway.proquest.com/openurl?url_ver=Z39.88-2004&res_
dat=xri:jjohnson:&rft_dat=xri:jjohnson:rec:20080218142229kw,
accessed 26 January 2018)   173
6.2 The first British advertisement for Helena Rubinstein's Hormone
Twin Youthifiers. ('An Amazing Discovery – A Triumph of
Beauty Science', *The Bystander*, 4 May 1932, 245.)   180
6.3 A 1936 advertisement for Dubarry's Nuglandin Cream, printed in
the high-end British periodical *The Tatler*. ('Nuglandin Cream',
The Tatler, 4 March 1936, 35.)   184
6.4 A typical advertisement in the British press for Number Seven
products. ('Loveliness that Defeats the Years',
WBA/BT/11/45/1/1/10, c.1938, Boots Company Archive).   188

Acknowledgements

There are too many people to thank.

My colleagues, past and present, in the School of Philosophy, Religion and History of Science at the University of Leeds, particularly those in the Centre for the History and Philosophy of Science, have been singularly supportive, and the best critical friends. I thank particularly Graeme Gooday, Jon Topham, Greg Radick, Claire Jones, Adrian Wilson and Mike Finn, whose insightful contributions have helped to shape my ideas in ways which I would never have considered.

Over the course of the last few years, countless fellow researchers have offered helpful and hugely constructive suggestions, comments and critiques when I took this material on the road. I am grateful to all who attended sessions at meetings around the world, and especially to my compatriots on the New Generations in Medical Humanities programme, who put up with periodic babbling about skin creams and testicle transplants for a year when the project was in its germinal stages.

I have been fortunate enough to secure support from the Arts and Humanities Research Council and the Wellcome Trust, whose financial assistance has been critical in enabling this programme of research. Further support from the School of Philosophy, Religion and History of Science covered reproduction rights for the images so critical to this story.

Staff at the Boots Company Archive – in particular Sophie Clapp and Judith Wright – have been unfailing in their support for this research, guiding me through their collections and offering that winning combination of expertise and tea so generously. Similarly, I would like to thank Alan Humphries and Joanne Bartholomew from the Thackray Medical Museum in Leeds, whose insight into their electrotherapy collections first inspired me to pursue the topic. As ever, librarians and archivists at Wellcome Library, Unilever Archives, the Mass Observation Archive, British Library and National Library of Scotland have made the process of research incredibly enjoyable.

There are too many others whose ideas and suggestions have been instrumental in shaping this book for the better, but at the risk of omission I would like to thank Nick Hopwood, Mark Jackson, Vanessa Heggie and Iwan Morus for their reflections, all of which opened up productive new avenues of inquiry.

I would also like to thank Lucy Rhymer, Emily Sharp, Lisa Carter and their colleagues at Cambridge University Press for being enthused by the project from the outset, and for their patience during the completion of the manuscript, as well as two anonymous readers who provided detailed and extremely constructive suggestions for improvement.

Finally, the book would have come nowhere near completion without the love and support of my family, especially my partner, Kristina, my mum, Gillian, and my son, Elliot, who gives joyous, daily reminders about what real youthfulness looks like. Thank you.

1   Introduction

In 1941, in the teeth of a second unprecedented and devastating global conflict, George Orwell published an essay, 'The Art of Donald McGill', which included a critical commentary on the saucy British seaside postcard.[1] He used these ubiquitous features of costal visits as a window into British social relations. Orwell considered the postcards to be highly revealing, even if they were possessed of 'an utter low-ness of mental atmosphere', as they inspired a feeling of 'indefinable familiarity' through reliance on the conventions of sex, marriage and politics, with the humour of drunkenness and 'inter-working-class snobbery' featuring heavily in the genre. Sex, marriage, drunkenness, home life and 'inter-working-class snobbery' were mainstays of the genre.[2]

Amongst his witty and irreverent critique of these postcards, which led a 'barely legal existence in cheap stationers' windows', Orwell also reflected on the appearance of signs of ageing, made visible in themes explored by McGill, which it is important to quote at length:

One of the few authentic class-differences ... still existing in England is that the working classes age very much earlier. They do not live less long, provided that they survive their childhood, nor do they lose their physical activity earlier, but they do lose very early their youthful appearance ... It is usual to attribute this to the harder lives that the working classes have to live, but it is doubtful whether any such difference now exists as would account for it. More probably the truth is that the working classes reach middle age earlier because they accept it earlier. For to look young after, say, thirty is largely a matter of wanting to do so. This generalization is less true of the better-paid workers ... they are more traditional, more in accord with the Christian past than the well-to-do women who try to stay young at forty by means of physical-jerks, cosmetics and avoidance of child-bearing. *The impulse to cling to youth at all costs, to attempt to preserve your sexual attraction, to see even in middle age a future for yourself and not merely for your children, is a thing of recent growth and has only precariously established itself.*[3]

---

[1] The piece appeared in *Horizon*, a short-lived but influential periodical which during its run from 1940 to 1949 included contributions from W. H. Auden, T. S. Eliot and Barbara Hepworth. See Orwell, *The Art of Donald McGill*.
[2] Orwell, *The Art of Donald McGill*.   [3] Ibid., emphasis added.

At the heart of this remarkable reflection on the social conventions surrounding ageing and the life course is Orwell's characterisation of defying ageing as a relatively recent phenomenon, which encompassed exercise, skin care and – at least for women – remaining child-free. Implicit in his commentary is a division of rejuvenation practices on grounds of both gender and class; men are discussed in the context of military service, where of those registering 'the middle- and upper-class members look, on average, ten years younger than the others'. Meanwhile, women were seemingly concerned with actively warding off the onset of signs associated with ageing, at least in part, to maintain their attractiveness; relatedly, '[s]ex-appeal vanishes at about the age of twenty-five. Well-preserved and good-looking people beyond their first youth are never represented [in postcards].'[4] Finally, for Orwell, the ability of someone over the age of thirty to achieve continued youthfulness was mostly dependent on their motivation – the implication here was that the products, procedures and habits necessary to preserve youthful appearance were available, accessible and effective in bringing about the desired effects.

Orwell's perspective on rejuvenation in Britain was linked to its emergence as a major social phenomenon over the preceding decades. In 1937, for example, the famous Blackpool illuminations featured "The Rejuvenator" (see Figures 1.1 and 1.2) – a magical device, created from lights, by which the elderly, infirm and disabled were transformed to become lithe, agile and youthful. Pamphlets, books, magazine articles, skin care products, surgical procedures and electrical appliances dedicated to the pursuit of agelessness came to prominence in interwar Britain in a way that was unforeseeable at the outset of the twentieth century. In an increasingly visual climate populated by photographs and film, the need to maintain markers of youthfulness gained greater social and cultural significance. The fantastical possibilities of rejuvenation also found expression in various forms of fiction, from novels to Hollywood films. This trend also manifested at a local level. For example, the 1935 film 'Quest for Youth', produced by members of the Tees-side Cine Club, highlighted a particularly middle-class anxiety associated with being unable to keep up with the 'young crowd'. In the film, an ageing woman's attempt to recapture her youth with the aid of a new chemical anti-ageing substance – known only as '596' – proves unsuccessful, although ultimately she is able to reconcile herself to having only one period of "true" youthfulness, having found the supposed miracle of modern science to be wanting.[5]

---

[4] Ibid.

[5] 'Quest for Youth', dir. C. Roeder, Tees-Side Cine Club, 1935. The nomenclature of '596' was undoubtedly a conscious mirroring of the hyperbolic curative expectations associated with Salvarsan – a new drug brought to market in the early 1910s as the first effective treatment for syphilis, and which medical practitioners hailed widely as the harbinger of a therapeutic revolution, and which was also known simply as compound '606'.

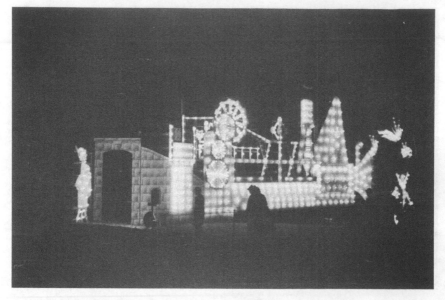

Figure 1.1 'The Rejuvenator', as presented in the 1937 Blackpool
Illuminations.
Source: Bolton Council Records, 1993.83.04.35

The visibility of rejuvenation and the myriad strategies for achieving it was
not unique to Britain, yet it has been uniquely neglected. *The Cult of Youth*
focusses on the British case in a period characterised by major social shifts
elsewhere in Europe and the United States, where the significance of health
and efficiency movements and their connection to ageing has long been
recognised. For interwar Germany, for example, Geoffrey Cocks and Michael
Hau have implicated the rise of youth culture and the impact of political
upheaval in the emergence of a highly racialised aesthetic which determined
desirable qualities of health and beauty in both men and women.[6] Against the
backdrop of what Carsten Timmermann identified as a 'crisis of medicine' in
the Weimar era, this was realised through the popularisation of mass physical
culture and dietary changes and underpinned gendered understandings of the
ideal functionality of male and female bodies.[7] In part, the significant move

[6] Cocks, *The State of Health*; Hau, *The Cult of Health and Beauty in Germany*; Usborne, *The
Politics of the Body in Weimar Germany*. For more on the emergence of physical prowess and
youthfulness in interwar Germany, see Jensen, *Body by Weimar*.
[7] Timmermann, 'Rationalizing "Folk Medicine" in Interwar Germany', 459–82. For a comprehensive account of how female bodies came under the gaze of the medical profession in a new way
in the first half of the twentieth century, see Mitchinson, *Body Failure*.

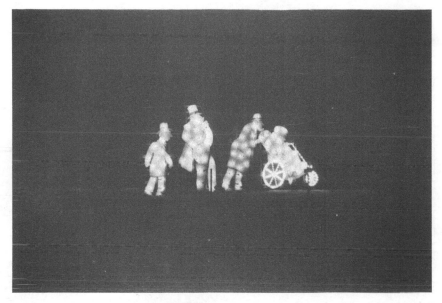

Figure 1.2 Elderly, infirm and disabled figures awaiting rejuvenation in the 1937 Blackpool Illuminations.
Source: Bolton Council Records, 1993.83.04.36

away from adherence to mainstream medicine in interwar Germany can be seen as a wider rejection of mechanism, accompanied by a concurrent reengagement with holistic concepts of mind, body and self.[8] Simultaneously, as Chad Ross has noted, the increasingly popular concept of *Nacktkultur* 'offered every German ... the possibility of establishing and regulating her or his own health; no doctors or other medical professionals were necessary'.[9] Whilst the interwar context of the Weimar Republic and subsequent National Socialism of Germany has therefore been the subject of a number of studies highlighting its supposed exceptional focus on rejuvenation at the level of the society, these ideas also gained considerable currency elsewhere.[10]

---

[8] Timmermann, 'Constitutional Medicine', 717–39. For a more general account of holism in German science during the Weimar period, see: Harrington, *Reenchanted Science*; Ash, *Gestalt Psychology*.

[9] Ross, *Naked Germany*, 83.

[10] Jensen, *Body by Weimar*; Ross, *Naked Germany*. Similar movements also gained traction elsewhere in Continental Europe and, to a lesser extent, in Britain. See: Tumblety, *Remaking the Male Body*; Jobs, *Riding the New Wave*; McDevitt, *May the Best Man Win*. A roughly analogous study for Britain, though concentrating more on the female body, is Zweiniger-Bargielowska, *Managing the Body*.

Meanwhile, the United States has been characterised as the cradle of commerce, where marketing and advertising campaigns for skin care products and fringe electrotherapy devices were pioneered and where dietary and exercise regimes became part of national culture, with other countries eventually following suit.[11] Work by Jessica M. Jahiel and Julia Rechter has revealed how the American Medical Association mounted a concerted campaign to discredit those peddling fringe rejuvenation practices, products and procedures, whilst also highlighting the extensive influence of rejuvenation-driven endocrinology on popular discourse about bodies, gender and sex.[12] Although the British Medical Association was far more cautious about publicly denouncing rejuvenation practitioners, major figures in the United States such as the physical culture advocate Bernarr Macfadden and the high-profile, fraudulent gland-grafter John R. Brinkley had almost exact analogues in Britain in exercise guru Eugene Sandow and controversial aesthetic surgeon Charles E. Willi. Debates about the authenticity of rejuvenation treatments and the credentials of their purveyors lay at the heart of public discourse; publications promoting these therapies sat at the intersection between medical text-books, popular scientific tracts and unashamed self-promotion and advertising.

Spanning national boundaries yet understood and practised in an almost impossible variety of ways, rejuvenation was inescapably associated with the scientific possibilities and social anxieties of the interwar period. Around the turn of the twentieth century the mainstream scientific ideas of August Weismann, Jacques Loeb and Alexis Carrel had provided complementary reasons to suppose that mortality and senescence were not necessarily an essential consequence of life.[13] In an era scarred by conflict and financial depression the prospect of enhancing youthfulness for economic, social and military security was appealing from the level of the individual to the state. Although the goal for some in seeking rejuvenation was a prolongation of life, arguably a more pressing imperative was to preserve youthfulness for as long as possible, overcoming senescence and enabling citizens to lead active, productive lives into older age.[14] The desire to retain physical and mental acuity had inspired Mrs Theodore Parsons – Matilda I. Cruice Parsons – to

---

[11] Verbrugge, *Active Bodies*.

[12] Jahiel, 'Rejuvenation Research'; Rechter, 'The Glands of Destiny'.

[13] Weismann's 1893 theory of heredity had emphasised the continuity of the germplasm. Weismann, *The Germ-Plasm*. In the early 1900s, Carrel was certainly part of mainstream science, and although his work on cellular immortality would later be widely discredited, we should resist the temptation to label him as anything other than a part of the established scientific community in the period in question.

[14] In this respect, parallels with the far more recent phenomenon of active ageing are striking. The World Health Organisation defines active ageing as 'the process of optimizing opportunities for health, participation and security in order to enhance quality of life as people age . . . [enabling] people to realize their potential for physical, social, and mental well-being throughout the

publish a wide-ranging popular book on the subject in 1912, *Brain Culture through Scientific Body Building*. Parsons was Physical Director of Schools in Chicago at the time, and she advocated the expansion of routinised physical education, whilst deriding existing programmes of competitive sport.[15] Her ideas were not taken up widely at the time, but her message of the virtues of movement for women had greater resonance following the US declaration of war on Germany on 6 April 1917. As reported in the *Pittsburgh Press* just four days later, in a speech in New York Parsons argued that '[t]he best part of a woman's life begins at forty', exhorting women to 'train for the special duties which may devolve upon them in war time'.[16] This, the first use of the phrase 'life begins at forty', later popularised by Walter Pitkin in his seminal 1932 manual *Life Begins at Forty*, exemplified a pressing and new need for older women and men, and returning soldiers, to extract the maximum possible value from their bodies for the benefit of their families and wider society.

In the case of Britain, we know already from the work of Kay Heath that the later Victorian period saw the emergence of middle age as a genuine time of anxiety. Rather than heralding maturity and experience, by the end of the nineteenth century the onset of middle age was accompanied by new fears of degeneration.[17] Similarly, across a large body of work, Margaret Gullette has revealed through analysis of literary sources the depth of concerns about ageing and the construction of a 'decline narrative' that dominated discussions of midlife and old age throughout the twentieth century on both sides of the Atlantic.[18] In *Declining to Decline*, Gullette identifies a deeply engrained master narrative of bodily decline across the life course, not actual loss of physical and mental capacities, as being responsible for our negative experiences and perceptions of ageing.[19] Set against this backdrop, *The Cult of Youth* uncovers a key role for commercial strategies which both responded to and reshaped experiences of ageing and our efforts to combat it during the turbulent socio-economic events of the first half of the twentieth century.

It is a near-fruitless task to determine whether any of the numerous different methods of rejuvenation which are contained in these pages had any perceptible effect on health or longevity, even though some of the ideas which I explore – such as caloric restriction, fasting and regular exercise – are

lifecourse and to participate in society'. World Health Organisation, 'What Is Active Ageing?', 2019, www.who.int/ageing/active_ageing/en/.

[15] Parsons, *Brain Culture*.

[16] 'Now Is the Time for All Women to Train for the Duties that War Time May Bring', *The Pittsburgh Press*, 10 April 1917, 20.

[17] Heath, *Aging by the Book*.

[18] Gullette, *Safe at Last in the Middle Years*; Gullette, *Aged by Culture*.

[19] Gullette, *Declining to Decline*, 4.

currently held up as effective methods for the prolongation of life.[20] Rather, my focus is on the motivations of would-be rejuvenators, how they attempted to persuade consumers to both literally and figuratively buy into their ideas, and what this can tell us about our changing relationship with ageing and old age. This is an account of how and why anxious agers tried a range of ways to slow, stop or reverse the ageing process, focussing on transformations during and around the interwar period.[21] Such efforts were a conscious attempt to subvert the established, intractable, linear life course of the Western tradition, which codified specific features of childhood, adolescence, adulthood and old age, as outlined by Steven Mintz in *The Prime of Life*.

Mintz argues that late nineteenth-century America witnessed the concretisation of old age as a definite life stage, marked by cognitive decline and social isolation.[22] We might, then, be tempted to read the popularity of attempts to rejuvenate ageing and ailing bodies in the first half of the twentieth century as indicators of a societal response to concerns about the social burden of under-productive human units. However, the events explored in *The Cult of Youth* also took place in a biomedical paradigm informed by Alexis Carrel's claim in 1912 that he had been able to keep tissues derived from a chicken alive, under laboratory conditions, far beyond the natural life span of the animal, and before the Hayflick limit – first mooted in 1961 and coined as a term in 1974 – seemed to confirm the inescapability of mortality.[23] Allied to the work of Carrel, would-be rejuvenators of the interwar period were able to draw on a range of emerging and highly fashionable scientific ideas about bodily function, including the vying physiological control mechanisms of the endocrine and nervous systems, and the seemingly extraordinary power of tiny quantities of vitamins to govern metabolic processes. As Hyung Wook Park has recently noted, a new and supposed scientific mastery of both early and later life in the decades around 1900 promised to make biological ageing a contingent phenomenon rather than a necessary feature of life. This represented a concerted attempt to understand the conditions of ageing as a distinct set of physiological, pathological and social circumstances, and was professionalised in the

---

[20] Omodei and Fontana, 'Calorie Restriction and Prevention', 1537–42; Spindler, 'Biological Effects of Calorie Restriction', 367–438.

[21] Chandak Sengoopta has characterised the 1920s as 'the decade of rejuvenation', not just in Britain but throughout the Western world. Sengoopta, 'Dr Steinach Coming to Make Old Young', 122–6.

[22] Mintz, *The Prime of Life*.

[23] For Carrel's original publication, see: Carrel, 'On the Permanent Life', 516–28; Hayflick and Moorhead, 'The Serial Cultivation of Human Diploid Cell Strains', 585–612. Historical treatments of rejuvenation in its myriad forms in this transformative period have been notably lacking. Eric J. Trimmer – himself a proponent of rejuvenation, as exemplified by his 1965 book, *Live Long and Stay Young* – stands as one of the only contributors to consider multiple forms of rejuvenation. See: Trimmer, *Rejuvenation*; Trimmer, *Live Long and Stay Young*.

emergence of the scientific and medical specialties of gerontology and geriatric medicine respectively.[24]

Such efforts came against an increasing awareness of, and resistance to, the concept of senescence and the natural ageing process. As Thomas Cole has explored, focussing on middle-class culture in Europe and North America, the two centuries preceding World War One saw the life course undergo gradual but profound changes as a result of increasing secularisation, scientific developments and a focus on the individual.[25] Here I trace how the effects of these shifts associated with ageing impacted on the ways in which social groups attempted to mitigate its effects and show how scientific claims about rejuvenation were presented by manufacturers and figures of supposed expertise both within and beyond the mainstream medical and scientific communities.

As well as the optimistic biomedical atmosphere cultivated by apparent breakthroughs, such as those associated with Carrel, intergenerational anxieties, including the powerful worry in *fin-de-siècle* Britain that young boys had been failed by their fathers, contributed to the sense of moral panic around lost youth and youthfulness in the early twentieth century.[26] 'Contraventions of the moral law' were for many as much a source of concern as the biological ageing process.[27] The increasing life span in North America and Western Europe, though also visible in other parts of the world, brought with it admiration for public health reforms of the nineteenth century, whilst also increasing concerns about the potential social and cultural upheaval engendered by radical demographic changes. Following World War One, with many of the supposedly healthiest and fittest young men killed during a destructive and heavily technologised conflict, gaze turned quickly to various levels of society – the race, family and individual – as a possible source of social, economic and biological regeneration. As Ina Zweiniger-Bargielowska has noted, the decline in family size in Britain during the first decades of the twentieth century provided a critical backdrop to a so-called depopulation panic. This translated into more generalised worries about the changing role of women in society, a decline of fertility and virility in men, and the future economic productivity of the nation.[28] Meanwhile the call from David Lloyd George to both restore the physical fitness of the nation and to 'give elderly folk a pension and a snug home' spoke to concerns about the extent to which younger men and women could both remain economically productive into later life and expect a secure, healthy retirement.[29]

The craze for rejuvenation did not, however, emerge solely in response to social anxieties, although concerns about the fitness of society, its fertility and

---

[24] Park, *Old Age, New Science*, especially 36–41.   [25] Cole, *The Journey of Life*.
[26] Olsen, *Juvenile Nation*.   [27] Bodley Scott, *The Road to a Healthy Old Age*, 7.
[28] Zweiniger-Bargeilowska, *Managing the Body*, 257.   [29] Lloyd George, 'Foreword', 5.

productivity were important motivating factors. These concerns were coupled with critical changes in scientific understanding of humans and animals from the first decade of the twentieth century, as well as the publication of a wide range of manuals designed to improve everyday health and ward off the onset of old age. There was also a strong continuation of late nineteenth-century traditions, such as domestic electrotherapy, vegetarianism and the emerging therapeutic approach termed organotherapy which depended on the work of Charles Brown-Séquard, modified during the early decades of the twentieth century.[30] The financial crash and Great Depression which followed were also fundamental, transforming the economic and social conditions within which rejuvenation operated. The resulting proliferation of self-help and domestic health manuals, in both the United States and Britain, provided fertile ground for manufacturers to promote new products and reconfigure existing therapies.[31]

Internationally, the proliferation of ideas about rejuvenation and how it might be achieved was uneven. Major centres of rejuvenation research, such as Paris and Vienna, which hosted figureheads in the field – Serge Voronoff and Eugen Steinach, respectively – acquired a reputation which stretched far beyond medical science; they became associated elsewhere with youthfulness, vigour and a reconfiguring of social norms. Both were places of scientific research where new procedures were rejuvenating the aged, but also sites of societal flourishing which promised to banish lassitude, old age and infirmity.

Chandak Sengoopta has argued that 'the history of rejuvenation research, like the history of science in general, reveals a complex interplay of rationality, gullibility and sheer folly.'[32] Focussing primarily on the work of medical practitioners and biologists – especially Elié Metchnikoff, Eugen Steinach and Serge Voronoff – Sengoopta's sphere of interest covers professional and public life of scientific rejuvenation, almost exclusively hormone treatments which came to prominence in the interwar period. On this basis he asserts that

---

[30] Organotherapy, for example, was a source of great inspiration for the hormone rejuvenators of the early twentieth century and the subject of the 1902 Hunterian Oration at the Hunterian Society in London, delivered by Arthur T. Davies, the son of noted English physician Herbert Davies. See Davies, 'The Hunterian Oration on Organo-Therapy', 1089–96. For more on Brown-Séquard, including his own account of the physiological effects of injecting fluids extracted from the testicles of animals (Brown-Séquard himself never claimed to have produced rejuvenating effects from his procedures), see: Brown-Séquard, 'The Effects Produced on Man', 105–7; Celestin, *Charles-Edouard Brown-Séquard*. As Jessica Jahiel has argued, organotherapy gained far greater traction in Europe than in the United States, although the situation in Britain is arguably different again, with less commitment to the ideas behind and practice of this brand of therapy. Jahiel, 'Rejuvenation Research', 86.

[31] Currell, 'Depression and Recovery', 131–44.

[32] Sengoopta, 'Rejuvenation and the Prolongation of Life', 55.

the 1920s was 'the decade of rejuvenation', a period dominated by public fascination with the quest to live longer, healthier and more youthful lives.[33] Angus McLaren's wide-ranging study, *Reproduction by Design*, likewise focusses closely on interwar Britain as a site where concern about the relationship between reproduction, fertility and modernisation combined to produce new forms of professional and public fascination with the human body and its longevity.[34] Sources from the period, however, suggest that attempts to restore or preserve youthfulness were far more wide-ranging, cutting across a swathe of lifestyle factors, medical interventions and devices. For example, in *Life Begins at Forty*, published at the outset of the self-help boom in 1932, Pitkin argued that the clear boundaries 'between youth and age' were fading in consequence of 'the Machine Age', citing changing habits in diet, employment, leisure, exercise and family life amongst numerous factors and motivations for remaining young and vigorous.[35]

The significance of this historical moment for rejuvenation in the United States has been recognised by Julia Rechter who argues that '[w]hile there were few entirely negative assessments of rejuvenation experiments published in the teens and twenties, by the 1930s, more skeptical reports began to proliferate. ... It was a collection of factors, cultural and scientific, which caused a dampening of popular enthusiasm for the hormones in the 1930s.'[36] However the story is even more complex than the varied and subtle landscape of hormone treatments and their impacts painted by Sengoopta, Rechter and other scholars, including Nelly Oudshoorn; hormones were just one aspect of a diverse range of strategies claimed to slow, stop or even reverse various aspects of the ageing process, from the appearance of wrinkles to a loss of sexual potency.[37] Only when we expand our view to consider how endocrinology intersected with and inspired other forms of rejuvenation can we get a more complete picture of the significance of hormones and their social and biological significance. Indeed, as McLaren has suggested, it was a period during which 'discussions of sexuality, reproduction, endocrinology, eugenics and environmentalism were hopelessly entangled', to which we must add a range of other factors, including commercialism, economic productivity, the invisible electrical forces at work in matter, and demographic stability.[38]

Meanwhile, other scholarly accounts, such as Helen Small's consideration of the relationship between ageing and philosophical thought, have

---

[33] Sengoopta, 'Dr Steinach', 122.   [34] McLaren, *Reproduction by Design*, 2.
[35] Pitkin, *Life Begins at Forty*, 4.   [36] Rechter, 'The Glands of Destiny', 214.
[37] Sengoopta, *The Most Secret Quintessence*; Oudshoorn, *Beyond the Natural Body*.
[38] McLaren, *Reproduction by Design*, 2.

disregarded the importance of rejuvenation as a social, biological or intellectual phenomenon.[39] Whilst Small creates a series of illuminating relationships between ageing and aspects of philosophy not generally considered to be of relevance, the marginalisation of rejuvenation therefore leaves a significant aspect of human ageing unexplored.[40] Such approaches, perhaps informed by the status of rejuvenation as a key part of popular culture, do not therefore take into consideration what light attempts to retain or recapture youth might shed on social attitudes towards ageing and the aged.

Discussions about rejuvenation during this transformative period were not peripheral to either mainstream scientific practice or social debate. They touched on some of the most pressing issues of the day, such as the fitness of populations, economic productivity and the nature of ageing, beauty and sexuality. In 1926, at what was arguably the height of the craze for rejuvenation, for example, a prominent advocate, Carl Ramus, wrote that 'the aging process which so soon depreciates and mars human bodies is not Divine Dispensation or Natural Necessity but a *chronic disease*'.[41] Others contended that the necessity of scientific rejuvenation arose from an environment where 'anxiety or over-fatigue' caused premature ageing of the skin, accompanied by a loss of beauty.[42] These were not new concerns – even a cursory glance at mid-nineteenth-century texts such as *Hufeland's Art of Prolonging Life* (1849) reveals 'prudent physical education ... sleep ... [and] mental tranquillity' amongst a host of common factors promoting a long and healthful life – but they were transformed in reciprocal relationships with innovations in medical science, commercialism and socio-economic upheaval.[43]

To achieve a comprehensible account of an era which witnessed a rapid and chaotic expansion of rejuvenation methods, some rational selection is clearly required. I take as an important part of my inspiration an early, authoritative and comprehensive text on the subject, Hermann Weber's *On Longevity and Means for the Prolongation of Life*. In this work, first published in English in 1919 and prefaced by Sir Clifford Allbutt, Weber concluded with 'the more important advice' for achieving a rejuvenated state. His advice included 'regular daily walks, rise, respiratory and other exercise ... moderation in eating, drinking, and all bodily enjoyments' and means 'to promote a healthy condition of the skin'.[44] Later the same year, hormonal intervention joined these long-standing non-naturals in spectacular fashion as a possible means of being rejuvenated, whilst both vitamin science and endocrinology, in turn,

---

[39] Significant works in the field which do not include consideration of rejuvenation in relation to ageing include: Cole, Van Tassel and Kastenbaum eds., *Handbook of the Humanities and Aging*; Steans, *Old Age in European Society*; Johnson and Thane eds., *Old Age from Antiquity*.
[40] Small, *The Longer Life*.   [41] Ramus, *Outwitting Middle Age*, vi.
[42] Willi, *Facial Rejuvenation*, viii.   [43] Wilson ed., *Hufeland's Art of Prolonging Life*, viii.
[44] Weber, *On Longevity*, 261.

inspired the development of a huge range of new rejuvenating skin care products from the late 1920s. Accordingly, five major methods which aspiring rejuvenators of the early twentieth century sought to harness – hormone treatments, electrotherapy, skin care, dietary regimes and exercise plans – dominate the story.[45] Whether bodies were being suffused with electricity or deprived of food for days on end, interwar Britain was a place where homes became laboratories for self-experimentation to test both the fantastical and modest claims which physicians, entrepreneurs and companies made for their products.

The case of rejuvenation also serves to further erode any lingering meaningful distinctions between 'mainstream' and 'alternative' approaches to medicine, and even some aspects of scientific practice.[46] One might expect that the scientific establishment generally presented a highly sceptical face to claims about elixirs of life, philosophers' stones and techniques for everlasting youth, yet many promoters of rejuvenation techniques and therapies were part of and gained traction within the orthodox scientific community.[47] Indeed, some of the foundational work in modern endocrinology emerged from research into hormonal rejuvenation which, shortly after being hailed by a significant cross-section of researchers and practitioners, became little more than a whipping child of medical hyperbole. Similarly, the variety of new rejuvenating electrotherapy devices available for purchase through the interwar period mirrored many earlier developments in mainstream, professional electrotherapy, and near-identical devices were pressed into service in clinics and major hospitals.

There has been a remarkable persistence of different rejuvenation methods over time, and the resulting marketplace is largely cyclical; as the popularity of one therapy or product wanes, another takes its place, often drawing on centuries-old mythology for marketing or manufacturing. The place and period with which this book is principally concerned – Britain between the world wars – offers just a glimpse into the world of rejuvenation.[48] In an era which

---

[45] 'Fighting Father Time: A Beauty Parlour Peep', 27 July 1922, www.britishpathe.com/video/fighting-father-time-a-beauty-parlour-peep.

[46] Cooter ed., *Studies in the History of Alternative Medicine*.

[47] For example: Elié Mechnikoff (1845–1916), discussed in more detail in Chapter 3, received the Nobel Prize for Physiology or Medicine – jointly with Paul Ehrlich – in 1908; Alexis Carrel (1873–1944), whose work on transplantation and in vitro tissue longevity we have already encountered briefly, and who reappears in Chapter 2, received the Prize in 1912. Aspects of the modern field of 'anti-ageing medicine' – beyond my purview here, but highly significant later in the twentieth century – have recently been explored by Aimee Medeiros and Elizabeth Siegel Watkins. See Medeiros and Watkins, 'Live Longer Better', 333–59.

[48] For more general accounts of British interwar social, political and economic culture, see: Constantine, *Social Conditions in Britain*; Bingham, *Gender, Modernity and the Popular Press*.

Richard Overy has identified as being populated with 'despair or helplessness or sober pessimism', particularly amongst higher social classes and those most at-risk in a context of a possible collapse of social order, or even the human race, the small cross-section of selected rejuvenation theories, products and practices which gained popularity during this period offer important insights into how youthfulness came to be so highly prized.[49]

The central driving question is this: How and why did different rejuvenation strategies come to prominence in interwar Britain in the way they did, and what was their impact on public and professional understandings of youth and ageing? This question touches on historical constructions of the body, the impact of global conflict on gender relations, the changing relationship between youth and beauty, the commercial world of rejuvenation products, and how our modern understanding of ageing was, at least in part, shaped by our anxieties about and hopes for both individual and societal rejuvenation. Whether taken collectively or individually, methods of rejuvenation represented a desire to escape impending catastrophe, a process which was accelerated by encounters with commercial interests and scientific discovery. The intended audiences of these products reflected a diversity of engagement with rejuvenation: for upper-middle-class and upper-class women, the salons of Elizabeth Arden promised sanctuary and refuge from the hectic pace of modern life, whilst small adverts in local newspapers offered pills to alleviate loss of sexual potency in working-class men affected by euphemistic conditions such as nervous exhaustion and loss of vitality.

By mapping these historical shifts, this book outlines a synthetic sociocultural history of the body and its relationship with emerging scientific knowledge in physiology, endocrinology, dietary science and electricity, bringing together a diverse range of literature which has previously considered different rejuvenation strategies and scientific disciplines in isolation. The boundaries between the five areas considered here were and remain fluid; in the case of cosmetics, for example, hormone creams blurred the lines between the endocrine and the aesthetic, the marketing literature of electrotherapy devices made claims about removing wrinkles, and major skin care manufacturers lauded a proper diet and regular exercise as essential habits for a younger-looking complexion. Different modes of rejuvenation were cast in highly gendered terms depending on the intended audience, and the marketing strategies both drew upon and influenced public views about the extent to which male and female bodies shared similarities over the life course.

The structure and function of individual bodies lay at the heart of rejuvenation discourse and practices, yet attempts to achieve rejuvenation were also

---

[49] Overy, *The Morbid Age*, 360.

active at the level of society. The influence of eugenic ideas in the early twentieth century saw youthfulness equated with fitness and beauty, while the atrocities of World War One fuelled the imperative for nations to preserve the health, vitality and fertility of their populations.[50] At the same time, technical developments in domestic electronic products and increasing consumer comfort with the power of electricity not just in homes but on bodies saw the emergence of a raft of products into the marketplace.[51] Britain was by no means unique as a site of rejuvenation – indeed many of the approaches were shared across Europe and the United States – yet it was precisely this lack of a single dominant approach to rejuvenation which marks the case as being one of particular interest. When it came to rejuvenation, national boundaries were highly porous; the ideas, practices and material culture associated with rejuvenation circulated globally. At the centre of this narrative were commercial imperatives: the battle for intellectual ownership of anti-ageing was waged predominantly in public by entrepreneurs, enterprising figures from science and corporate interest, all of whom claimed a high degree of expertise about human physiology, the ageing process and desirable aesthetics.

It is the marketplace of rejuvenation – its origins, reach, audiences and impacts – which forms the heart of this story. What emerges is a complex matrix of ideas and actors that shaped the expansion of popular and commercial interest in retaining or regaining youth. Manufacturers drew on both novel and long-standing scientific ideas about bodily vitality and beauty to construct elaborate claims for their devices and preparations. The use of these anti-ageing strategies can therefore tell us a great deal about historical attitudes towards both natural and 'premature' ageing, 'mid-life', and the emergence of modern gender roles, revealing the reasons why particular methods were seen as the most efficacious in producing the desired result, whether that was literal youth or simply youthful appearance. In the process, we see that the fragmentary and prescribed 'modern' life course identified by Michael Anderson as emerging particularly from the 1940s to the 1970s was driven as much by products targeted at particular demographics (such as the under-thirties or over-fifties) as changes in the timing of major life events, such as marriage, retirement and death.[52]

---

[50] Nye, 'The Rise and Fall of the Eugenics Empire'; Logan, *Hormones, Heredity and Race*; Dyck, *Facing Eugenics*; Turda, *Modernism and Eugenics*; Day, 'The Ideological Development of Physical Activity'; Dowbiggin, *The Sterilization Movement*.

[51] The extension of electrification of the domestic and medical spaces was largely a continuation of Victorian practices. See: Gooday, *Domesticating Electricity*; Loeb, 'Consumerism and Commercial Electrotherapy', 252–75; Elliott, 'More Subtle than the Electric Aura', 195–220; Morus, *Shocking Bodies*. For the parallel case of the emergence of electrical modes of thought and practice in the United States, see de la Peña, *The Body Electric*.

[52] Anderson, 'The Emergence of the Modern Life Cycle', 69–87.

Rejuvenation: Social, Physiological, Aesthetic

What exactly did rejuvenation mean to audiences in the early twentieth century? On the one hand, rejuvenation was a purely biological process, whether operating at the level of the organism, organ, tissue, cell or even individual molecule. This rejuvenation was and remains concerned with the reversal of the ageing process to create a youthful state; a classic example from our period is the hormonal research of Eugen Steinach and Serge Voronoff, whose surgical interventions were held up by their acolytes as means through which youth might be recaptured. However, rejuvenation had an equally important and subtly different meaning: the restoration of the *appearance* of youth. Whilst a reversal of the physiological ageing process might therefore have had the accidental consequence of creating a more youthful appearance, this was not its primary aim. Yet rejuvenation could also be achieved by manipulation designed to change the face and body without altering the underlying biology in a significant way.

It is also important to stress that there existed both slight and total differences both in practice and ideology between rejuvenation and longevity. It is certainly true that many of the enthusiastic disciples of rejuvenation who populate this book also sought to extend lifespans (whether their own or that of others). However, a quest for rejuvenation did not necessarily translate into a desire for life extension.[53] An obvious example might be rejuvenators whose principal preoccupation was with restoring the youthful appearance of their skin; their mission to present a young face to the world was almost wholly unconnected to adding literal years to the lifespan or extending the youthful portion of life.

We must also remember that, in addition to human beings, rejuvenation can affect numerous other biological entities as well as inanimate objects. Primates, salamanders' tails, the economy, urban spaces and careers can all be rejuvenated: refreshed and restored to new life.[54] When we take this into account, we see that *The Cult of Youth* is not about explaining the diffuse *idea*, but the *practices* of a quite particular type of rejuvenation associated with humans and their search for youthfulness. The process of youth-seeking touches on numerous themes across biomedicine, economics, culture and society. Manufacturers and advocates of rejuvenation strategies mobilised the latest scientific claims about the ageing process to court consumers.

---

[53] A number of major scholarly works do not consider this distinction. See, for example: Boia, *Forever Young*; Haycock, *Mortal Coil*. These dual aspects of anti-ageing – rejuvenation and longevity – are often conflated in contemporary accounts. See, for example, de Grey, *Ending Aging*. De Grey is one of the most high-profile advocates of human rejuvenation and transhumanism.

[54] 'Rejuvenation', *Oxford English Dictionary Online*, Oxford University Press, 2017.

In doing so they laid claim to scientific authority, drawing on a wide range of research from across multiple disciplines. The market surrounding rejuvenation was a battleground for expertise about ageing, skin and the human body, where science was used as a tool to establish credibility.

Rejuvenation was and remains deeply entwined with money, ownership and profit. We know that there existed a close and deep relationship between the worlds of medicine and commerce in the early twentieth century, yet anti-ageing products occupied a unique place within this sphere.[55] Although many purveyors of rejuvenatory wares were undoubtedly committed to providing a valuable service to the anxious ager, rejuvenation opened up distinctive commercial spaces. Enterprising individuals sought to exploit small niches in the market, and aspiring multinational corporate entities such as Boots, Elizabeth Arden and Ponds all unleashed a raft of new products and accompanying promotional campaigns in an effort to establish market dominance. While the United States is often taken to be the paradigmatic example of commerce and market capitalism in this period, Britain shared many features of advertising and promotion. This built on the increasing visibility of cosmetic preparations from the late nineteenth century and formed the basis of an ongoing and large market in anti-ageing products.

The diverse forms of rejuvenation also appealed to very different cross-sections of post–World War One British society, dependent on both class and gender. Whilst the expensive and high-profile gland-grafting procedures pioneered by surgeons Steinach and Voronoff found favour amongst a small enclave of wealthy higher-class clients, nourishing skin foods and domestic electrotherapy devices appealed to a broader middle class for whom rejuvenation was an aspirational possibility, especially in an age of nervous disorders and concerns about economic and social productivity.[56] More everyday, mundane products such as toilet soaps and vitamin supplements also drew on themes of youthfulness, attempting to remould daily bathroom habits. As Chandak Sengoopta and others have uncovered, although hormone treatments were limited almost exclusively to men in the 1920s, radiation therapy for women also offered parallel treatment in order to restore lost fertility through

---

[55] See, most particularly: Ueyama, *Health in the Marketplace*; Jones, *The Medical Trade Catalogue*; Digby, *Making a Medical Living*; Stark, 'Introduction: Plurality in Patenting', 533–40. Much research in this area has focussed on medical practice, whilst devices and products aimed at a non-specialist audience have received less attention, although the excellent recent special issue of *Social History of Medicine* on the theme of 'Medicine in the Household' goes some way to redressing this imbalance. See Bivins, Marland and Tomes, 'Histories of Medicine in the Household', 669–75.

[56] High-profile individuals who underwent surgical rejuvenation treatment included Sigmund Freud in 1926 and the poet W. B. Yeats in 1934. See: Foster, *W. B. Yeats*, 496–500; Wyndham, 'Versemaking and Lovemaking', 25–50.

means other than surgery.[57] This was far from a dichotomy, however, as we see extensive use of hormones in skin care products as well as a significant effort from manufacturers of electrotherapy equipment to appeal to potential consumers regardless of sex or gender. Proponents of various dietary regimes likewise made claims for the universal benefits of their systems, although the purported results in men and women were often considered to be very different. Forms of exercise were also frequently gendered; communal exercise for women emerged as a major national movement in Britain, exemplified by the founding in 1930 of the Women's League of Health and Beauty, an organisation which placed as much emphasis on the development of healthy character as on the maintenance of a youthful physiology through organised physical movement. Cosmetics manufacturers also attempted to capitalise on the strong links between skin health and overall well-being by establishing their own exercise routines, and in some cases salons, dedicated to physical activity.

Cultural outputs of many different kinds, including film, novels and artworks, also echoed prevailing attitudes towards rejuvenation.[58] Almost all reinforced highly gendered views of the ageing process; in many cases the overwhelming narrative was of women seeking to retain (or regain) their beauty and charm, or the male quest for sexual rejuvenation to restore fertility, virility and sexual potency. These were not just passive responses to the anti-ageing climate; rather, they played an active role in constructing the terms of public discussions about the possibility and desirability of rejuvenation. One notable contribution which this genre of rejuvenation literature made to public discourse was the reinforcement of the purported sexual danger which was posed by rejuvenated older men. The returning of a youthful libido in these aged individuals was widely regarded as a moral aberration which restored unwelcome, unnatural desires and presented a hazard to the stability of social order. The high-profile descent of fictional male characters into this debauched state after their successful rejuvenation served to warn readers of the negative consequences of such radical and sudden restoration of youth.[59]

---

[57] Eugen Steinach pioneered both a surgical procedure for men and radiation therapy for women, with both claimed to produce rejuvenating effects, whilst Serge Voronoff's male rejuvenation procedures had their origins in animal experiments using female specimens. See Sengoopta, *The Most Secret Quintessence*, especially 92 and notes on 262–63.

[58] For some noteworthy examples, see: Gayton, *The Gland Stealers*; Atherton, *Black Oxen*; Mills, *Phoenix*; Smith, *The Glorious Pool*; Gloag, *Winter's Youth*. From later in the period Aldous Huxley explored what he took to be the American obsession with youth and youthfulness in *After Many a Summer*. Catherine Oakley's recent doctoral research has revealed a fascinating sub-genre of rejuvenation-related fiction in both print and film; Oakley, 'Vital Forms'.

[59] See, for example, the failed male rejuvenation explored in C. P. Snow's novel, *New Lives for Old*, published anonymously in 1933. Snow, *New Lives for Old*; Oakley, 'Sexual Rejuvenation and Hegemonic Masculinity'.

'One Alone Is Not Sufficient': Multiple Methods for a Younger You

A history of methods of rejuvenation must necessarily be selective. Nevertheless, the five areas considered here – hormones, electricity, skin care, diet and exercise – are a reflection of approaches to rejuvenation which found most favour in Britain at the time. Other factors recognised as having a restorative effect included sleep, long since recognised as a restorative, which was claimed again in the interwar period as an essential enabler of vitality. However, unlike the methods which occupy the bulk of my attention here, sleep was far more strongly linked with maintaining general health in older age rather than combating the process of ageing per se. Sleep, together with other popular methods of restoration such as the use of radiotherapy belts and other similar products, as well as a continued engagement within society beyond retirement or withdrawal from public life, might represent an area for future inquiry.[60]

We begin with hormones, whose significance in the rejuvenation craze of the early twentieth century has already been widely recognised. In *The Most Secret Quintessence of Life*, Chandak Sengoopta charts the importance of hormones in underpinning interpretations of the gendered body, as well as the ways in which bodily control was reconceptualised. As part of this, he argues that the work of surgical rejuvenators Eugen Steinach and Serge Voronoff, as well as their forerunners, represented attempts to recapture vitality and virility, especially sexual potency, over and above rejuvenation. Much of the focus of Sengoopta's excellent work is on the expensive, sensational and highly visible surgical interventions of Steinach and Voronoff.[61] In Chapter 2 I argue that the chief impact of these individuals and their methods was not in the attempted rejuvenation of a small number of wealthy clients, but in the popularising of the concept of rejuvenation itself, and not just through modifications of the endocrine system. I use this account to provide the springboard to an argument which recurs throughout the book: that the principal effect of the extraordinary attention afforded to hormone rejuvenation in both the popular and medical press was to create a renewed fascination with rejuvenation. This in turn opened a commercial and ideological space of public credibility (and credence) in which other means of securing enhanced youthfulness were able to flourish. Manufacturers of hormone-based products, distinct from the specialised and professional intervention of the surgical rejuvenators, attempted to capitalise on a wave of interest, which went far

---

[60] In her current research, Lucy Santos is exploring the development of products – many of them rejuvenating – which relied on the mysterious and powerful action of radium.

[61] Sengoopta, *The Most Secret Quintessence*.

beyond the social elites treated by Steinach and Voronoff. Hormonal rejuvenation consequently expanded to cover mainstream domestic products such as
hormone tablets, running alongside the more visible but far smaller world of
celebrity rejuvenation through specialist surgery.

As well as promoting specific medical interventions, many of the most high-
profile rejuvenators also emphasised the importance of correct diet, the subject
of Chapter 3. The benefits of effective skin care or exercise routines, they
argued, could only be realised if the body was receiving appropriate nourishment. Building on the metaphor of 'feeding' the skin, numerous different diets
were held up as paragons of rejuvenatory practice. Excessive consumption of
oily foods, overindulgence, immoderate drinking habits and a diet based
around high meat and protein intake were widely castigated, with leading
authorities, both scientific and popular, advocating instead for a range of
suitable options, including vegetarianism, periodic fasting, abstention from
alcohol and dietary regimes based on the supposed virtues of individual foods
and extracts, from carrots and other miracle vegetables to vitamin and mineral
supplements tailored to the body. Noted personalities within the dietary literature promoted the benefits of a diet consisting of raw and unprocessed foods,
particularly fresh fruit and vegetables, as the science of nutrition uncovered the
importance of specific chemical vitamins which appeared to perform essential
functions in the human body. The function-specific vitamins and minerals
(Vitamin E for the skin, Vitamin C for the teeth) gradually displaced products
characteristic of the nineteenth century, such as kidney and liver pills which
had been based as much on a latent and persistent humoral understanding of
the body as on physiological processes. All became tied up with the quest of
maintaining youthful vigour and energy, forming an important strand of
activity for the would-be rejuvenator.

In Chapter 4 I move to examine a major competing model of bodily control
in the early twentieth century: electrical control. Whilst the discovery of
successive hormonal actions had given rise to a categorisation of the male
and female bodies as distinctively different, electrical models of control
emphasised similarity; a common underlying power source and control mechanism, coupled with increasing comfort with electrical technologies and the
seeming benefits of their use, supported the view that electrical energy acted as
a vital force. Discoveries which further deepened our understanding of the
importance of electrostatic forces for the interaction and composition of matter
also gave strength to theories which placed electricity at the heart of the body,
particularly when coupled with crucial developments in neurology in the late
nineteenth century. I argue that these products associated with electrical
rejuvenation represented a powerful confluence between the emerging domestic force of electricity and the societal fascination with rejuvenation possibilities. The popularity of electric products from the nineteenth century, such as

belts and body combs, persisted, and these devices were reconfigured as rejuvenating appliances. Advocates of domestic electrotherapy expanded their claims of efficacy; everything from nervous conditions such as neurasthenia and 'debility' through to rheumatism and lumbago was amenable to electrical cure, although in this was now a strong emphasis on alleviating ailments associated with old age and bodily degeneration, such as greying hair and wrinkles.

To preserve the body and prevent decay, another complementary method of maintaining youthfulness was a comprehensive programme of exercise. Chapter 5 explores a number of different forms of rejuvenating activity, from group fitness classes which emphasised collective social responsibility of remaining athletic to individual exercise regimes which recommended keeping fit by continuing everyday physical tasks such as walking and housework. This period was also characterised by an increasing appreciation for the natural world, and pursuits such as rambling sought to promote both enjoyment of and benefit from outdoor activities. The rise of environmental treatments for conditions such as tuberculosis as well as the popularity of heliotherapy reflected the belief that exposure to nature led to improved physical health, spiritual well-being and increased vitality. Leading figures within the physical culture movement drew on their own transformations – often from weak child to strong adult – to highlight the universal and apparently limitless potential within all human bodies. For authors, trainers and rejuvenators exercise was generally one strand of a broader strategy, frequently coupled with dietary management and, in the case of women, the use of appropriate forms of skin care.

The outwardly visible signs of ageing were also amenable to prevention and treatment by skin care products, which form the basis of Chapter 6. Although humans have modified their skin for millennia, the immediate aftermath of World War One saw a fascination with fashion and appearance which extended far beyond clothing to the body. Numerous creams, soaps and cosmetic products emerged on the market, promising optimistic yet believable results for the anxious ager. Advertisements codified for women (and it was almost exclusively women) the key markers of ageing, such as wrinkles and lines, and promised at least to stave them off a little longer, and at best to reverse the ageing process altogether. These products vied for women's attention in newspapers, magazines and salons, some of which were dedicated to assisting the pursuit of youthful beauty. Manufacturers and retailers made claims to scientific authority and attempted to ally this with the lived female experience of products as the gold standard of efficacy. In this chapter I examine how companies deployed imagery, testimonials and other strategies to persuade consumers that rejuvenating skin care products were effective, safe and desirable. Powerful metaphors of 'feeding' the skin and its underlying tissues borrowed extensively from dietary advice, and the enduring popularity of so-called skin foods highlighted the resonance of these messages with users.

These approaches to rejuvenation were themselves far from homogeneous; almost all drew on heavily gendered narratives of the ageing process and the key markers of youthfulness and the life course. Even those entrepreneurs who railed against such gender distinctions and claimed more universal efficacy for their treatments and regimes drew on these mythologies to appeal to a broad base of everyday medical consumers. Through the book I therefore gradually build up a picture of interlocking practices, all of which drew to varying degrees on prevailing scientific and sociocultural ideas about ageing, youth and health. The advocates of these multifarious practices were as varied as the systems of rejuvenation which they endorsed, yet there was often substantial overlap, with specialists in one particular area of rejuvenation also highlighting the importance of other factors. For example, advertising pamphlets for a range of skin care products, distributed by the British retail chemists Boots during the 1930s, noted that '[t]he condition of the skin depends so much, of course, upon the whole process of living; a correct diet, a normal amount of suitable exercise, adequate rest, the care of internal conditions and personal hygiene.'[62] Skin care products in particular became simply one component in a lifestyle calculated to promote health and the cultivation of youthful appearance. As another brochure noted, '[t]he most scientifically blended preparations are unable to produce the results they claim if these things are neglected or uncorrected.'[63]

On the one hand, entrepreneurs attempted to corner the market with distinctive offerings, insisting that their own methods were vastly superior to that of others. On the other, commercial entities positioned their products as a vital enhancement to other forms of rejuvenatory practice. It is far from clear in most cases what motivated these concerned parties to promote specific methods; whilst the search for rejuvenation was a quest common to a range of scientists, physicians and entrepreneurs, their decisions to advocate different means were based on a combination of commercial, scientific and ideological factors.

Many of the practices associated with rejuvenation which gained substantial traction in the interwar period had significant heritage, in many cases reflected in the persistence of the non-naturals as sources of longevity and youthfulness. For example, the standard-bearer of English longevity in the early modern period, Thomas Parr (also known as Old Tom Parr or even simply Old Parr),

---

[62] 'Beauty', Boots Company Archive, Nottingham (hereafter Boots Archive), A30/1, 1.
[63] 'Beauty Treatment Paper No.1. Activities of Staff Training School and Demonstrators', Boots Archive, 331/1, 1.

was venerated, both during his lifetime and long after his death, by proponents of dietary moderation for his temperate habits.[64]

Whatever the basis for the often hyperbolic but always confident claims which surrounded rejuvenation products, the visual and rhetorical culture which accompanied their advertising was laden with references to mythical cups of life, images of highly stylised and almost impossible beauty, and a sense of moral duty to remain young, fit and healthy. The visual and material culture of rejuvenation was in many ways just as significant as the competing scientific theories of ageing in shaping the landscape of practices. Advertisements trumpeted the eminent realisability of both exterior perfection and internal harmony; women were urged to treat the use of products designed to maintain a youthful visage as a necessary task, a duty, rather than an optional extra. Indeed, if we are to look for roots of current perspectives on youthfulness in advertising, the early twentieth century saw the emergence of many features of 'modern' ageing, when wrinkles, fine lines and sagging throats became concretised alongside the long-standing markers of grey hair, hearing loss and declining fertility as key signs of ageing. In many, but not all, cases, those who advocated means of achieving rejuvenation held old age to be a highly undesirable period of decline, frustration and dogmatism.[65]

Historians have much to learn from examining rejuvenation in its historical context; each set of practices was rooted in concepts of biological ageing, perceptions of the male and female life course, social values and capital ascribed to the elderly and aged, management and limits of the human body, and the scope of scientific expertise and authority, all the while harnessing and subject to influence by commercial interests through advertising. In contrast to the view of Jon Savage, who claims that in the decade following World War One '[y]outh became an abstract concept, detached from biology', I argue that biological research into rejuvenation was a critical motivating factor behind the obsession with youth.[66] Such scientific work was, of course, viewed through the lens of a milieu which amplified and transformed public perceptions of ageing, vitality and youthfulness, yet new models of biological ageing and the life course remained fundamental, and many of precisely the same sociocultural factors identified by Savage drew on aspects of biological thought.

---

[64] For a historical account of Parr's life, see Taylor, *The Old, Old, Very Old Man*.

[65] Bernard Hollander, who we will encounter principally in Chapter 4, quoted Francis Bacon with admiration in his 1933 text on rejuvenation: '[m]en of age object too much, consult too long, adventure too little, repeat too soon, and seldom drive business to the full period, but content themselves with a mediocrity of success.' Hollander, *Old Age Deferred*, 20. With noted differences between the sexes, Hollander continued that '[t]he old man may become peevish, mean, tyrannical, exacting, querulous, and grumbling ... [though] some old men, and especially old women, become more benevolent with advancing years.' Hollander, *Old Age Deferred*, 23–24.

[66] Savage, *Teenage*, 183.

Following this approach, and charting a broad shift across gender, *The Cult of Youth* begins with hormones, the most widely studied form of twentieth-century rejuvenation, and ends with skin care, where numerous disparate scientific ideas about ageing were reconfigured into products suitable for everyday domestic use.

2   Hormones, 1918–1929

In broad terms, and with notable exceptions, the historical literature has characterised attempts to understand control and management of the human body from the seventeenth to the mid-twentieth century into periods dominated by a focus on anatomy, physiology, electricity and hormones.[1] For example, the refutation of the expected primacy of neurological mechanisms in the secretion of pancreatic juices by Bayliss and Starling in 1902 ushered in a focus on what they termed 'an entirely different order of phenomena': blood-borne chemical messengers, termed hormones by Starling in 1905.[2] Reflecting on this in the early 1930s, Sir Edward Sharpey-Schafer – one of the chief architects of endocrinology – termed this chemically based biology of the body the 'New Physiology'.[3] Popular discourse mirrored this shift in the supposed mechanism of bodily control. As Serge Voronoff, one of principal advocates of hormone rejuvenation, noted in a 1926 interview with *Scientific American*, 'the brain was found to be not the controlling centre of life, but a peculiar combination of grey flesh, capable of producing thought only when properly controlled by the chemical action of the liquid from the thyroid glands.'[4]

Although historical accounts of rejuvenation in the interwar period have focussed heavily on the supposed dominance of hormone treatments, arguably the most significant impact of these was to expand existing but smaller-scale medical and commercial opportunities for a range of other potential

[1] For examples of studies which have focussed on some of these specific elements, characteristic of certain periods, see: Foucault, *The Birth of the Clinic*; Geison, *Michael Foster and the Cambridge School*; Senior, 'Rationalising Electrotherapy'; Ueyama, 'Capital, Profession and Medical Technology', 150–81; de la Peña, *The Body Electric*; Morus, *Shocking Bodies*; Petitt, 'Becoming Glandular', 1052–76.

[2] This remark came from Bayliss and Starling's full publication of results: Bayliss and Starling, 'The Mechanism of Pancreatic Secretion', 327. Earlier in the year they had issued an abridged version of their findings. Hirst, 'Secretin', 339. Starling introduced the term 'hormone' in the first of his Croonian Lectures to the Royal Society: Starling, 'The Croonian Lectures', 339–41.

[3] Sharpey-Schafer, 'Endocrine Physiology', 484.

[4] 'Can Old Age Be Deferred?', *Scientific American*, October 1925, 226–27, 226. This was reprinted far further afield, even appearing in Australian newspapers: 'Can Old Age Be Deferred?' *The Adelaide Advertiser*, 22 January 1926, p. 22.

rejuvenating and therapeutic strategies. The 1920s might have been the decade of rejuvenation in terms of endocrinology-inspired surgical interventions, but in many ways it was just the starting point for a far longer-lived industry built around hyperbolic claims of youthfulness. As Morris Fishbein, that American dismantler-of-quacks-in-chief, noted in his telling 1925 intervention on the subject – *The Medical Follies* – the publication of 'Rejuvenation Through Experimental Revivifying of the Senescent Puberty Glands' by Eugen Steinach, marked 'the opening gun in the great international scramble for priority recognition in the alleged discovery of the profound secret of restoring lost youth and youthful vigor'.[5]

By the late 1930s almost all mainstream medical and scientific professionals had adopted Fishbein's view. A. J. Carson, writing in 1939, decried 'the spectacular pseudo-science of "rejuvenation" via the route of the gonad hormones or gonad implantation'.[6] The long-term failure of rejuvenation methods based on hormone treatments might tempt us to view the effects of this sensational and controversial episode in the history of medicine as tightly constrained, something of an interwar fad. However, considering these developments as part of wider trends in anti-ageing culture enables us to see that, far from constituting a niche and fringe scientific movement, the brief period for which hormones appeared to offer salvation from ageing and infirmity (especially, though not exclusively, for men) provided a transformative platform which enabled rejuvenation to occupy an accepted space in everyday life. Nor had the gonads vanished from view; in the same volume as Carson, Edgar Allen argued that '[p]remature ageing of female genital organs ... follows removal of the ovaries or their damage by X-rays ... whilst [t]herapy with ovarian hormones replaces destroyed or lagging ovarian endocrine function, induces growth of genital organs and restoration of menstrual function.'[7] With the menopause regarded at the time as a key milestone in determining the progression of female ageing, what other explanation could there be but a close, causative and reciprocal relationship between endocrine function and senescence?

This chapter outlines the work of key figures involved in practising and promoting surgical methods of hormone rejuvenation, before moving to consider the wider social and commercial landscape surrounding such practices. In contrast to those historical accounts which have generally emphasised the relatively rapid shift from shock and cautious enthusiasm to outright hostility and derision towards practitioners and advocates of hormone rejuvenation, what we see instead is a set of highly plural responses. Many of these were as

---

[5] Fishbein, *The Medical Follies*, 161.   [6] Carson, 'The Thyroid, Pancreatic Islets', 363.
[7] Allen, 'Female Reproductive System', 429.

concerned with the extrapolation of conclusions observed in animal models to humans as the spurious nature of those claims.

'Even a Cabbage May Be Steinached': Endocrinology and Surgical Intervention

In 1923, the already famous German-American poet and author George Sylvester Viereck (1884–1962) published a popular science treatise entitled *Rejuvenation: How Steinach Makes People Young* under the pseudonym George F. Corners, an alias which he used on just the one occasion.[8] In the book, Viereck made clear his admiration for Eugen Steinach (1861–1944), the Austrian physiologist and endocrinologist who pioneered an eponymous rejuvenation operation. Steinach, Viereck contended, could add 'several years, possibly decades, to the economic life of the patient', critically, 'at the height of their maturity and experience!'[9] From Viereck's perspective the process of rejuvenation was not about extending lifespan, rather it was 'a charm to wean us from the vulgar habit of growing old.'[10] Rejuvenation through simple, surgical means could enhance productivity, vitality, youthfulness and energy amongst the aged and the prematurely ageing. As one might imagine, in the eugenic heyday of the interwar period in both Europe and the United States, this was a welcome claim.

Viereck's fervently held views were not outliers, but rather entirely commensurate with many members of the mainstream scientific community; his claim that 'cabbages, lasting two seasons ordinarily, may last five, if their reproductive function is checked by radioactivity' was the sole departure from rejuvenatory orthodoxy (though radioactivity was itself a force deployed by many rejuvenators of the time).[11] As *Time* magazine reported, 1923 also saw the Russian-born Parisian surgeon Serge Voronoff (1866–1951) acclaimed at the International Congress of Surgeons in London, 'when 700 of the world's leading surgeons applauded the success of his work in the "rejuvenation" of old men'.[12] According to the report, the inflation of Voronoff's own claims in a hysterical press was largely responsible for negative perceptions of his findings, and the opinion amongst the medical community was 'growing more lenient as increasing numbers of surgeons in various countries are experimenting with these methods'.[13]

---

[8] Wolff, *Magnus Hirschfeld*, 396.   [9] Corners, *Rejuvenation*, 49.   [10] Ibid., v.
[11] Ibid., vii.
[12] 'Medicine: Voronoff and Steinach', *Time*, 30 July 1923, http://content.time.com/time/sub scriber/article/0,33009,727231,00.html, accessed 26 June 2017.
[13] 'Medicine: Voronoff and Steinach'.

Steinach, held up by Viereck within the community of rejuvenation researchers, has been the subject of considerable historical scholarship, alongside the equally significant figure of Voronoff.[14] It is, however, in some ways misleading to consider the two together. In the first place, whilst Voronoff qualified as a surgeon and performed rejuvenating procedures himself, Steinach was in essence a laboratory scientist, working with animals, who gave his name to an operation practised on humans by others.[15] Additionally, the introduction of animal material into patients by Voronoff stood in contrast to the procedure of Steinach, where no transplantation took place. In the long term it was arguably Steinach, not Voronoff, who gained the more significant recognition from professional medical and scientific practitioners, whereas Voronoff's introduction of primate tissue into humans was the more sensational practice. Finally, Steinach's legacy in endocrinology was assured – he was nominated several times for the Nobel Prize in the 1920s and 1930s – whilst Voronoff has been characterised by historians as a 'charlatan' who carried out 'expensive, dangerous and useless grafts'.[16] However, when we consider the initial reception and lasting effects of their work, we see that both Steinach and Voronoff played critical roles in popularising the idea of rejuvenation beyond their professional specialisms.

Voronoff

> In recent times the whole world has observed with interest the experiments of the Russian doctor Voronoff.[17]

Serge Voronoff was born in Shekhman in the Tambov Governorate of Russia in 1866. His father was a cantonist, or "Nicholas soldier" – a Jewish distiller who was conscripted to serve in the army of Czar Nicholas I; his mother Rachel Esther-Lipsky.[18] He began his medical training in Paris in 1884, and later made the acquaintance of Alexis Carrel (1873–1944). Several authors have claimed that, variously, one was a pupil of the other or that Voronoff met Carrel when the former was still a student, but this is highly doubtful given that Carrel did not move to Paris until after he had completed his medical training

---

[14] Understandably, both Steinach and Voronoff have also acted as magnets for popular writing, much of which sensationalises their work without proper consideration of the wider historical context. See, for example: Cooper and Lanza, *Xeno*, especially 24–26; Real, *Voronoff*.

[15] 'Medicine: Rejuvenation', *Time*, 10 December 1923, http://content.time.com/time/subscriber/article/0,33009,717158,00.html, accessed 26 June 2017.

[16] Wyndham, *Norman Haire*, 88.

[17] 'The Truth about Vitamins and Sunlight', *The Times*, 22 May 1928, xxxvii.

[18] 'Voronoff Called to Turkey to Improve Breed of Sheep through Gland Grafting', *Jewish Daily Bulletin*, 29 January 1928, 1; Augier, Salf and Nottet, 'Le Docteur Samuel Serge Voronoff', 163–71.

at the University of Lyon in 1900 and, in any case, emigrated to the United States via Canada in 1903–04.[19] Likely far more significant was Voronoff's proximity to Charles-Édouard Brown-Séquard who was one of the most prominent figures in the proto-endocrinology field of organotherapy and whom Voronoff referenced in glowing terms in many of his publications.

A native of Mauritius, Brown-Séquard had himself trained as a physician in Paris in the early 1840s before an eventful trans-Atlantic career which included posts at the Medical College of Virginia (Richmond), National Hospital for the Paralysed and Epileptic (London), École de Médecine (Paris) and a Professorship in Physiology and Neuropathology at Harvard.[20] By the time that Voronoff arrived in Paris, Brown-Séquard had already attracted notoriety for his claim that by injecting the testicular extract under his skin he had caused a rejuvenation.[21] As has been noted by Laura Hirshbein, the idea of the spermatic economy – a staple assumption in the late nineteenth century that men possessed a finite store of bodily energy which could be depleted through masturbation and excessive sexual activity – underpinned the supposed treatment, though many of his colleagues were dismissive of the 'Brown-Séquard Elixir'.[22]

Voronoff's ideas were unquestionably rooted in the potency and influence of the sex glands, in both men and women. On these seemingly all-powerful vehicles for secretion he wrote:

It pours into the stream of the blood a species of vital fluid which restores the energy of all the cells, and spreads happiness and a feeling of well-being and the plenitude of life throughout our organism ... The idea of capturing this marvelous [sic] force, of placing it at our service when its natural source begins to dry up as we advance in age, had haunted my mind for a number of years.[23]

Charting a clear lineage from the work of Brown-Séquard, Voronoff argued that the reason for the failure of his compatriot's ideas in clinical practice was that the glandular extract did not contain the '*active element*' required to produce a true, lasting rejuvenation.[24] In a move clearly designed to assert

---

[19] Schneider, *Quality and Quantity*, 272. Voronoff later claimed that he learned transplantation techniques from Carrel, although this is doubtful given that Carrel was seven years his junior (Carrel's year of birth is incorrectly given in Roy Porter's *Blood and Guts* as 1884; Porter, *Blood and Guts*, 127). Chandak Sengoopta notes that Voronoff and Carrel met while the former was a student, but does not suggest a formal educational relationship. See: Sengoopta, *The Most Secret Quintessence*, 95; Cuperschmid and de Campos, 'Dr Voronoff's Curious', 1–24.

[20] Laporte, 'Charles-Édouard Brown-Séquard', 363–68; Loriaux, *A Biographical History of Endocrinology*, 123–25.

[21] Borell, 'Brown-Séquard's Organotherapy', 309–20.

[22] Hirshbein, 'The Glandular Solution', 278. The title of Hirshbein's excellent study is in some ways indicative of the ways in which historians have systematically interrogated hormonal rejuvenation at the expense of exploring other popular methods.

[23] Voronoff, *Life*, 60.   [24] Ibid., 62, original emphasis.

the importance of surgery over the use of extracts, he claimed that the liquid derived through trituration of the sex gland 'changes very rapidly, loses its properties and may even become toxic'.[25]

He drew extensively on his experiments with animal models in which the process of grafting appeared to restore both the vigour of youth *and* reproductive potency.[26] For example, as Voronoff reported, he carried out a graft on a male ram on 7 May 1918, implanting four sections of testicular material (which, collectively, amounted to an entire organ) into the 'vaginal tunic', a membrane situated around the inside of the scrotal sac. In consequence, 'he [the ram] no longer looked afraid ... [h]is bodily carriage had become magnificent, he behaved in a lively, aggressive manner' and, after being 'isolated in a small stable, together with a young ewe-lamb', sired a 'vigorous lamb' born the following February.[27]

The exploits of Voronoff's rams were critical to his earliest report on male grafting which he delivered to the *Congrés Français de Chirurgie* in Paris on 8 October 1919.[28] Subsequent presentations of his findings indicate that he soon switched to consider the effects of glandular interventions in primates and humans. For example, in one of his earliest presentations to a British audience, at the sixth triennial meeting of the International Surgical Society, held at the Royal Society of Medicine in July 1923, Voronoff focussed on his specific method rather than the supposed rejuvenating effects, and he was perpetually fascinated with the minutiae of the surgical procedure. These remarks followed the success of Banting and Best's successful isolation of insulin the previous year and Tuffier's claimed positive results in the case of grafting of human ovaries.[29] This created a professional environment within which the interest in and promise of hormones had been only recently renewed. Nevertheless, Voronoff noted multiple difficulties, including the expense of having to use mature rather than young monkeys and the fact that not only whole testicles but also smaller portions appeared not to grow successfully.[30] He claimed a wide range of clinical outcomes for his procedures; 'not only was there a subjective appreciation by patients, but such physiological phenomena as lowered blood pressure, loss of weight in obese subjects, production of better

---

[25] Ibid.

[26] Although I do not propose to investigate this here, Voronoff and Steinach's claims to be pioneers in this field were contested by Lydston, who claimed priority over both in demonstrating the effects of transplanted sex glands. See 'Transplantation of Sex Glands', *British Medical Journal*, 12 March 1921, 42.

[27] Voronoff, *Life*, 74.   [28] Faure, *Congrès Français de Chirurgie*.

[29] McLaren, *Reproduction by Design*, 84; 'Ovarian Transplantation or Grafting', *British Medical Journal*, 26 November 1921, 909–10.

[30] 'International Congress of Surgery. Inaugural Session', *British Medical Journal*, 21 July 1923, 121–24, 124.

vision ... new growth of hair, etc., had been demonstrated.'[31] Whether a function of selective reporting or of Voronoff's actual choice of topic for the audience of distinguished surgeons, sex and fertility – prominent motivating factors – did not feature.

His contribution to the meeting provoked discussion on a range of aspects of endocrinology, including insulin therapy and the role of the pituitary gland, whilst the Paris-based English surgeon Ivor Back endorsed Voronoff's findings.[32] Back (1879–1951) was far from a fringe practitioner. A member of the Royal College of Surgeons, he read Natural Sciences at Cambridge before completing his medical training at St. George's Hospital in London and taking a leading role in the Royal Army Medical Corps during World War One. He was one of only two London-based medical practitioners noted as having observed first-hand Voronoff's grafting operations by 1925, the other being Leonard Williams.[33]

In common with many rejuvenators of the period, Voronoff was quite clear about the object of his interest: 'natural physiological death, and not ... death arising from accident, malady or aggression by the stronger'.[34] As part of his work Voronoff also went far beyond the biological, making assertions about the nature of old age itself. From his perspective, for example, women 'are more fearful of old age' than men, and '[t]he period when a woman definitely loses the capacity for becoming a mother marks for her the beginning of old age.'[35] He was, however, keen to distance his work from the terminology of 'rejuvenation'; in 1923 when the American surgeon and grafting enthusiast Max Thorek delivered a lecture on the subject in Paris, Voronoff agreed with him that 'the application to the operation of the term "rejuvenation"' was misleading.[36] Despite having extrapolated from his earlier findings in rams to humans, Voronoff did not abandon his interest in or exploitation of animal models. Indeed, at least as late as 1928, he continued to use dogs in order to understand more fully the factors behind the action of grafted testicular material and to refine the analogous procedure for potential patients.[37]

Other practitioners, including Richard Müsham and Carl Pariser – both based in Berlin – took up methods akin to those used by Voronoff in the early 1920s, yet explicitly aligned their work more closely with Steinach. The exploits of both Müsham, a clinician at the Virchow Hospital, and Pariser, physician at the nearby Woltersdorfer Schleuse sanatorium, attracted interest

---

[31] Ibid., 124.   [32] Ibid., 124.   [33] Voronoff, *Rejuvenation by Grafting*, 10.
[34] Voronoff, *Conquest of Life*.   [35] Ibid., 183 and 185.
[36] 'Gland-grafting. American Surgeon's Method', *The Times*, 24 October 1923, 13.
[37] Voronoff, *Conquest of Life*.

from *The Lancet*, 'when organotherapy is being strongly condemned in this country by some of our leading thinkers'.[38]

Amongst these 'leading thinkers' was Ernest Starling. At the same time as Voronoff was able to secure at least a modicum of public support from some high-profile members of the mainstream medical community in Britain, Starling, arguably the most significant figure in the development of endocrinology, provided a very different response. Without naming Voronoff, Steinach or any other purveyors of supposedly rejuvenating procedures, Starling – in a 1923 review of Benjamin Harrow's popular book *Glands in Health and Disease* – warned that '[s]ensationalism and imagination have not only rushed ahead of the ascertained facts but have also opened the way to a shameless exploitation of the uneducated curiosity that has been aroused. ... Charlatanism finds an easy and profitable prey in the curious and uneducated.'[39] Strangely, however, in the very same year Starling delivered the Harveian Oration to the Royal College of Physicians, in which he presented a rather different assessment of Steinach's work. In his address, entitled 'The Wisdom of the Body', Starling noted that Steinach's findings were 'perfectly reasonable and follow, as a logical sequence, many years' observation and experiments in the field'.[40]

Criticism of Voronoff came from a variety of perspectives. Writing in the *English Review*, L. C. Dundas Irvine – surgeon-lieutenant with the Royal Naval Volunteer Reserve and later specialist in rheumatic fever – argued that atherosclerosis, one of the principal physiological effects of age, could not be reversed by any kind of glandular activity. However, this was largely an issue with Voronoff's extrapolation from animal models to humans; Dundas Irvine did not rule out such transformative effects taking place in lower animals.[41]

Neither was it the case that those who originally poured scorn on Voronoff's ideas and methods steadfastly refused to engage. One early sceptic, William Belfield, a general practitioner based in Chicago, continued to explore the possibilities of the endocrine system along similar lines. Writing in 1925, he confessed that the 'irrational attempt at an impossible "rejuvenation" may emerge from the disrepute of its infancy, and develop into a valuable means for relieving ailments that are not now associated with gonad deficiency.'[42]

---

[38] 'Testicle Transplantation', *The Lancet*, 3 February 1923, 244–45, 245.

[39] S[tarling], 'Hormones', 695. Benjamin later showed an appreciation for Steinach – 'a first-class biologist' who did 'much fine work' – yet for him rejuvenation through gland grafting or other surgical means only served 'to entertain newspaper readers'. Harrow, *One Family*, 30.

[40] Starling, 'The Wisdom of the Body', 690. As if to underline the eugenic implications of the rejuvenation debate in Britain, Starling, argued that 'if longevity is our goal it is not medical science we must look to but eugenics.'

[41] Dundas Irvine, 'Rejuvenation: A Reply', 167–71.

[42] Belfield, 'Some Phases of Rejuvenation', 1242.

By 1927, even cautious, conservative outlets in the United States, such as *Nature*, were claiming that it might be possible, through surgical refinement, to 'prolong the span of life'.[43] Others noted that the modification or coupling or glandular methods with other strategies – such as through the application of electricity or ultra-violet light – might also yield improved results.[44]

Voronoff's continued publications were aimed almost exclusively at a popular audience, yet they aroused considerable interest amongst the medical community. His 1926 work, *Étude sur la Vieillesse*, was translated into English as *The Study of Old Age and my Method of Rejuvenation* the same year and presented a large number of cases, in both animals and humans.[45] Far from confirming the futility of his efforts to achieve rejuvenation in man, a reviewer for the *British Medical Journal* noted that 'the value of his work must be determined by clinical results rather than theoretical arguments. No longer can it be suggested that his deductions are based on insufficient material.'[46] The issues with the book lay not in the lack of evidence but in Voronoff's failure to translate the subjective, clinical experience or to 'analyse the thousand cases of animal grafting and the 600 human experiments, and to tabulate the results'.[47]

Steinach

Nothing is more difficult than to assess the clinical results of ligature of the vas [deferens] in man.[48]

If Voronoff drew a decidedly mixed response from medical communities, there was arguably far less public controversy surrounding Steinach's methods which, critically, did not necessitate the use of animal tissues in humans (but still rested on earlier experimental work with animal models). Eugen Steinach (1861–1944) was born to Jewish parents in the Austrian province of Vorarlberg and followed in the tradition of his father and grandfather, both physicians, by studying physiology and embarking on a research career. After time in Innsbruck, Geneva and Prague, where he focussed principally on teaching duties and research into the physiology of the eye, Steinach settled in Vienna in 1912 when he was appointed to lead the physiology division of the prestigious Institute for Experimental Biology of the Imperial Academy of Science,

---

[43] 'On Rejuvenation', *Nature* 119 (1927), 396–97, 397.

[44] Schneider, 'The So-Called Rejuvenation Treatment', 49–74; Schneider, 'Some Suggestions on Reactivation', 722–36.

[45] Voronoff, *The Study of Old Age*.

[46] 'Voronoff's Method of Rejuvenation', *The Lancet*, 26 February 1927, 446–47, 446.

[47] Ibid., 447.   [48] Walker and Lumsden Cook, 'Steinach's Rejuvenation Operation', 225.

also known as the Vivarium.[49] The new posting, which came when Steinach was already fifty-one years of age, opened two critical opportunities. The first was to concentrate almost solely on research, given that the Vivarium was not a teaching institution; the second was to collaborate closely with the long-standing Vivarium researcher Paul Kammerer (1880–1926) who had been based there for a decade by the time of Steinach's arrival.

Drawing on his previous experience of noting that cattle, bred by his grandfather, seemed to exhibit significantly altered physiological and behavioural patterns once castrated, Steinach took advantage of his newfound experimental freedom to better understand why these changes took place. His earliest work in this regard plotted a very explicit connection between 'sexual disposition' and sex glands. As *The Lancet* reported, dismissively, in 1917 Steinach claimed to have 'changed the sexual disposition of small mammals by implanting, as the case might be, an ovary into a young male or testicular substance into a young female'.[50] Prior to this, his work had been discussed in the British medical press primarily in regard to the effects of manipulating the sex glands on puberty and the function of the prostate gland.[51] The culmination of his research in his early years at the Vivarium was a book of rather different focus: *Verjüngung durch experimentelle Neubelubung der alternden Pubertätsdrüse* (*Rejuvenation by Experimental Revitalisation of the Ageing Gland of Puberty*), which appeared in 1920.[52] Drawing on the work of G. Frank Lydston, an American urologist who had carried out a number of transplantation procedures of the sexual organs in men, and his own colleague in Vienna, Robert Lichtenstern, Steinach noted that having performed ligation of the vas deferens – a procedure we recognise today as vasectomy – on elderly rats, they appeared to regain some of their former youthful features, including significant weight gain as a result of increased

---

[49] Södersten, Crews, Logan and Soukup, 'Eugen Steinach; Walch, *Triebe, Reize und Signale*. Steinach had previously carried out investigation into the physiology of the male sex glands, but only shortly before his appointment at the Vivarium had he begun to explore the links between glandular activity and sexual characteristics. For examples of these earlier studies, see: Eugen Steinach, 'Untersuchungen zur vergleichenden Physiologie der männlichen Geschlechtsorgane insbesondere der accessorischen Geschlechtsdrüsen', *Pflügers Archiv* 56 (1894), 304–38; Eugen Steinach, 'Geschlechtstrieb und echt sekundäre Geschlechtsmerkmale als Folge der innersekretorischen Funktion der Keimdrüsen', *Zentralblatt für Physiologie* 24 (1910), 551–66. Steinach's early work on the eye was reported in the British medical press. See, for example, 'Comparative Physiology of the Iris', *The Lancet*, 22 November 1890, 1112.

[50] 'The Internal Secretion of the Reproductive Glands', *The Lancet*, 3 November 1917, 687.

[51] 'The Function of the Prostate', *British Medical Journal*, 5 June 1909, 1382–83; 'Physiology', *British Medical Journal*, 3 October 1914, 586–87. Chandak Sengoopta has also argued that Steinach's theories of sexuality, developed in this period, played a fundamental role in 'anchoring' the activism of Magnus Hirschfield, who was able to claim that homosexual men were 'a distinct, autonomous group of organically feminized men'. Sengoopta, 'Glandular Politics', 445.

[52] Steinach, *Verjüngung*.

appetite, heightened levels of physical activity and a restored drive to mate, leading to higher fertility, at least at the population level.[53]

In Britain, *Verjüngung* itself received comparatively little attention – it was, for example, not reviewed in either *The Lancet* or *British Medical Journal* – despite Sengoopta's claim that '[i]t caused an immediate uproar' owing to Steinach's collaboration with Lichtenstern. Lichtenstern had extended the animal-bounded procedure to human patients.[54] Instead, the British medical community was as much interested in the priority dispute between Lydston, Steinach and Voronoff in their discovery of the effect of transplantation of sex glands as the likely consequences of these claims; initially, at least, they were rooted in debates about the nature of sexuality over and above rejuvenation.[55] Steinach's assertion at a meeting of the Biological Society of Vienna in early 1921, that 'by causing a proliferation of these [interstitial] cells [of the sex gland,] rejuvenation of the organism can be produced in a marked degree', brought rejuvenescence into focus.[56] Following this, and the subsequent race to replicate Steinach and Lichtenstern's findings, discussion moved quickly to the likelihood that they had identified a method which could restore vitality in older men.

Accounts which seemed to provide striking confirmation of the success of Steinach's methods in animals continued to appear in the British medical press throughout the early 1920s. Many were based around individual cases; for example, in findings reported in *The Lancet* in April 1922 (published first the preceding month in *Zeitschrift für Sexualwissenschaft*), the Danish sexologist, eugenicist and forensic clinician Knud Sand (1887–1968) claimed that he had effected a rejuvenation in a senile German shepherd dog following 'resection of the left epididymis and right-sided vasectomy' – a procedure akin to the Steinach operation.[57] Subsequently, and like both Steinach and Voronoff, Sand expanded his purview to humans, and in 1923 reported on 'the rationale, technique, and the results' of eighteen such cases. His procedure was more complex than that of Steinach, yet he still relied extensively on subjective reports from his patients, collected between three and twenty-one months after the operation. Presenting a digest of the findings, *The Lancet* noted that rejuvenation had 'an apparently irresistible appeal to elderly persons whose waning virility renders them disconsolate and fretful'; of Sand's findings, 'the method is evidently in such an early, experimental stage that its unreserved advocacy is not at present warranted.'[58]

[53] Sengoopta, *The Most Secret Quintessence*, 83; Steinach, *Verjüngung*, 30.
[54] Sengoopta, *The Most Secret Quintessence*, 84.
[55] 'Transplantation of the Sex Glands', *British Medical Journal*, 12 March 1921, 42.
[56] 'Vienna (from our own Correspondent)', *The Lancet*, 26 February 1921, 454.
[57] 'A Canine Rejuvenation Experiment', *The Lancet*, 29 April 1922, 857.
[58] 'Steinach's Operation', *The Lancet*, 24 February 1923, 393.

One of the most extensive reflections on Steinach's work came from a dedicated article – 'Steinach's Rejuvenation Operation' – jointly authored by Kenneth M. Walker and J. A. Lumsdem Cook. Walker was Hunterian Professor at the London-based Royal Northern Hospital, Lumsden Cook an Assistant Medical Officer at St Mary Abbots Hospital, and together they outlined Steinach's claims and considered critical responses, paying particular attention to the relationship between the results in animals and human cases. Rather than an outright rejection of this possible means of rejuvenation, Walker and Lumsden Cook acknowledged that 'there is insufficient material on which to base a decision as to the value of vasoligature as a means of treatment in man.' At the same time, they recognised that 'whatever the verdict concerning this clinical problem may be the results, obtained by Steinach in his animal experiment are certainly of the greatest biological interest.'[59]

This was at odds with the Vienna correspondent of the *British Medical Journal* who, just one year later, reflected on the 'original enthusiasm over the boon conferred upon mankind by Prof Steinach and his collaborators', which had by then 'given way to profound silence'.[60] Others still, such as Swale Vincent, professor of physiology at the University of London and a clinician at the Middlesex Hospital, decried the attention afforded to hormones. In his Ingleby Lectures delivered at the University of Birmingham in 1921, Vincent argued that

current views on the whole subject of internal secretion demand a severely critical examination, for no other branch of physiology is littered with so many vague, unproved, and, in many case unprovable hypotheses. A newly-coined word appears every few months; the term 'hormone' is in everybody's mouth.[61]

In many respects, it was this frenzied dedication to the hormonal cause which long outlasted the claims of supposed rejuvenation rooted in the endocrine system. Two years later, on 9 January 1923, Vincent introduced a discussion on 'The Present Position of Organotherapy' at a meeting of the Royal Society of Medicine. Here, he began by delivering a 'cold douche of scepticism' over the efficacy of gland-derived treatments, yet he also stated 'that it was too early to appraise the value of these rival claims [of Steinach and Voronoff], or to express a positive opinion as to the results which might be expected to follow either of the methods.'[62]

A significant number of authors across both Europe and North America explicitly rejected Voronoff's claims whilst at the same time endorsing the

---

[59] Walker and Cook, 'Steinach's Rejuvenation Operation', 226.
[60] 'Vienna (from our own Correspondent)', *The Lancet*, 28 March 1925, 683.
[61] Vincent, 'The Endocrine Functions', 303.
[62] 'Medical Societies. Royal Society of Medicine. Section of Therapeutics and Pharmacology', *The Lancet*, 20 January 1923, 130–32, 130 and 132.

practice of the Steinach operation. One such individual was the German physician and rejuvenation advocate Peter Schmidt. Even as early as 1924, when the efficacy of Voronoff's methods did at least remain a possibility in the minds of many medical practitioners, subject to more extensive verification, Schmidt argued that the advent of Steinach's procedure had effectively supplanted the necessity for any kind of gland grafting. For Schmidt, the grafting of donor animal tissue had 'obvious disadvantages' and was of a fundamentally different nature; the Steinach operation had 'nothing whatever in common with those [experiments] of Voronoff on monkey glands, although it is often confused with that work, even in the profession'.[63] After these remarks, Voronoff was a virtual absentee from Schmidt's account, which presented eighty-four cases of the vasoligature operation which he had carried out, as well as selected examples from other surgeons. Collectively, Schmidt claimed that his cases demonstrated the central tenet of Steinach's thesis, namely that '[i]ncrease in hormonopoiesis [production of hormones] in individuals with signs of old age, premature or not, partial or total, causes a regeneration which may be termed rejuvenation.'[64] Tellingly, this hormonopoiesis was 'independent of the formation and excretion of procreative cells', demonstrating a clear break with the sealed spermatic economy advanced in the latter decades of the nineteenth century.[65]

By presenting and describing a series of cases of successful rejuvenation through surgical means, Schmidt clearly hoped to sway doubters amongst the medical profession and lend credibility to the Steinach operation. However, reviews of his work indicate that in some circles it had the opposite effect. Rather than enhancing support for Steinach's idea, *The Theory and Practice of the Steinach Operation*, in the words of a reviewer writing for the *British Medical Journal*, 'very much weakened' such a claim.[66] In other quarters the jury was still out. An earlier review in *The Lancet* praised Schmidt for documenting cases 'in which no very definite results were obtained' in addition to accounts of stunning success. Although the reviewer in this case noted that Schmidt was an 'ardent partisan' for the views of Steinach, the clinical results spoke for themselves, and the book was 'one of the best scientific expositions of the subject available for British readers ... [which] should prove of interest to all who are prepared to adopt an unprejudiced attitude towards its subject-matter'.[67]

In his later work, *The Conquest of Old Age*, published in 1931, Schmidt reiterated his support of Steinach and critique of Voronoff. The method of testicular grafting favoured by the latter, he argued, 'cannot be regarded as an

---

[63] Schmidt, *Theory and Practice*, x and xiii.   [64] Ibid., 36.   [65] Ibid.
[66] 'Steinach's Operation', *British Medical Journal*, 4 April 1925, 662–63, 663.
[67] 'The Steinach Operation', *The Lancet*, 4 October 1924, 702.

ideal one'.[68] Schmidt, in common with some of the more fervent advocates of rejuvenation, such as Jean Frumusan, went further in his claims than Steinach and practitioners of the eponymous procedure. Whilst Harry Benjamin – the New York surgeon who grew to prominence performing the Steinach operation on both men and women – was reluctant to link interventions in the sex glands with lifespan, Schmidt had no such qualms. His rejuvenation doctrine was summed up as 'more life in each year and more years in each life'; the Steinach operation could, he claimed, not only restore lost vigour but also extend lifespan.[69]

Schmidt's reporting of numerous cases also highlighted a perpetual challenge for rejuvenation advocates: How to present cases of failure without delegitimising or undermining their claims of efficacy? Both Voronoff and Steinach fell foul of this in the eyes of medical commentators by not including unsuccessful cases in their publications, with others, such as the auto-experimenting Maximilian von Zeissl, praised for communicating instances where the procedures seemed to produce no perceptible results. Zeissl, who pioneered the use of Salvarsan in cases of venereal disease in Germany, was sixty-nine years old when he submitted himself for section of both vasa deferentia – an operation analogous but not identical to the Steinach operation – in 1922.[70] The report was originally published in *Wiener klinische Wochenschrift* before being taken up by *The Lancet* in an article entitled 'An Unsuccessful Steinach Operation' which commended the 'praiseworthy candour' of Zeissl in making the negative results of his procedure available.[71] Later other outlets, including the *Indian Medical Gazette*, also looked favourably on Zeissl, reporting his experience alongside others and also declaring the premature end to Steinach's other notable procedure – female rejuvenation through diathermy and X-rays.[72]

The mobilisation of Zeissl's case to sow doubt about the efficacy of the Steinach operation was not without riposte, however. This came in the form of a letter from the American psychologist Edward Wheeler Scripture, who noted that there were fundamental differences in the procedure reported by Zeissl and that described by Steinach. Scripture, then based at the West End Hospital for Nervous Diseases in London, contended that '[t]he case reported ... cannot be called an "unsuccessful Steinach operation," as no Steinach operation was performed.'[73] In a lecture to the Medical Section of the British Psychological Society just a month previously, Scripture reported Steinach as arguing that

---

[68] Schmidt, *Conquest of Old Age*, 39.   [69] Ibid., 301.   [70] 'The By-Effects of Salvarsan', 4.
[71] 'An Unsuccessful Steinach Operation', 1154.
[72] Diathermy is discussed in more detail in Chapter 4. 'The Results of Attempted Rejuvenation', *Indian Medical Gazette*, September 1925, 436.
[73] Scripture, 'An Unsuccessful Steinach Operation', 1206.

'psycho-analysis (as well as all psychic treatment) ... alters the internal secretions and thereby influences the bodily and mental character.' He went on to note that, given the seeming connection between hormone therapy and psychoanalysis, there was the 'possibility of curing a portion of the countless cases of anxiety neurosis (including hysteria) by a simple inexpensive surgical operation', namely the Steinach operation.[74]

Seeding Rejuvenation beyond Steinach and Voronoff

Critical to the success of Steinach and Voronoff in stimulating debate within the medical profession was a small but fervent clutch of disciples. For Steinach this was, of course, necessary, given that he was not able to carry out the procedures in humans himself. Voronoff initially ensured that his own practices remained more opaque, keeping his techniques largely secret before producing a comprehensive, illustrated account in 1927.

Amongst the most high-profile advocates of rejuvenation was Paul Kammerer. Kammerer was and remains a controversial scientific figure whose experimental work on forms of Lamarckian inheritance has been categorised as at best misguided and at worst entirely fraudulent.[75] In 1924, just two years before committing suicide in the face of accusations of falsifying results – claims which he strenuously denied – Kammerer published *Rejuvenation and the Prolongation of Human Efficiency,* drawing on the sensational results of his Vivarium colleague, Steinach, and the science of rejuvenation, which he claimed was 'forging ahead on the road to victory'.[76] In this text, Kammerer identified 'intensified eagerness and capacity to work' as one of the most significant benefits to rejuvenation, which he took to be literally 'regained youth'.[77] Rejuvenation was a process which involved wholesale physiological change: the disappearance of wrinkles, alleviation of deafness, improvement in eyesight, restored appetite, luxuriant hair growth, as well as reawakening of the dormant libido.[78] Indeed, for Kammerer the 're-awakening of the most tender feelings in man which, with the growing re-strengthening of the patient, are almost invariably intensified to an actual possibility to live up to the gratification of his desires'.[79] The restoration of sexual desire through means of rejuvenation was therefore accompanied by a parallel return of virility and potency, with a hormonal rebalancing cited as the principal cause.

Just as the Steinach operation had tended to treat male and female bodies as fundamentally different – anatomically, hormonally and sexually – Kammerer

[74] 'Vienna: Some Recent Medical Work', *British Medical Journal,* 18 November 1922, 988–99, 999.
[75] Bowler, *Evolution,* 265–66.   [76] Kammerer, *Rejuvenation,* vii.   [77] Ibid., 95.
[78] Ibid., 96–97.   [79] Ibid., 101.

highlighted the 'much greater obstacles' faced when attempting to rejuvenate women.[80] He endorsed Steinach's view that this might be achieved through the use of X-ray treatments, and also highlighted the utility of ultra-violet treatments, whether through exposure to natural sunlight or through the use of bespoke UV lamps, such as the Quartz Light or Alpine Sun Lamp, which would 'reawaken the joy of life and the urge to live and love'.[81]

However, although we might be tempted to read Kammerer's work as an enthusiastic endorsement of scientific rejuvenation for all, his first suggestion was in fact to combat ageing through 'proper living'; the Steinach operation was, for Kammerer, the option of last resort.[82] This is, perhaps, especially surprising given that Kammerer was a collaborator of Steinach in Vienna: both worked at the Vivarium and held similar goals of integrating the emerging sciences of endocrinology and genetics.[83]

Nor was Kammerer alone in arguing that, for the most part, old age was best attained by natural means. The French physician and author of popular books on rejuvenation, Jean Frumusan, highlighted the erroneous practice of ascribing the age of a person to 'the almanac'. Rather, he argued, age should be defined according to the physiological state of 'tissues, viscera, the great nervous and arterio-venous system and by their results which form the physical and moral personality'.[84] Kammerer's position reflected an increased emphasis on biological rather than chronological age, though this distinction would only become more concretised later in the twentieth century.[85]

In Britain one of the chief prophets of rejuvenation treatment was the Australian-born sexologist Norman Haire (1892–1952).[86] An early advocate of birth control who had arrived in London in 1919 and quickly established a flourishing Harley Street practice, Haire's work reveals that he saw a particularly English anxiety about public discussions of hormone rejuvenation. He noted in his 1924 commentary, *Rejuvenation*, that

[s]o much general misapprehension and ignorance exists concerning Rejuvenation ... In America it has received more attention, and on the Continent has been very fully treated by both medical and lay writers. In England, when one speaks of Rejuvenation, even educated people will say, 'Oh, yes, I know. Monkey glands. The thyroid, isn't it?'[87]

Just as Haire acted as promoter-in-chief for the Steinach operation, putting it into practice in Britain, so too Voronoff had his own champion: Leonard

---

[80] Ibid., 111.   [81] Ibid., 111 and 133.   [82] Ibid., 134.
[83] Logan, *Hormones, Heredity, and Race*, 4.   [84] Frumusan, *Rejuvenation*, 34.
[85] Moreira, *Science, Technology and the Ageing Society*.
[86] For a comprehensive analysis of Haire's life and work, see: Wyndham, *Norman Haire*; Crozier, 'Becoming a Sexologist'.
[87] Haire, *Rejuvenation*, 5–6.

Williams (1861–1939). Williams was a medical officer in the employ of the Legal and General Assurance Society who embraced Voronoff's approach to understanding the role and function of the sex glands in rejuvenation and defended not only the surgeon's ideas but also his motivations. In the face of what he saw as misleading representations of Voronoff's work in the British medical press, Williams visited Voronoff in December 1922.[88] Following this meeting, where he observed an operation on a male patient and conversed with the surgeon, Williams was convinced that 'the internal secretion of the male gonad can accomplish miracles.'[89]

In subsequent years Williams published further and expanded his remit from the hormone surgery of Voronoff which first piqued his interest. As we will see in Chapter 3, Williams was very much in line with his contemporaries in recommending a diet of moderation as a sure way of preserving 'health, efficiency, and longevity of the community'.[90] This, he argued in his 1924 book, *The Art and Science of Living*, was the foundation of 'the case for a simpler life'; pursuing the 'quest of health and efficiency', he argued, would enable humans to avoid the 'petty luxuries which we have ignorantly and arrogantly embraced'.[91] For Williams, the pure biology espoused by the likes of Darwin and Huxley had become obscured by the elevation of the human mind amongst professional scientists who should instead 'recognise that it is useless to study man as he now shows himself; they must study, not the gentleman or the bourgeois, but the genus homo.'[92]

Williams – ostensibly a medical assessor for an insurance company, yet conventionally trained at Glasgow University and a member of the Royal College of Physicians – embodied the somewhat territorial spirit adopted by the medical profession on matters of ageing. His commentaries, which were rooted in the hard rejuvenation procedures of Voronoff, extolled 'the curative effects of sunshine' and castigated the fashion for 'tight corsets', all the while bemoaning 'the most fantastic and foolish defiance of Nature's laws' represented by 'present-day food'.[93] It is sufficient to note here, then, that Williams's purview had widened significantly, far beyond his original interest in hormone rejuvenation. By 1929 he had become even more specifically focussed on the ageing process, beyond simple health and efficiency. In his short book, *Growing Old Gracefully* – just forty-eight pages long – he articulated a vision of longevity which was almost entirely detached from medical intervention. Diet, exercise, fresh air and work were critical to preserve 'an old age unhampered by impaired efficiency'.[94] Tight clothing was again in Williams's firing line as he argued that the continued fashion for a

---

[88] Williams, 'Testicular Grafts', 130.   [89] Williams, 'Endocrines, Vitamins', 1011.
[90] Williams, *Science and Art*, 8.   [91] Ibid., 7 and 10.   [92] Ibid., 18.
[93] Williams, *Science and Art*, 20–21.   [94] Williams, *Growing Old Gracefully*, 8.

clost-fitting collar worn by men over fifty years old contributed 'very largely to the baldness, deafness, and defective sight which characterise advancing years'.[95] This concern with numerous factors affecting the ageing process was later expanded still further as Williams turned his pen to a range of topics, producing well-received books on emanotherapy (treatment using radon) and obesity amongst others.[96]

For all the focus on the sex glands in the early interwar period, within a decade even Steinach's own focus had shifted. In the spring of 1928 he announced that he no longer held the view that the gonads were the sole arbiter of bodily youthfulness; rather, he claimed that the 'germinal glands', the testes and ovaries, had a 'secretive alliance with the pituitary gland'.[97] The implication of other structures within the endocrine system from one of the principal architects of hormone rejuvenation represented not a wholesale *volte face*, but a recognition that there was more to the biological aspects of the ageing process than expiring testicles. The procedures carried out by surgeons and practitioners such as Steinach, Voronoff and Haire were just one aspect of hormonal rejuvenation in the interwar period. However, their work also served to open a far more long-lasting niche in the marketplace for products such as the hormone-containing skin creams and dietary supplements, discussed in later chapters, aimed at less wealthy and high-profile, but still affluent, clients.

Given the divergence of attitudes and practices even amongst those who pioneered and advocated rejuvenation, can we say anything substantive about their work as a collective? First, it is noteworthy that the rejuvenators placed huge reliance on the case history as a form of evidence, and in particular the subjective, reported experience of patients, followed up over many months. The functional unit was the successfully rejuvenated older person, and such instances were invariably accompanied in both medical and public discourse with fulsome extramedical details, such as occupation, character and lifestyle habits. To pick just one of Schmidt's cases illustrates the point. The patient was described as a '[h]ighly-placed State official (in foreign parts)' who had 'never felt sure of himself'. Sexual activity was almost beyond him and, even '[i]f he succeeded in performing coitus, the orgasm was very difficult to achieve'. Seven months after ligature of the right vas deferens according to the Steinach method, his skin was 'firmer and better lined with fat ... far more lively and cheerful'. Further, he had 'become enterprising' and was able to

[95] Ibid., 12.
[96] Humphris and Williams; 'Emanotherapy', *Indian Medical Journal* 72:7 (1937), 448; Williams, *Obesity*.
[97] 'Science: Rejuvenation', *Time*, 23 April 1930.

'play his part better in society'.[98] As we will see in later chapters, however, hormone rejuvenators were far from unique in relying on the individual case history; examples which drew on diet, electrotherapy, exercise and electrotherapy also made extensive reference to such features.

Second, the before-and-after images of Voronoff, Schmidt and Steinach were illustrative of the importance placed on visual documentation of rejuvenation. As we have already seen, the supposed clear transformation experienced by Voronoff's patients was mobilised to constitute a powerful form of visual testimony about the efficacy of testicular grafting. Voronoff reproduced some images across numerous publications through the 1920s. Both Steinach and Schmidt employed similar and even more startling techniques (see Figures 2.1 and 2.2). Whilst enhanced sexual proficiency was widely recognised as a key indicator of rejuvenation success, an increase in weight through improved musculature and strength was also critical in demonstrating a return of youthful physical fitness and bodily prowess.[99] In the view of most medical commentators these forms of evidence were sufficient only to provide proof for the laity. For example, an editorial in *The Lancet* responded to Voronoff's recent publication of *Greffes Testiculaires* by noting dryly that 'a few observations by means of ergographs, fatigue experiments, blood-pressure records, and basal metabolism investigations would have been of greater value to the scientist than photographs of old gentlemen fencing and carrying bags upstairs.'[100]

Wider Politics and Perceptions of Hormone Rejuvenation

Grafting of glands is still on its trial.[101]

During the 1920s, Voronoff's xenotransplantation of slivers of monkey testicle into aged and prematurely ageing men and reports on instances of the Steinach operation served to heighten the physiological allure of monkey glands, hormones and the biological possibility of bodily renewal in the public imagination. Their practices kept members of the medical profession alert to the possibility that these methods might be effective, but more importantly they also acquired a deep cultural resonance. Cultural outputs such as a large number of fictional accounts of rejuvenation, including novels like Gertrude Atherton's *Black Oxen* (1923, as well as its accompanying film of the same

---

[98] Schmidt, *Conquest of Old Age*, 159–60. Intriguingly, Schmidt noted that the 'hereditary equipment' of the patient 'was obviously defective', yet 'it was possible to give him a useful impetus from the endocrine side.' Schmidt, *Conquest of Old Age*, 60.

[99] Ibid., 165–68.

[100] 'Testicular Grafting', *The Lancet*, 18 November 1922, 1079–80, 1080. Voronoff did, in fact, report on reductions in blood pressure in some of his subjects but did not aggregate these into a systematic analysis, and his general claims were extracted from specific cases rather than the organised investigations typical of medico-scientific enquiry.

[101] 'Gland-grafting', *The Lancet*, 1 May 1926, 920.

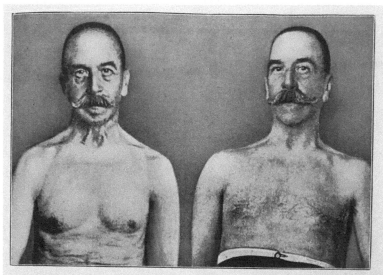

FIG. 1.   MAN AGED 66 ON DAY OF   FIG. 2.   SAME MAN THREE MONTHS
            OPERATION   LATER
            (From E. Steinach's material, shown in the Ufa Film)

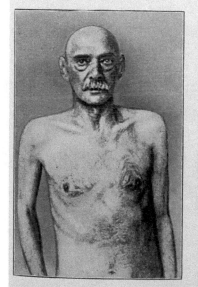
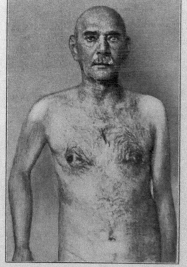

FIG. 1.   MAN AGED 74 ON DAY OF   FIG. 2.   SAME MAN FOUR MONTHS
            OPERATION   LATER
            (From E. Steinach's material, shown in the Ufa Film)

Figure 2.1 Before-and-after images of two patients featured in the
Steinach Film.
(Peter Schmidt, *The Conquest of Old Age*, 1931, plate XXXV.)

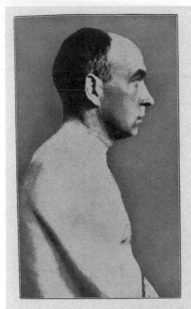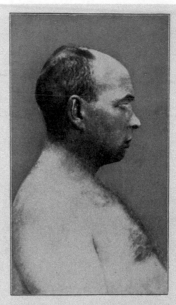

FIG. 1. ON DAY OF OPERATION   FIG. 2. THREE MONTHS LATER
(Case A.10. Text, pp. 165 *et seq.*)

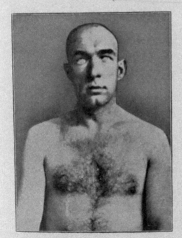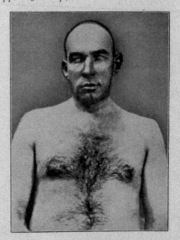

FIG. 1. ON DAY OF OPERATION   FIG. 2. THREE MONTHS LATER
(Case A.10. Text, pp. 165 *et seq.*)
(From Peter Schmidt's material)

Figure 2.2 Before-and-after images of a thirty-four-year-old technician, one of Peter Schmidt's patients. Schmidt noted that the patient had become impotent as a result of premature masturbation from the age of eight. Restoration of sexual potency was combined with 'muscular energy' and such objective indicators of successful rejuvenation as being able to 'now lift and carry a burden of about 200 lbs', which was previously impossible, as well as weight gain of 28 lbs.
(Peter Schmidt, *The Conquest of Old Age*, 1931, plate XXXVII.)

year) and Bertram Gayton's *The Gland Stealers* (1922) provided playful, imaginative spaces for continued rejuvenation discourse.[102] This enabled everyone from advertisers to politicians to mobilise the concept of rejuvenation for commercial gain and to provide satirical commentary on aged and decrepit organisations, individuals and ideas. The medium of educational and instructive films was also critical in promoting the procedures and findings of Steinach and Voronoff both in Britain and elsewhere. For example, in his 'Medical Review of Soviet Russia' – a series of articles published throughout the mid-1920s in the *British Medical Journal* – W. Horsley Gannt noted that a series of films to promote 'personal hygiene' included one entitled '"Rejuvenation", explaining the Voronoff and Steinach operations'.[103] Cartoonists and commentators also relished the opportunity (see Figure 2.3), with the influence of rejuvenation spanning across class and social context. Speaking in the House of Lords on 20 June 1927, the Duke of Marlborough commented 'that while Professor Voronoff has produced a formula for the prolongation of the life of the individual, at present His Majesty's Ministers seem undecided as to the formula to be applied for the prolongation of the corporate existence of this House.'[104]

Indeed, alongside the supposedly wondrous results of the procedure and the figure of Voronoff himself, who took on a quasi-mythical status in the popular imagination, the 'monkey gland' and its effects also assumed huge cultural significance. At the height of the rejuvenation craze in 1923, for example, the famous bartender of the Ritz Hotel in Paris, Frank Meier, whose notoriety ensured that he was known simply as 'Frank of the Ritz', developed a new cocktail entitled 'The Monkey Gland'.[105] According to the *Washington Post*, the drink consisted of 'half and half gin and orange juice, a dash of absinthe, and a dash of raspberry or other sweet juice. Mix well with ice and serve only with a doctor handy. Inside half an hour the other day Frank purveyed forty of these, to the exclusion of Manhattans and Martinis.'[106] The Monkey Gland was also known as 'The McCormick' after Harold McCormick, the millionaire

---

[102] See, for example, Oakley, 'Vital Forms'; Oakley, 'Sexual Rejuvenation and Hegemonic Masculinity'. These works of 'rejuvenation fiction' continued through the 1930s, with examples such as M. E. Mitchell's *Yet in My Flesh* (1933), John Gloag's *Winter's Youth* (1934), Thorne Smith's *The Glorious Pool* (1934), and Aldous Huxley's *After Many a Summer* (1939).

[103] Gantt, 'A Medical Review of Soviet Russia', 340. Gantt himself was former Chief of the Medical Division of the American Relief Administration, based in Leningrad.

[104] 'House of Lords Sitting', 20 June 1927, 20th Century House of Lords Hansard Sessional Papers, Series 5, Vol. 67, 765.

[105] Meier was the author of a legendary text on cocktails and mixing. According to this, Meier himself had later amended the recipe to replace absinthe with Pernod. See Meier, *The Artistry of Mixing Drinks*, 35.

[106] 'New Cocktail in Paris Is the Monkey Gland', *Washington Post*, 29 April 1923, 43.

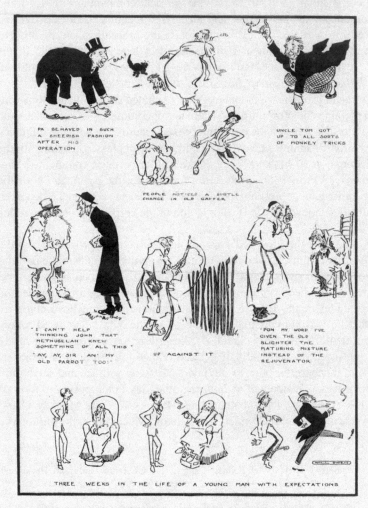

Figure 2.3 An imagination of the social consequence of rejuvenation in a number of contexts, from the pen of the illustrator Will Owen (1869–1957). These and other images reflected public fascination with various aspects of hormone rejuvenation, such as the relationship between humans and animals, the battle between man (exemplified here by Serge Voronoff) and natural death, and rejuvenation 'gone wrong'. ('When All the World Is Young', *The Sketch*, 15 October 1919, 75.)

former husband of Edith Rockefeller, who following their divorce in 1921 was one of the first of Voronoff's patients in Paris.[107]

As well as the human implications of Voronoff's work with goats, sheep and other animals, the economic prospects of being able to rejuvenate livestock were also taken seriously. For example, in March 1927, Sir Harry Brittain, the Conservative MP for Acton, enquired of the Minister of Agriculture, Walter Guinness, whether he was aware of the outcome of Voronoff's grafting experiments in livestock. Guinness responded that a 'small Commission of scientific men' were scheduled to examine the rejuvenated animals at the 'Government Breeding Station in Algeria' in October or November.[108] Politicians and scientists alike continued to take Voronoff's claims seriously, or at least agreed that they warranted serious attention, with further questions of this nature – on everything from wool production to old-age pensions and support for older workers – a regular feature in Parliament.[109] After repeated calls, the Commission was brought together by the Ministry of Agriculture and Fisheries and the Board of Agriculture for Scotland, and included Francis Crew, Chair of Animal Genetics at the University of Edinburgh, and W. C. Miller of the Royal Veterinary (Dick) College.[110]

Sensationally, the so-called super-sheep (as described in *The Times*) also attracted the attentions of delegations from Argentina, Italy, Spain and Czechoslovakia.[111] After visiting Algiers and inspecting first-hand the animals which had been subject to treatment by Voronoff, the Commission offered its

---

[107] McCormick, *Family Record and Biography*.

[108] 'Commons Sitting', 21 March 1927, 20th Century House of Commons Hansard Sessional Papers, Fifth Series, Vol. 204, 22.

[109] 'Commons Sitting', 12 July 1927, 20th Century House of Commons Hansard Sessional Papers, Fifth Series, Vol. 208, 1932. In the context of a major debate about the extent to which the Widows, Orphans and Old Age Contributory Pensions Act (1925), the first contributory state pension scheme, Cecil L'Estrange Malone, Independent Labour MP for Northampton, highlighted that pensions were not paid out in the event that non-pensionable individuals were deemed too old to work. In the same debate, highlighting the ubiquity of Voronoff and rejuvenation in public discourse, the Labour MP for Wellingborough, William Cove, argued that 'Members opposite if and when they are senile can afford to consult Dr. Voronoff and get a rejuvenation of monkey gland. My old gardener could not afford that, and, although he has worked all his life and paid contributions for 12 years since the health insurance scheme began, he is denied the old age pension.' 'Commons Sitting', 22 February 1928, 20th Century House of Commons Hansard Sessional Papers, Fifth Series, Vol. 218, 1681.

[110] *Sixteenth report of the Board of Agriculture for Scotland*, 37.

[111] '"Super-sheep". Dr Voronoff's Experiments', *The Times*, 11 November 1927, 15. In response to the article two members of the Commission, Marshall and Crew, noted that they reserved judgement on whether policy changes should be made in light of their findings. Marshall and Crew, '"Super-sheep"', 21. This discussion mirrored an earlier episode from 1923 when an exceptionally aged former racehorse was 'operated on according to Professor Steinach's method of rejuvenation' in the hopes of 'becoming a youngster again'. The horse in question was described in the press as an 'inoculated super-horse'. See 'The Inoculated Horse', *Rugby Advertiser*, 20 February 1923, 4.

findings in the spring of 1928. The report was largely inconclusive, with the Commission refusing to be drawn on whether they had secured proof that Voronoff's method was either effective or ineffective.[112] For example, as reported in the *British Medical Journal*, having been presented with the rejuvenated bull, Jacky, who had been 'discarded as useless in 1922, when 17 years of age', the Commission was informed that Jacky had, since being grafted with freshly testicular material, 'sired nine calves . . . and the operation was repeated, apparently with some success'.[113] It was unclear, however, that other factors, such as diet, natural fertility (Jacky was considered to be an exceptional case) and proper experimental control, were considered adequately, and the members of the Commission were clear that there were no reasons to suppose that Voronoff's method would be of economic significance for British stock breeders.

By the second half of 1928, the Board of Agriculture for Scotland was making the first of a lengthy series of independent efforts to test the efforts of Voronoff's procedures on sheep.[114] Their preliminary line of enquiry involved the use of thyroxin 'as an influencing agent in the growth of [the] fleece', a far departure from the gland grafting of animal testicular extract into ageing men in the fashionable climate of interwar Paris.[115]

Even after the publication of this report, in response to a further question in Parliament, Guinness revealed that plans were in place 'for carefully controlled experiments to test the claims made on behalf of Dr. Voronoff's work'. To allay fears about improper treatment of animals, Guinness was at pains to point out that 'experiments on living animals calculated to give pain are subject to licence and inspection by the Home Office under the Cruelty to Animals Act, 1876.'[116] This anxiety surrounding the experimental work of Voronoff also extended to humans, and was brought into focus when the surgeon visited England in the early summer of 1928. The radical Liberal MP for Lambeth North and frequent critic of Voronoff, Frank Briant, was particularly concerned that Voronoff would use the opportunity to further blur the lines between human and animal, and between male and female, by conducting 'dangerous and disgusting operations, which include the transfer of the organs

---

[112] Marshall, Crew, Walton and Miller, *Report on Dr Serge Voronoff's Experiments*; 'Commons Sitting', 21 June 1928, 20th Century House of Commons Hansard Sessional Papers, Fifth Series, Vol. 218, 1747.

[113] 'Voronoff's Experiments on the Improvement of Livestock', *British Medical Journal*, 24 March 1928, 505.

[114] These continued well into 1929: *Development Commission*, 71.

[115] *Seventeenth report of the Board of Agriculture for Scotland*, 32.

[116] 'Written Answers (Commons)', 13 March 1928, 20th Century House of Commons Hansard Sessional Papers, Fifth Series, Vol. 214, 1744.

of propagation from an ape to a woman'.[117] The *British Medical Journal* printed the parliamentary exchange between Briant and the controversial Home Secretary William Joynson-Hicks, who sought to reassure Briant that he had not issued Voronoff with a licence to practise vivisection.[118]

Elsewhere, the noted anti-vivisectionists Lizzy Lind af Hageby and the Duchess of Hamilton, who had co-founded the Animal Defence and Anti-Vivisection Society in 1903 and taken leading roles in the Brown Dog Affair in subsequent years, arranged a public meeting at Caxton Hall in Westminster on 8 June to declare the practices of Voronoff as 'dangerous, indecent, and cruel'.[119] At the meeting Dr Maurice Beddow Bayly – like Lind af Hageby and Hamilton a prominent member of the Society – described Voronoff's practices as 'a grave menace to the human race', and noted that 'serious risk of ape-like offspring was incurred by women through transplantation [of animal material].'[120] Beddow Bayly went into print in June 1928, decrying Voronoff's methods in a pamphlet published by the Animal Defence Society and warning of the 'ghoulish despoliation of the corpses of people who happen to die in hospitals', 'increase in prostitution, venereal disease and illegitimacy', and 'the risk to any woman … of a subsequent pregnancy resulting in semi-monkey offspring'.[121] This publication eventually drew him into correspondence with the founder of the Centenarian Club and enthusiastic rejuvenation commentator Maurice Ernest who in 1936 wrote to Beddow Bayly to request copies of his pamphlets.[122]

Indeed, the preoccupation with Voronoff's work as it applied to animals was a peculiar phenomenon of government and prominent anti-vivisection

---

[117] 'Commons Sitting', 14 June 1928, 20th Century House of Commons Hansard Sessional Papers, Fifth Series, Vol. 218, 1148; 'Commons Sitting', 13 June 1928, 20th Century House of Commons Hansard Sessional Papers, Fifth Series, Volume 218, 975. Briant continued to raise the matter in Parliament at regular intervals. See 'Written Answers (Commons)', 19 July 1928, 20th Century House of Commons Hansard Sessional Papers, Fifth Series, Vol. 220, 631.

[118] 'Medical Notes in Parliament', *British Medical Journal*, 23 June 1928, 1094–96, 1095.

[119] 'Protest against Dr Voronoff. Meeting Condemns Gland Treatment. "Degradation of Medicine"', *Manchester Guardian*, 8 June 1928, 13. For more on Lind af Hageby, Hamilton and the Brown Dog Affair, see: Kean, 'The "Smooth Cool Men of Science"', 16–38; Gälmark, 'Women Antivivisectionists', 1–32; Kean, *Animal Rights*; Lansbury, *The Old Brown Dog*.

[120] 'Protest against Dr Voronoff', 13.

[121] Bayly, *Dr Sergius Voronoff*, 4–5 and 7. Beddow Bayly's claim that Voronoff was responsible for desecrating bodies stands in sharp contrast to his acknowledged reliance on materials from animals; this whilst his contemporaries, including Lespinasse, Morris, Lydston and Kenneth Walker, used homografts from humans.

[122] M. Beddow Bayly to Maurice Ernest, 20 August 1936, interleafed in Bayly, *The Gland-Grafting Operations*, held at the British Library, UIN: BLL01012798038. Ernest was less-than-favourably impressed, replying that Beddow Bayly was 'using religious prejudice and anti-vivisectionist sentiment in trying to depreciate the value of biological experiments'. Maurice Ernest to M. Beddow Bayly, 24 August 1936, interleafed in Beddow Bayly, *The Gland-Grafting*.

activists, despite the broad acknowledgement of the effectiveness of such procedures in lower animals. For example, one of Beddow Bayly's principal anxieties about gland grafting was that 'it was bound to have an effect on the human race.' In a lecture to the London College of Physiology in early 1929, he expressed considerable concern that it might lead to the 'terrible possibility of the production of a new race ... more bestial than anything which had yet afflicted humanity'.[123] Nor was the anxiety of anti-vivisectionists restricted to the public arena. Surgeons sympathetic to gland-grafting were also faced with an environment in which, as the Birmingham-based surgeon Hamilton Bailey noted, 'anthropoids are scarce and antivivisectionists abound', preventing rigorous testing of this 'method full of promise'.[124]

Beddow Bayly, concerned not just at the endorsement by some medical practitioners but also the continued public fascination with the subject, also penned an article for *The Graphic* – 'The Menace of Dr Voronoff' – which claimed that his supposed rejuvenation came 'at the price of losing human characteristics'.[125] The article was a direct response to an interview with Voronoff which was published the previous month, and lamented 'this cult which ... has penetrated to every quarter of Western civilisation'.[126] Nor was Beddow Bayly alone in objecting to Voronoff's conclusions on anti-vivisectionist grounds. The Bristol-based campaigner Maurice L. Johnson, who had earlier attacked the Pasteurian therapy for rabies as being responsible for causing more cases than it prevented or treated, was one such voice.[127] Johnson condemned 'the fatuous speculations of vivisectors' and argued that Voronoff turned his patients into 'a sort of organic and functional mosaic by grafting the glands of monkeys into them'.[128] Others, such as members of the emerging British Theosophist tradition, considered that 'the engrafting of a portion of such a gland, from a lower and amoral animal, may effect a change in the psychic attributes of a human being.'[129]

These attitudes towards Voronoff's methods were therefore deeply rooted in pre-war moral ideals, anxieties about social degeneration, opposition to vivisection and religious concerns about the mixture of human and animal.[130]

[123] 'Monkey Glands', *The Scotsman*, 13 February 1929, 13.   [124] Bailey, 284.
[125] Bayly, 'The Menace', 147.   [126] Ibid., 147.
[127] For earlier correspondence in which Johnson provided spirited critique of vivisection, see: Maurice L. Johnson, 'Treatment of Hydrophobia', *Hereford Times*, 16 April 1910, 16; Maurice L. Johnson, 'Anti-Vivisection', *Western Daily Press*, 17 December 1907, 9; Maurice L. Johnson, 'Rabies', *Wells Journal*, 14 October 1897, 6.
[128] Maurice L. Johnson, 'Abolition of Old Age', *Western Daily Press*, 3 December 1919, 3.
[129] 'Monkey Glands Effects. "Harmful," says Derby Lecturer', *Derby Daily Telegraph*, 5 February 1929, 5.
[130] For more on the anti-vivisection movement, see French, *Antivivisection and Medical Science*.

Such responses created a sceptical public environment for his work, even as many British medical practitioners were giving a cautious welcome to some of his findings. The spectre of monkey gland treatments roused similar feelings of apprehension and revulsion as those incited by forms of evolutionary theory which formed a cornerstone of public scientific debate in the second half of the nineteenth century.[131]

The context of late nineteenth century biological and medical science was also critical in informing the reception of hormone rejuvenation procedures elsewhere. For example, in Australia, the cover illustration (see Figure 2.4) of the satirical 1925 song 'Be Rejuvenated' – penned by lyricist Annie Salter and composer W. R. Barwick – showed a youthful Darwin-like figure dancing exuberantly with a young flapper girl amongst palm trees, watched over by smiling monkeys. In a clear reference to the introduction of animal material into humans, the song expressed a longing to 'feel like Tarzan', and exhorted 'front row baldies' to 'say goodbye to hobble sticks and gout'.[132] Similarly, when George Viereck, who we encountered earlier as a disciple of Steinach, interviewed Voronoff for *The Graphic* in March 1929, the double-page feature was accompanied by images of cavorting primates laughing at unsuspecting old and infirm men approaching a statue which represented the elixir of youth.[133] Such anxieties intersected closely with fears about racial degeneration, articulated by Beddow Bayly, whilst another image from the same article suggested that the Voronoff procedure was an upper-class fad, scorned by others who favoured a simple life as a sure means of ensuring continued health and youthfulness. The accompanying caption read:

'Do you,' I asked, 'believe I Signor Voronoff's monkey-operation to renew youth?' The peasant woman laughed. 'The sunshine, the air, my food and my happiness are all I need to remain young,' she said.[134]

In the United States, meanwhile, one of the key constituencies to embrace the possibilities of rejuvenation were adherents of so-called New Thought. Emerging originally from the writings of the American mesmerist and healer Phineas Quimby, who practised animal magnetism across the country during the mid-nineteenth century, New Thought drew on both religious and meta-physical tenets in order to emphasise the importance of self-healing.[135] Such an optimistic and pragmatic view of health was a natural vehicle through

---

[131] See, for example: Bowler, *Charles Darwin*; Paul, 'Darwin, Social Darwinism and Eugenics'.
[132] Salter and Barwick, *Be Rejuvenated*, 2–3.
[133] 'Gland of Hope and Glory', *The Graphic*, 30 March 1929, 486–87.   [134] Ibid., 486.
[135] For more on Quimby and his significance as a source of inspiration for New Thought, see Pickren and Rutherford, *A History of Modern Psychology in Context*, 93.

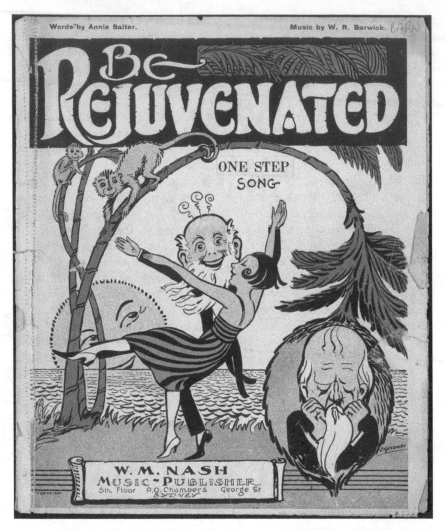

Figure 2.4 A rejuvenated old man, bearing a striking resemblance to an aged Charles Darwin, dances with a young flapper on the cover illustration of the satirical song, 'Be Rejuvenated'.
(Annie Salter and W. R. Barwick, *Be Rejuvenated*. Sydney: W. M. Nash, 1925, front cover.)

which to promote rejuvenation, both before and after the work of leading European rejuvenators.

Writing in 1919, for example, the Californian teacher Jessie Millard English (1860–1935), 'a graduate of several of the best schools of suggestive healing', articulated a set of aphorisms and affirmations designed to promote bodily 'renewal and rejuvenation'.[136] English was one of several advocates of New Thought who used the cultural resonance of rejuvenation to popularise their own ideas. Her system relied on positive affirmation – the aphorisms included exhortations to '*think* my body into *Health*', but also to 'drink for cleanliness, purity, fairness of flesh and freshness of complexion' and 'exercise *more* and eat *less* of rich foods'.[137] Conventional aspects of everyday practices of diet and exercise were therefore acknowledged to be of significance, even for advocates of New Thought.

Both regional and national British newspapers scampered to report incidences of supposed rejuvenation by hormonal means. In this context there was rather less caution, as publications throughout the country first hailed 'perpetual youth and length of life in comparison with which Methuselah would be considered quite a youth' – the supposed promises of Voronoff's grafting procedure.[138] Similarly lauded was Steinach's 'important discovery': the 'remarkable claim to the discovery of the secret of youth' or even, as reported in the *Sheffield Independent*, 'perpetual youth', in 1920.[139] Indeed, by this stage the grafting of simian glands onto humans was so well publicised that several publications had to make it clear that the 'reported discovery [of Steinach's method(s)] seems to be quite distinct from the grafting of a gland from a monkey.'[140] Notwithstanding the cautious optimism of some in the medical community, the *Dundee Courier* proudly proclaimed that the 'general opinion' on the efficacy of Steinach's methods was 'very favourable', with patients regaining 'physical capacities ... youthful appearance and a capacity for work'.[141] An editorial, reprinted in at least four regional papers from Lanarkshire in Scotland to Suffolk in southern England, asserted that 'medical opinion is inclined to believe in its definite and practical results.'[142] In those

---

[136] English, *A Treatise on the Renewal*, 5. It is somewhat ironic that critics of rejuvenation would prefer to ascribe some of the mental and physical changes after to procedures to auto-suggestion – another object of mainstream medical ire – over the grafting of glands.

[137] English, *Renewal and Rejuvenation*, p. 21.

[138] 'The Old Young Again', *Western Gazette*, 17 October 1919, 10. This article was also reprinted in the *Western Advertiser* and, in an abridged form, in the *Yorkshire Evening Post*.

[139] 'Making Old Men Young: New Discoveries. Reported Proof of Two Methods', *Globe*, 9 July 1920, 7; 'Secret of Youth. Old Man Made Young Tells His Story. Joy of Life Restored', *Nottingham Evening Post*, 24 July 1920, 3; 'Perpetual Youth. New Discoveries by a Vienna Professor', *Sheffield Independent*, 10 July 1920, 1. For other reports, see: 'The Old Made Young Again', *Western Times*, 12 July 1920, 4; 'Making the Old Young. Testimony by Youth of Seventy', *Aberdeen Press and Journal*, 15 July 1920, 5; 'Making Old Men Young: A Youth of Seventy' *Motherwell Times*, 16 July 1920, 7.

[140] 'Making Old Men Young: A Youth of Seventy' *Motherwell Times*, 16 July 1920, 7.

[141] 'To Restore Youth of Men. Rejuvenation of Aged Glands', *Dundee Courier*, 12 July 1920, 4.

[142] 'Postponing Old Age', *Bellshill Speaker*, 29 October 1920, 1; 'Postponing Old Age', *Todmorden and District News*, 29 October 1920, 1; 'Postponing Old Age', *Arbroath Herald*, 29 October 1920, 2; 'Postponing Old Age', *Framlingham Weekly News*, 30 October 1920, 2.

national papers which covered the story, Steinach's results were hailed as 'sensational' after he 'succeeded in restoring mental and physical strength to aged human beings and animals'.[143] In a clear attempt to differentiate their work from the testicle grafting of Voronoff, Steinach and his colleagues 'expressly declared that in the experiments no organs were grafted from another individual'.[144]

The commercial side of rejuvenation too was visible at an early stage. Investment in the Steinach operation came as a group of financiers and physicians from the United States visited the biologist in Vienna in the autumn of 1920 in order to 'give a wider scope to the Professor's discovery' – effectively to scale up his activities.[145] Despite Steinach himself asserting in an interview in 1920 that his method was 'not to prolong life, but to prolong youth' – a key distinction between claims made by rejuvenators and advocates of life extension – many headlines continued to imply that patients could expect increased longevity.[146] Steinach and Voronoff, of course, were not alone in the public discussion of the endocrine system. Scientific luminaries such as Julian Huxley were at the same time extoling the power of hormones, and in particular those secreted by the thyroid gland, to produce remarkable physiological effects.[147] It is therefore a mistake to assume a binary distinction between proponents and practitioners of rejuvenation on one side and the mainstream scientific establishment on the other. Rejuvenators were, at least in part, successful in directing attention to their work and its supposedly miraculous results precisely because hormones constituted a genuine scientific explanation for bodily control. Indeed, reports in newspapers often conflated the Steinach operation with manipulation of the thyroid gland, reflecting both the ubiquity and interconnectedness of the endocrine system in the public imagination.[148]

Reports of successful cases were critical to the mission of rejuvenators. Largely centred on the experience of the patient – testimony was key – these also invariably commented on their social position. Many, but not all, were

As well as passing comment on the highly desirable nature of 'how to avoid the bill when old age comes', the article reflected on the rapid rise and fall in popularity of Elié Metchnikoff's 'sour milk cure for human ills', discussed more in Chapter 3.

[143] 'Old Made Young Again. Revival of Germ Glands. Vienna Doctor's Discovery', *The Sunday Post*, 11 July 1920, 12.

[144] 'Renewing Youth. Remarkable Results at Vienna', *Aberdeen Journal*, 12 July 1920, 5.

[145] 'Prolonging Human Life to 100 Years. American Financiers' Visit to Viennese Professor. Gland Discovery', *Evening Telegraph*, 13 October 1920, 4.

[146] 'The Doctor Who Makes Old Men Young. Claim to Prolong Youth, Not Life', *Yorkshire Evening Post*, 11 November 1920, 5.

[147] George F. Morrell, 'Youth Regained by Thyroid?', *The Graphic*, 11 December 1920, 22.

[148] 'Youth in Old Age', *Lincolnshire Echo*, 17 May 1921, 2; 'Youth in Old Age', *Buckingham Advertiser and North Bucks Free Press*, 21 May 1921, 3.

characterised as noteworthy members of high society. For example, Alfred Wilson was reported in the *Derby Daily Telegraph* as having experienced physical and mental rejuvenation through a Steinach operation, at the age of seventy-one, after a varied career as a 'sailor, stevedore, marine store dealer, shipbreaker, gold digger, ferryman, steward, and corporation contractor'.[149] Elsewhere he was described as a 'very rich Australian'.[150] Wilson's supposed rejuvenation case aroused great public interest owing to his untimely demise. So convinced was he of the success of the operation and its remarkable effect on him that he paid 85 guineas to hire the Royal Albert Hall for a night 'to lecture on his experiences and his rejuvenation'.[151] However, on the morning before he was due to deliver his address, Wilson was found dead in his bed, leaving organisers to hastily post a notice announcing that his talk – entitled 'How I was made twenty years younger by the method of Professor Steinach, of Vienna' – would now no longer take place.[152] The case was investigated by the Coroner, and reported in the high-profile *Pall Mall and Globe* (known for most of its run as the *Pall Mall Gazette*) amongst other publications.[153] During the proceedings, Wilson's physician, Dr Kennedy, testified that he could, in fact, find 'no signs of injury or an operation', not even a scar, during his post-mortem. Wilson's cousin also confirmed that the total cost of the operation was more than £700, including an extensive period of rehabilitation in Vienna.[154] Steinach's own verdict was apparently simple: '[h]e overdid it.'[155]

Another notable recipient of the Steinach operation was the recently knighted actor, director and producer Sir Charles Hawtrey (1858–1923). Following his death in late July 1923 it emerged that on 13 April Hawtrey had visited Dr Burchardi, the Viennese surgeon practising in London, after a protracted period of ill health.[156] Burchardi, described as far afield as

[149] 'The "Monkey Gland" Fiction. Second Youth due to a Simple Operation', *Derby Daily Telegraph*, 15 April 1921, 2.
[150] '"Eternal Youth", but Not Yet', *Western Morning News*, 14 May 1921, 4.
[151] 'Death Dictates. Tragic End of Man with a Mission. Rejuvenation after Gland-Operation', *Dundee Evening Telegraph*, 13 May 1921, 6.
[152] 'Death Dictates', 6.
[153] The case also made news headlines in several regional publications. See, for example: 'Thyroid Gland "Cure". Death of Man Who Said He Had Been Made 20 Years Younger', *The Citizen*, 14 May 1921, 3; 'Not Master of his Fate. How Death took Secret of "Young" Old Man. Mystery of an Operation', *Nottingham Evening Post*, 14 May 1921, 1; 'The Rejuvenation Theory. Death on Eve of Lecture', *Western Daily Press*, 14 May 1921, 7.
[154] 'Rejuvenated Man's Sudden Death. Doctor Finds No Trace of £700 Operation', *Pall Mall and Globe*, 13 May 1921, 2.
[155] 'Puzzled Professor. The Mystery of Rejuvenated Man's Death', *Nottingham Evening Post*, 16 May 1921, 1.
[156] 'News in Brief', *The Evening News*, 1 August 1923, 7.

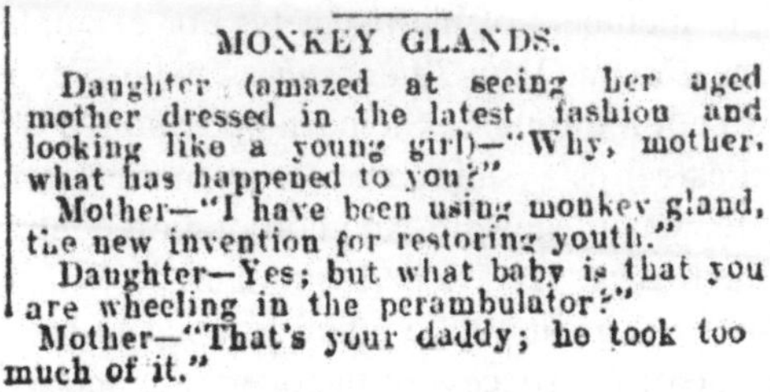

MONKEY GLANDS.

Daughter (amazed at seeing her aged mother dressed in the latest fashion and looking like a young girl)—"Why, mother, what has happened to you?"

Mother—"I have been using monkey gland, the new invention for restoring youth."

Daughter—Yes; but what baby is that you are wheeling in the perambulator?"

Mother—"That's your daddy; he took too much of it."

Figure 2.5 A sketch printed as one of the 'Prize Jokes' in the *Ballymena Weekly Telegraph*. Commentators expressed anxiety about misuse of rejuvenation procedures in an effort to realise a greater degree of youthfulness, and this can be seen in the case of other forms of rejuvenation, such as extreme fasting, overuse of skin care products and the elderly taxing themselves too much with vigorous exercise regimes.

('Prize Jokes' *Ballymena Weekly Telegraph*, 2 February 1929, 5.)

Singapore and Australia as '[o]ne of the busiest men in London', performed the procedure, apparently without success.[157]

Other early reported cases included 'a Parisian prominent in public affairs, with vitality exhausted by a life of hard work' who was rejuvenated by means of Voronoff's testicular graft operation, yet almost all cases, notwithstanding Steinach's development of a rejuvenation technique for women in the early 1920s, were men.[158] This polarisation of the rejuvenation debate did not go unnoticed amongst the British press. In 1922, the regular female columnist in *The Sphere*, Sylvania, focussed on this imbalance, yet provided an alternative narrative to the traditional view that the ageing woman suffered from a gradual loss of social capital. Concentrating on the importance of the figure of the grandmother – 'a precious possession … [whose] advice is sought and her opinions deferred to' – she argued that '[a]ge brings far more compensations to a woman than to a man, in spite of popular belief to the contrary.'[159]

As well as an object of fascination, rejuvenation was also a source of satire (see Figure 2.5). Exploring whether the process might be taken to extremes, several newspapers took up a humorous sketch, originating from the *Boston*

---

[157] 'Fear of Middle Age', *Straits Times*, 22 February 1923, 11; 'Monkey-Gland Warning. Sending Humanity Back to the Trees', *The Age*, 15 December 1923, 4. For other reports on Hawtrey's operation, see: 'Notes and Comments', *Portadown Times*, 3 August 1923, 6; 'Cross-Channel', *The Northern Whig*, 3 August 1923, 5; 'Epitome of News', *Diss Express and Norfolk and Suffolk Journal*, 10 August 1923, 3.

[158] 'The Old Young Again', *Western Gazette*, 17 October 1919, 10. The use of diathermy and X-rays to rejuvenate women will be considered in Chapter 4, relying as they did on electrical technologies.

[159] Sylvania, 'Madame and the Monkey Gland' *The Sphere*, 27 October 1922, iv.

Transcript, about a woman whose husband had supposedly 'overused' the Steinach method, resulting in her pushing him around in a perambulator.[160] This imagery of overindulgence at the fountain of youth also covered Voronoff's monkey glands later in 1920s. Indeed, even at an early stage in the public life of hormone rejuvenation methods, 'the industrious Steinach' was showcasing ways in which longevity might be loathed as 'a new form of frightfulness'. As the *Daily Herald* noted dryly in 1920, 'we poor Britons have already one example of perpetual youth in Winston Churchill. We don't want a second helping.'[161] At the same time, fictional imaginings of the implications of successful rejuvenation through a range of high-profile publications only served to heighten the mythology and dramatic allure of hormone treatments and monkey glands.[162]

Voronoff's use of monkey glands was, as might be expected, a gift for those who sought to send up both modern medical practice and decadent post-World War One society. For example, when asked what he suggested in order to make the British a more 'musical nation', the legendary conductor and impresario Sir Thomas Beecham (1879–1961) replied, '[t]ake out their brains, pickle them, add monkey glands, and let it simmer'.[163] Meanwhile, the *Northern Whig*, an influential and long-running Belfast-based newspaper, ran a story in 1928 about a long-lived family from Manitoba, Canada, in which a mother and her six children were all in receipt of the old-age pension, under the headline 'Monkey Glands Not Wanted'.[164] Such stories were commonplace, and the use of monkey glands as a byword for the prolongation of life illustrates just how ubiquitous Voronoff's principal rejuvenation ingredients were in the British psyche. They were synonymous with longevity but had also become – as Norman Haire noted – a vague and uncertain substitute for detailed discussion of rejuvenation procedures themselves.

Commercialising Rejuvenation

As well as a lively discussion in printed public forums, many members of the mainstream medical community had at least given rejuvenation the benefit of the doubt, in the absence of concrete evidence, for much of the 1920s. This

---

[160] 'How's This One', *Pall Mall Gazette*, 11 May 1923, 8; 'An Overdose', *Hampshire Advertiser*, 12 May 1923, 7; 'Alarming Possibilities', *Dundee Courier*, 14 May 1923, 8; 'Oh, Those Glands!', *Nottingham Evening Post*, 22 May 1923, 3; '"Mail" Mustard and Cress', *The Daily Mail*, 30 June 1923, 1.

[161] 'Not so Splendid, Really', *Daily Herald*, 10 July 1920, 3.

[162] See, for example, Tebbutt, 'Popular and Medical Understandings of Sex Change', 156–69.

[163] 'Making Us Music Lovers. Sir T. Beecham's Cure. By Monkey Glands. His Good Word for Leeds Audiences', *Leeds Mercury*, 23 November 1926, 6.

[164] 'Monkey Glands Not Wanted. Seven in One Family Quality for Old-Age Pensions', *Northern Whig*, 4 June 1928, 8.

came even as Steinach himself had begun to retract some of his more sensational claims by the end of the decade. However, public interest and credulity showed no sign of waning, particularly when, in December 1926, the Italian physician Francesco Cavazzi had announced that he had, by far more simple means, achieved the same results as Voronoff in rejuvenating men 'from the poorer classes' between the ages of fifty-six and eighty.[165] Initial responses to Cavazzi's findings, indeed, were themselves rooted in the assumed social groups – 'the bored and the bereaved, the vinegar-faced and the unemployed' – who might be supposed to most desire to avail themselves of such treatments.[166] In advertisements, women's magazines and the newspaper press, articles praising the sovereign physiological power of hormones and endorsing rejuvenation abounded, drawing inspiration from the original findings of Voronoff and Steinach, as well as subsequent investigations. For example, in early 1931, a major feature in *Britannia & Eve* – 'a monthly journal for men and women' which owed much of its focus to its forerunner, *Eve*, a 'Lady's pictorial' – claimed that

[t]he experiments of Voronof [sic] have proved that many symptoms of age are the result of failure on the part of certain endocrine glands to manufacture the necessary hormones. Professors Steinach, of Vienna, and Bloch in Berlin have carried experiments on this premise further and established that the introduction of certain endocrine gland products into the human system, not necessarily by operation, will, at any rate temporarily, arrest the process of age [sic].[167]

Amongst the companies who sought to profit from the attention lavished on hormones in the medical and popular press was British Glandular Products Ltd. (BGP), established in 1929. The promotional material for the company, consisting in a large part of a pamphlet entitled *The Essence of Life*, demonstrates just how tarnished the work of the leading interwar gland surgeons had become by the end of the 1920s. One of the principal claims was that

Medical Science in recent years has made great progress in the study of REJUVENATION, and the object of this Booklet is to convey to the laity as simply as possible, something of the means now adopted to impart in a natural and perfectly harmless manner, New Vigour, Vitality, and Youthful Energy to the Human organism.[168]

Despite this, only selected contributors to this area of physiological knowledge were mentioned in the booklet, including Leonard Williams, William Arbuthnot Lane and Charles Brown-Séquard; Steinach was credited with adding

[165] 'Doctors' Rejuvenation Claim. Restoring Vitality to the Aged', *The Evening Telegraph*, 15 December 1926, 8.
[166] 'New Faces for Old. Rejuvenation Claim – What May Happen – Some Perils and Some Advantages', *Sheffield Daily Independent*, 21 January 1927, 4.
[167] 'You are as Young and Fit as Your Glands', *Britannia and Eve*, 1 March 1931, 87.
[168] British Glandular Products, *The Essence of Life*, n.p.

'several years, possibly decades, to the economic life of the patient', yet Voronoff – whose scientific credibility had steadily waned through the 1920s – was absent.[169] Tellingly, by the early 1930s, both Williams and Lane had switched focus away from hormonal rejuvenation almost entirely, concentrating instead on lifestyle factors. Tablets aimed at both men (Testrones) and women (Overones) featured in the range of preparations offered by BGP, and these contained a dizzying array of extracts derived from, we must surmise, animal sources, including, in Testrones, suprarenal, prostate, cerebrin ('extracts of Brain substance') and albumen, and in Overones, 'Ovarian Substance, Corpus Luteum, Pituitary whole Gland, Thyroid'.[170] Although Testrones and Overones were the flagship products, other preparations included, for men, 'Virules', 'Prostalin' and the mysteriously named 'S.P. H.P. Tablets', whilst women could obtain 'special skin tonic tablets', 'special skin cream' and 'Miracle Hormone Cream'.[171] Other manufacturers, including G. A. Hutton, imbued their products with a similar range of ingredients, including dried ox brain, testes and prostate.[172] Female customers of Hutton could expect to ingest cows' ovaries and mammary gland as well as the seemingly universal ox brain.[173]

Some of the effects of Overones, as well as the expected 'organic regeneration and new physical vigour', were listed as 'quickening of step, brightening of eyes, more lustrous growth of hair, increased beauty of the skin'.[174] This was indicative of a transitional period for hormone-related products in the late 1920s when a rejuvenated exterior occupied just as significant a place in female rejuvenation as the actual physiological changes which might take place. These and other tablets also promised much by way of sexual rejuvenation, following the tradition of increased virility, potency and appetite reported in numerous cases of surgical interventions. Chief amongst the conditions in which men might notice improvement 'after two or three

---

[169] Ibid. We have already encountered Brown-Sequard in the context of his organotherapeutic work in the late nineteenth century. Leonard Williams was one of the most prominent British exponents of the organotherapy tradition in the early twentieth century but moved on to other matters by the late 1920s. See: Williams, 'The Present Position of Organotherapy', 255–56; Williams, 'The Interstitial Gland', 833–35. One of Williams's major contributions was to the understanding of linked action between thyroid and gonads in men and women. See Cobb, *The Glands of Destiny*, 93.

[170] British Glandular Products, *The Essence of Life*, n.p.

[171] 'Formulas of Some Glandular Preparations' in 'SEXUAL BEHAVIOUR 1939–1950', January 1939–December 1950, Mass Observation Archive (hereafter MOA), University of Sussex, Box 12-16-F, 2.

[172] 'Formulas of Some Glandular Preparations' in 'SEXUAL BEHAVIOUR 1939–1950', January 1939–December 1950, MOA, Box 12-16-F, 6.

[173] Formulas of Some Glandular Preparations' in 'SEXUAL BEHAVIOUR 1939–1950', January 1939–December 1950, MOA, Box 12-16-F, 6.

[174] British Glandular Products, *The Essence of Life*, n.p.

bottles' of Testrones were 'impotency, sterility, loss of virile tone, weakness, mental and physical apathy, premature aging, sexual indifference, sexual exhaustion, sexual inefficiency, sexual neurasthenia, diminished potency, nocturnal enuresis, sexual functional imbalance'.[175]

Hormone products such as these were not mere fads of the interwar period, but a longer-lasting theme in direct-to-consumer marketing. British Glandular Products celebrated their twenty-first anniversary in 1950 by issuing a promotional leaflet offering the still popular Testrones and Overones at their original prices.[176] In this publication, BGP noted that their Testrones tablets would have similar effects to 'those obtained by taking regular daily physical exercise'; in a significant departure from their interwar claims, BGP were not promising miracles, but a shortcut.[177] On 8 May of the same year, an unknown investigator arranged an interview with the chief pharmacist of the London-based Whipps Cross Hospital. The hand-written notes record that, at the outset of the interview, the interviewee noted: 'let's get one thing straight first. The only dried gland used in legitimate medicine is dried thyroid … any other dried gland is practically, if not totally useless'; in their view, '[t]his gland tablet, Prostalin, is just an aspirin tablet.'[178]

As well as BGP, the Middlesex Laboratory of Glandular Research was another entity established in the late 1920s, specifically to capitalise on the hormone craze.[179] Focussing more explicitly on their products as a means of restoring sexual functionality in men, the Middlesex company issued order forms which promised to post the selected goods in a 'PLAIN SEALED WRAPPER' so as to ensure discretion.[180] Like many competitors, the Middlesex company also devised specialised products for women and men. Some, for example, were claimed to contain 'high oestrogenic potency' and marketed specifically as treatments for impotence.[181] Similarly, 'Testonic' Brand Tablets promised to restore 'vital energy', and were supplied to retailers with

[175] British Glandular Products, *The Essence of Life*, n.p.
[176] British Glandular Products, '21st Anniversary Offer' in 'SEXUAL BEHAVIOUR 1939–1950', January 1939–December 1950, MOA, Box 12-16-G, 42-45.
[177] Ibid., 44.
[178] M.L. 'Interview with the Chief Pharmacist of Whipps Cross Hospital on some Glandular Preparations', 8 May 1950, in 'SEXUAL BEHAVIOUR 1939-1950', MOA, Box 12-16-F, 10-13, 10.
[179] For more on the Middlesex Laboratory, see: Middlesex Laboratory of Glandular Research, Ltd., *The Treatment of Impotence*. The company continued to trade until 1979. See 'Department of Trade', *The London Gazette*, 9 November 1979, 14064–66, 14066.
[180] Middlesex Laboratory of Glandular Research, 'To the Middlesex Laboratory of Glandular Research Ltd., Order Form', c.1929, EPH26, Wellcome Library.
[181] Middlesex Laboratory of Glandular Research Ltd., *The Treatment of Impotence*; Middlesex Laboratory of Glandular Research Ltd., *The Fires of Life Replenished*.

'[d]ignified and arresting Display Material', highlighting the obvious sexual relevance of the product.[182]

G. A. Hutton, the self-styled 'glandular specialists' based in London, made similar claims as other manufacturers about their scientific credentials, having carried out 'a profound study of the human body, particularly those conditions which bring about the ageing process'.[183] According to Hutton's promotional material, modern medical science had demonstrated that the process of rejuvenation 'was in some mysterious way entirely dependent on ... "ENDOCRINE" or "internally secreting" glands'.[184] Advertisements from later in the period reveal that the Hutton (Brand) Gland Tablets were aimed solely at men, highlighting that the consumer would be 'virile and vigorous' and make the 'nerves function efficiently'.[185]

A number of existing companies also sought to engage with this emerging market. Around 1930, the long-standing retail chemists Hancock & Co. put together a promotional leaflet detailing numerous 'foreign preparations' which were 'the logical outcome of the work of such savants as **Voronoff, Metchnikoff, Steinach** etc.'[186] These included not simply details of the likely effects of treatment using the remedies, but an elaborate justification for the focus on glandular extracts. According to their book of prescriptions designed to address conditions associated with ageing and general ill health,

[T]he achievement of longevity together with full enjoyment of mental and physical activity and the whole problem of staying young, or wooing back youth once it is lost, is a problem of the endocrine glands of the body. ... Youth lasts as long as the glandular system is properly nourished and stimulated. Old age, with its manifested symptoms of loss of life force, inactivity and general sluggishness, is not a wearing-out process, but a cessation of glandular activity, and is therefore both preventable and curable.[187]

Hancock marketed specific preparations for 'Longevity, Premature Senile Decay' (based on 'German research'), 'Sterility' (Italian), 'Muscular Atrophy' (French), 'Unsightly Elbows' (Japanese), 'Premature Greyness' (Russian) and 'Baldness, Thinning Hair and General Scalp and Hair Troubles' (Portuguese), amongst others. Tellingly, each was supplied in plain packaging, with directions for use provided separately, and the female audience which the manufacturer had in mind is suggested by their assertion that the containers 'may be left quite safely on the dressing table'.[188]

---

[182] '"Testonic" Brand Tablets', *Chemist and Druggist Supplement*, 2 May 1936, viii; '"Testonic" Brand Tablets', *Chemist and Druggist Supplement*, 11 January 1936, xi.

[183] *The New Way to Vitality*, G. A. Hutton and Co.: London, [1929], n.p., in 'SEXUAL BEHAVIOUR 1939–1950', MOA, Box 12-16-G.

[184] *The New Way to Vitality*, n.p., in 'SEXUAL BEHAVIOUR 1939–1950', MOA, Box 12-16-G.

[185] 'Need a Man Feel Prematurely Aged?', *Daily Herald*, 3 July 1936, 20; 'New Life for Every Man!', *The Stage*, 25 June 1936, 7.

[186] *Foreign Prescriptions*, 4, original emphasis.　　　[187] Ibid., 7.　　　[188] Ibid., 6.

The impact of surgical rejuvenation on the hormone product market was ongoing. For example, Bioglan Laboratories Limited was incorporated on 25 February 1932 as a manufacturer of pharmaceutical products and issued many pamphlets over subsequent years. These were aimed primarily at physicians, and claimed to draw in particular on 'the epoch-making discoveries since 1930' which had 'put endocrine medication in the forefront of modern therapeutics'.[189] The 1930s also saw the emergence of new anxieties about what might result from excessive manipulation of the glandular system. Advertising for the new product Bioserm – described on the front cover of a promotional pamphlet as 'biology's gift to women' – was careful to reassure potential users that '[i]t will not stimulate any glands, beyond the minute skin glands whose activity produces skin-health and skin-beauty'.[190] Other firms, such as the theatrical make-up innovator Ludwig Leichner's London operation, produced hormone tablets from the early 1930s specifically designed to restore or preserve beauty.[191] These were calculated to aid

the formation of new and perfect cellular tissue, which means nothing less than complete rejuvenation of the skin and of the outlines of the human body. The Medical Profession have tested and approved of Leichner Beauty Hormones and found that they may be taken regularly with perfect safety, as they will never give rise to adverse reactions of any kind.[192]

This shunning of cosmetics was replaced by a reliance on the supposed medical approval received by Leichner's, though this was an odd strategy given that their competitors had been exploring hormone-containing skin creams with some considerable success since the late 1920s.[193]

Other firms, such as Le Brasseur, who in the 1920s were amongst the leading manufacturers of contraceptive devices and 'pro-race goods, as recommended by Dr Marie Stopes', promoted Vi-vims tablets. These, they claimed, would restore 'lost vitality' and put 'life back instantly in weak glands', demonstrating the extent to which non-specific, underperforming glands had become synonymous with lack of sexual potency amongst a host of age-related indicators.[194] Tellingly, these small advertisements which appeared in local newspapers throughout Britain and Ireland highlighted the suitability of the remedy for both young and old, as they proclaimed 'age no barrier' in the efficacy of treatment, even producing a pamphlet entitled

[189] The Bioglan Laboratories Hertford, *Bioglan Hormone Compounds*, 1.
[190] Zenobé, *The New 'Bioserm'*, 10. For more on Bioserm and rejuvenation of the skin, see Chapter 6.
[191] 'Leichner Beauty Hormones', *The Chemist and Druggist*, 13 June 1931, 17–18, 18.
[192] Ibid., 18.   [193] For more on hormone creams, see Chapter 6.
[194] Le Brasseur Surgical Manufacturing Co. Ltd., *Le Brasseur's Revised List*; 'Weak Men, Get Vigour!', *Birmingham Mail*, 2 February 1939, 1.

Rejuvenation to accompany their range, which included an 'extra strong' version.[195] In contrast to many products, the promotional material did not claim to contain glandular extracts, only to *act* on glands lacking in vitality and sufferers 'from Nervous Exhaustion, Premature Decay, Loss of Vitality, and similar Nervous Complaints arising from overwork, late hours, or excesses of any kind', the latter clearly resonating with arguments about the dangers of overindulgence in its myriad forms.[196]

As well as intersecting with anxieties about sexual performance, hormone rejuvenation therapies also reconfigured the pathological nature of ageing. As the George E. O. Knight noted in his 1933 work *Sex and Rejuvenation*, 'recent discoveries point to the conclusion that the so-called diseases of natural and premature old age are really symptoms of a single disease – the disease of growing old, and that it occurs because the endocrine glands have been neglected.'[197] Knight was an intriguing character – a Fellow of the Royal Geographical Society who travelled extensively in Asia with the flamboyant William McGovern.[198] It was during his travels through Tibet, Assam, Sikkim, China and Manitoba that Knight encountered a plethora of 'curious' beliefs surrounding rejuvenation, including that 'the ingestion of the excreta of the Dalai Lama cures every known disease, and in addition has the effect of reactivating the old'.[199]

Sex and Rejuvenation was in many ways typical of a new form of rejuvenation publication, incorporating elements of advertising – in this case for the London-based 'Advanced Health Institute' – textbook, original scientific findings, history, moralising, philosophy and religion. Knight, like many others, strayed far from his established domain of disciplinary expertise. One of his arguments, for example, was that 'priests who are not permitted by their Church to marry are either abnormally fat or abnormally lean' – a sign of 'disturbances to potency' and therefore a key indicator of premature old age.[200] Knight embodied a hybrid attitude towards rejuvenation and glandular activity which included both scientific and commercial aspects; elements of commercial interest were central in the construction of a rejuvenation marketplace which ran from the cost of surgical procedures through to hormone preparations designed for use in an everyday, domestic setting.

---

195 'Weak Men, Get Vigour!', *Birmingham Mail*, 21 January 1939, 2, original emphasis. This campaign ran throughout the 1930s and was consistent in claiming that Vi-vims could promote vitality and vigour. By 1939, for example, the *Birmingham Mail*, to take just one example, was running weekly advertisements for the product.

196 'A Free Cure for Weak Men. "Vi-vims" Bring New Life', *Sporting Times*, 28 February 1925, 7.

197 Knight, *Sex and Rejuvenation*, 9.

198 They were joined for one particular journey through Tibet by the geologist Frederick Fletcher, as well as William Harcourt, a cinematographer. See McGovern, *To Lhasa in Disguise*.

199 Knight, *Sex and Rejuvenation*, 8.   200 Ibid., 17–18.

Professional and public discourse surrounding hormone rejuvenation in the early twentieth century was a muddy affair, despite occasionally scathing interventions such as that handed down in 1930 by Jan Boeke, Director of the Laboratory of Embryology and Histology at the University of Utrecht. In a pair of lectures organised by the Chadwick Trust on 'The Histological Basis of Health', Boeke took aim not only at the methods and findings of Voronoff and Steinach, but also at the desirability of these reported outcomes, arguing that they had demonstrated 'no evidence whatsoever of rejuvenescence', and that, in any case, 'a reawakening of the sexual instinct ... [was] far from desirable in the aged.'[201] That Boeke felt the need to deliver such a damning verdict supposedly long after both his principal targets had been discredited speaks volumes about the ongoing public, if not professional, lure of rejuvenation. In contrast to the clear-cut case of 'paradigms in conflict', identified by Jessica M. Jahiel for the medical community of the United States in this period, rejuvenation constituted a fluctuating landscape of credulity and persuasion, dismay and optimism which spanned both the medical and lay press.[202]

Legacy and Conclusion

On 15 August 1948, the English photographer and designer Cecil Beaton wrote to his then-lover, the actress Greta Garbo, describing his experiences in Paris during the summer. As well as commenting on the extreme poverty endured by residents in the French capital and the violent pro-Communist riots besetting the city, Beaton also noted that three prominent members of the Parisian artistic set – Jean Cocteau, Georges Auric and Paul Eluard – had undergone rejuvenation treatment. In the case of Cocteau and Auric, this was 'successful', whilst Eluard's procedure had been unsuccessful.[203]

Although the early interwar period was without doubt the most significant in terms of the visibility of hormone rejuvenation procedures and practices (and their attending public and professional discourse), their influence was by no means confined to this period. Indeed, beyond the obvious persistence of rejuvenation operations such as those carried out in Paris in the summer of 1948, Barbara Marshall and Stephen Katz have noted that the 'cultural significance [of hormone rejuvenation] has continued throughout the twentieth century to the present day.'[204] Likewise, Chandak Sengoopta has argued that hormone replacement therapy (HRT) shared many common assumptions about

---

[201] Boeke, 'The Histological Basis of Health', 220.
[202] Jahiel, 'Rejuvenation Research and the American Medical Association'.
[203] Cecil Beaton to Greta Garbo, 15 August 1948, Papers of Sir Cecil Beaton, A2/14a/40, St. John's Library, Cambridge.
[204] Marshall and Katz, 'From Androgyny to Androgens', 79.

the physiological role of hormones in maintaining health and youthful functionality.[205] However, it was neither simply the continued resonance of the idea of hormone rejuvenation nor its reconfiguration in practices of HRT which continued into the second half of the twentieth century. Hormones also underpinned efforts to create and sell a diverse range of new rejuvenation products, many of which relied on direct action through the skin.

For example, on 18 March 1949, the Dutch pharmaceutical firm Organon Laboratories opened a new factory in Motherwell.[206] Employing a workforce of 400, including 'between 35 and 40 biochemists', the opening was conducted by the Secretary of State for Scotland and MP for Clackmannan and Eastern Stirlingshire, Sir Arthur Woodburn. In his comments, Woodburn wished the enterprise 'long life', apt words for a facility which manufactured synthetic hormones; guests at a celebratory lunch included Sir Andrew Davidson, Chief Medical Officer for Scotland and C. A. Oakley, Scottish Regional Controller of the Board of Trade.[207]

Organon has been producing a wide range of hormone and vitamin products since at least the mid-1930s.[208] Yet aside from products such as Lydiol, an oral contraceptive, one of Organon's most successful products was Endocril, described by the company as 'the first cosmetic hormone cream produced by specialists in hormones'.[209] This was marketed well into the 1950s even at a time when the Merchandise Committee at Boots, under advice from their internal Medical Department, decided against introducing a similar product.[210] As we shall see in subsequent chapters, hormone rejuvenation procedures, popularised by the disciples of Steinach and Voronoff and amplified by a press and publics eager to entertain the possible consequences of success, had a profound influence which stretched far beyond the confines of endocrinology, later hormone-based therapies and even sex and gender identities in the interwar period. Significant private and public debate about the effects of rejuvenating hormone treatments continued long after most mainstream scientific figures had dismissed the efficacy of such procedures, as prominent

---

[205] Sengoopta, 'Transforming the Testicle'. For more on hormone replacement therapy and its relation with rejuvenation treatments in the American context, see Watkins, *The Estrogen Elixir*.

[206] For a detailed historical account of Organon's activities, products and popularity across its first fifty years from its founding in 1923, see Tausk, *Organon*.

[207] 'New Factory Opened', *Motherwell Times*, 18 March 1949, 6.

[208] 'Remedia Nova', *Retail Chemist*, January 1934, 10.

[209] 'Lyndiol', [1960s], PP/RJH/A.5/1, Wellcome Library; 'Lyndiol 2.5', October 1965, PP/RJH/A.5/2, Wellcome Library.

[210] For more on this, see Chapter 6. Merchandise Committee Minutes, 31 March 1953, 'No7 Extra Rich Skin Food Product File', Boots Archive, 843/24.

researchers, including the much-vaunted Masters and Johnson, periodically rehabilitated the field.[211]

In very different ways, Steinach and Voronoff highlighted the possibilities of rejuvenation afforded by surgical intervention in the endocrine system, specifically in relation to the production of sex hormones. Although the moral and evolutionary concerns associated with Voronoff's use of animal tissues did not attend Steinach and those who practised his procedure, critiques based on efficacy and reliance on the power of 'suggestion' were rife amongst the medical literature. Away from professional medicine, anxieties about the introduction of glandular materials from monkeys and the resexualising of older men provided legitimate and pressing cause for social concern. Voronoff was at once satirised as a demonic adherent to the Darwinian relationship between man and primates and lauded by eugenicists for providing a means of increasing the overall physical and mental fitness of human stock by artificial means. Whilst it is certainly the case that emerging specialists in endocrinology benefitted from the close attention on their discipline, most sought to downplay the likelihood of the rejuvenators having discovered a panacea for human ageing. Instead, they gave cautious welcome followed by summary dismissal in the face of increasing evidence, preferring to allow the more fantastical narratives to remain at arm's length in the popular press.

Both Leonard Williams and Paul Kammerer mobilised the language and imagery of efficiency. This reflected what Anson Rabinbach identified as an imperative to 'conserve, deploy, and expand the energies of the laboring body'.[212] As we will see throughout the remainder of the book, such conceptions of how bodies were organised, how they functioned and the extent to which medical science could intervene to prevent their natural wastage underpinned arguments mobilised by almost all proponents of rejuvenation therapies. Under this view, aged and prematurely aged bodies – both male and female – were treated in much the same way as inefficient ones, pathologising the ageing process itself and promoting a view of bodily typicality. Normal bodies were defined in relation to their functionality and productivity; bodies which fell short of this threshold were considered impaired, and the prospect of overcoming such shortcomings through medical intervention offered a tantalising glimpse of a future society uninhibited by the limitations of the human lifecycle.

Meanwhile, Tim Armstrong, in his broader treatment of the relationships between modernism, technological change and bodies, has argued that the process of male sexual rejuvenation through the Steinach operation was credible owing to 'two interlocking traditions of thought relating to male

---

[211] Masters, 'Sex Steroid Influences'; Masters and Johnson, 'Sex and the Aging Process'.
[212] Rabinbach, *The Human Motor*, 2.

sexuality: the idea of the "spermatic economy" and, less directly, of seminal energy', as well as the procedure being 'a response to contemporary fears ... of masculine decline'.[213] Whilst these were undoubtedly central factors in the popularity and desirability of being Steinached during this period, the flourishing diversity of approaches to rejuvenation which coexisted with those founded on hormonal principles suggests that there was little, if any, consensus within British public discourses about how bodies functioned. In the immediate post-war period some commentators such as Mary H. Youde, who advocated the importance of mysterious 'human vegetable magnetic rays' in rejuvenation, even began to 'doubt if they [Voronoff's efforts to transplant "Monkey Glands"] ever got beyond the experimental stage'.[214]

As we shall see in subsequent chapters, the use of the language of both hormones and rejuvenation to underpin claims of rejuvenatory efficacy became staple in advertising materials for a huge range of products promoting human health and wellbeing. It is insufficient to dismiss the practitioners of procedures such as the Steinach operation as quacks or charlatans, even though some achieved notoriety in this field on spurious grounds or with fabricated medical credentials.[215] Such characterisations obscure the centrality of these figures in establishing the possibility of recapturing lost youth in popular discourse. A lively press picked up and circulated the sensational accounts of individual rejuvenation, propagating a positive view of the operations of Steinach and Voronoff, with articles often reprinted extensively through local press outlets. Having established the significance and extent of public debate around hormone rejuvenation, as well as its commercial expansion through the interwar period, we move next to dietary habits. These were reconfigured in relation to rejuvenation in the immediate aftermath of World War One, where manufacturers elaborated a hormonal-vitamin complex as the mechanism by which many foodstuffs and dietary products acted on the body to counteract the ageing process.

---

[213] Armstrong, *Modernism, Technology, and the Body*, 147 and 149.
[214] Ellison [Youde], *The Key to Rejuvenation*, n.p.   [215] Brock, *Charlatan*.

3   Diet, 1918–1929

Old age may be 'frosty,' but it would certainly be 'kindly,' if in earlier life we lived upon a suitable diet.'[1]

The study of dietetics should be looked upon as very nearly, if not quite, as important as the study of therapeutics. ... How often are insomnia and other neuroses due to the tea and egg for dinner so dear to the feminine heart, and how much brain fag may not be put down to the coffee and roll for lunch of a busy city man?[2]

A leading article from the *British Medical Journal*, published on 21 May 1904, claimed that dietetics and so-called scientific feeding had been overlooked by physicians despite clear links between diet and physical degeneration.[3] Such assertions about the significance of diet for health were commonplace during the first decades of the twentieth century, both in Britain and elsewhere.[4] As well as groups such as the anti-vivisectionist and theosophical Order of the Golden Age, established in 1895 to promote 'a natural and hygienic dietary as a preventive of Disease, a practical remedy for Physical Deterioration, and an efficacious way of lessening human suffering and sub-human pain', eminent medical authorities devoted significant attention to the role of food and health.[5] James Crichton Browne, for example, noted that the 'question of food is one of primary importance, far more than education,' whilst noted surgeon Sir Henry

---

[1] Webster, *Beauty and Health*, 8.
[2] 'The Food Question in Health and in Disease', *British Medical Journal*, 21 May 1904, 1208.
[3] Ibid.
[4] For some of the most prominent discussions on this topic, see: Brown, *Scientific Living for Prolonging the Term of Human Life*; Lorand, *Health and Longevity through Rational Diet*; 'Metchnikoff's Theory of Longevity', *Scientific American* 98, 16 May 1908, 347; Whittaker, 'Alcoholic Beverages'; Child, *Senescence and Rejuvenescence*.
[5] Abramowski, *Fruitarian Diet*, opposite title page. The Order was a product of the burgeoning anti-vivisection movement in Britain at the close of the nineteenth century. They had a distinctive approach to promoting a natural, lightly cooked vegetarian diet, and ran a successful periodical *The Herald of the Golden Age*, which was a key voice within the early twentieth-century food reform movement. See: Gilheany, *Familiar Strangers*; French, *Antivivisection and Medical Science*.

Thomson argued that 'more than half the disease that embitters life is due to avoidable errors of diet.'[6]

One hundred years later, writing in 2004, a group of clinicians and biomedical scientists, Gemma Casadesus, George Perry and James A. Joseph, led by Mark A. Smith, Professor of Pathology at Cape Western Reserve University, provided a cautious summary of the evidence for specific dietary intervention to promote long life. They concluded their review by noting that 'the good [long and healthy] life is not marked by extremes of diet but rather by a balance in metabolism.'[7] The group focused exclusively on recent literature from the late 1980s through to the early 2000s, but throughout the twentieth century the vexed question over the relationship between diet, health and longevity occupied medical and lay writers and commentators, not to mention a swathe of emerging dietetic and nutrition specialists. For some, balance was critical, whilst others claimed for their favoured foodstuffs or extracts a level of influence over the body more than any medical panacea. That we are still uncertain of the exact mechanism of how diet influences physiological ageing says less about the issue than the fact that a huge range of longevity and reducing diets has come to dominate the marketplace, with specialised products supplementing texts, television programmes and classes.[8]

Set against the backdrop of a range of social factors, such as food insecurity during World War One and the development of vegetarianism as both a dietary and social movement, this chapter explores and explains how diet and dietary innovation were increasingly mobilised as a form of rejuvenation therapy. Specific diets, including so-called rational fasting, were combined with an increasingly scientised view of food and its preparation to promote ways of eating for youthfulness. When combined with expanding practices of professional advertising and promotion, they created a new marketplace for rejuvenation diets and dietary-related products. The links between health and food, and even longevity and food, were of course extant long before the interwar period, reflecting a lineage traceable in the Western tradition through Ancient medicine, Galen's "four basic things" and the non-naturals. However, just as the emergence of hormones as an explanatory physiological component of bodies created a disruption of existing rejuvenation practices, so the relationship between food and ageing was radically reconfigured.

---

[6] 'Reviews', *The Citizen*, 29 January 1911, 2.

[7] Casadesus, Perry, Joseph and Smith, 'Eat Less, Eat Better', 215.

[8] For overviews of dieting and obesity, see: Foxcroft, *Calories and Corsets*; Oddy, Atkins and Amilien eds, *The Rise of Obesity in Europe*. Peter N. Stearns's now-classic *Fat History* established a strong link between consumption and the bodily aesthetic, highlighting how 'unnecessary aging' in the middle-aged, brought on by excessive fatness, could be seen 'at the waistline'. Stearns, *Fat History*, 17.

Habits of eating and diet were intimately connected with the perceptions of age in the human body in the interwar period. We know from the work of Tenna Jensen, for example, that institutional dietary regimes were heavily reliant on 'societal perceptions of ageing and age-related food habits' in interwar Denmark.[9] The link was even stronger, however, amongst some of the highest-profile advocates of rejuvenation therapy, such as Serge Voronoff and Eugen Steinach. Both noted the links between rejuvenation and appetite but remained unsure as to whether weight gain or loss was the most appropriate indicator of success. For example, Voronoff noted in one particular case that 'a loss of weight of 7 kilos' was indicative of a return of the 'well-being and of joy' associated with restoration of youthfulness.[10] At the same time, and perhaps paradoxically, both and he and Steinach highlighted an increased appetite as one of the expected outcomes of their procedures.

New products and the emerging science of nutrition reconfigured and provided renewed justifications for habits of eating in the interwar period. However, just as significant were methods of living and eating which promised to rejuvenate through moderation and abstention. The effect of strictly limiting food intake was already well known by the turn of the twentieth century. As the noted physician Hermann Weber (1823–1918) put it in his 1903 lecture to the Royal College of Physicians, later published through numerous editions as *On Longevity and Means for the Prolongation of Life*, 'the want of moderation is opposed to the prolongation of life.'[11] This approach took on a new sense of urgency in the period around World War One, dictated by the relatively limited availability of luxury food items during and after the conflict. The so-called cult of reducing – examined for the British case by Ina Zweiniger-Bargiolewska – was linked not just to dietary habits but also to exercise, sleep and work.[12] However, when we shift the focus from health and the maintenance of a healthy body to rejuvenation and a search for recapturing youthfulness, what patterns of change can we identify in the reconfiguration of dietary practices?

In this chapter I argue that the advent of new forms of nutritional science and dietary innovation, fuelled primarily by the emergence of vitamins as objects of dietary fascination, imbued with far-reaching physiological properties akin to hormones, reshaped the marketplace connected to the consumption of food.[13] This encompassed not just foodstuffs themselves but the manner of

---

[9] Jensen, 'The Importance of Age Perceptions', 159.
[10] Voronoff, *The Study of Old Age*, 106.   [11] Weber, *On Longevity*, 119.
[12] Zweiniger-Bargielowska, *Managing the Body*. See also, Zweiniger-Bargielowska, *The Culture of the Abdomen*.
[13] This takes further the argument which I have made elsewhere, that dietary modification was an essential component of far more wide-ranging rejuvenation strategies. As we shall see in later chapters, vitamins served not only as dietary supplements but as active agents promoting youth through the medium of skin creams. Stark, 'Replace Them by Salads and Vegetables'.

their nutritional composition, preparation and exclusion, the food and nutritional extracts marketed through newspapers and magazines, popular dietary texts and dietary trends (dismissed by many in the medical press as 'fads' or 'faddism'). In contrast to the supposed quick fix offered by hormone surgeries, advocates of everyday dietary modification highlighted the superiority of such a natural system as a means of achieving rejuvenation over the artificial surgical intervention, mirroring somewhat the present-day debate about the desirability of bariatric surgery.

We begin by considering how Steinach and Voronoff – principal architects of hormone rejuvenation craze – wove subtle but substantial and revealing references to eating practices into their publications and case reports, before moving to explore how the social environment of the interwar period and vitamin science reconfigured dietary advice and enabled manufacturers to capitalise on claims for their vitamin-rich foods and supplements.

Fuel for the Glands: Appetite and the Endocrine System

The advocate of Steinach's methods, Paul Kammerer, noted in his enthusiastic endorsement of rejuvenation in 1924: 'animals that have been subjected to vasoligature [the Steinach operation] develop a voracious appetite soon after the operation.'[14] Kammerer argued that this was equally the case in humans, and articulated that even more specific changes in eating were to be observed. For example, in one case, following vasoligature, 'the patient does not crave very rich and appetizing dishes', yet 'even scanty rations of cheap food were assimilated so thoroughly that even a part of the ration which before had not sufficed to retard a progressive diminution in weight, now proved more than sufficient to bring about a gain of weight.'[15] The gaining of weight, particularly through the laying down of additional fat deposits, was celebrated by Kammerer as an indication of success in cases of the Steinach operation. It sat alongside other subjective signs such as 'general buoyancy, new joy in life and work, mental and physical ability to work, improved memory ... and greater endurance' as markers of a rejuvenation.[16]

Like Kammerer, Peter Schmidt recorded the centrality of diet for rejuvenation in his treatise on cases of rejuvenation from numerous authors, originally published in German in 1928.[17] The English translation, considerably expanded and updated, appeared as *The Conquest of Old Age* in 1931. In the text, Schmidt outlined seventy pages of case histories, drawn from both his own practice and that of fellow exponents of the Steinach operation from throughout Europe and North America, including Harry Benjamin (United

---

[14] Kammerer, *Rejuvenation*, 83.   [15] Ibid., 92–93.   [16] Ibid., 160–61.
[17] Schmidt, *Das überwundene Alter.*

States), Knud Sand (Denmark), Norman Haire (England) and a single case originating from Steinach himself.[18] Across these diverse practitioners there was clear appreciation in their records of the importance of increased weight following rejuvenatory vasoligature and a close connection between appetite and senility.

In the sole case overseen by Steinach and his collaborator Lichtenstern, in which the two performed a vasoligature on 10 February 1919, the seventy-one-year-old patient reported that, nine months after the operation, 'my appetite has become so keen that I find it very difficult to satisfy my hunger in the food conditions now prevailing [in post-war Vienna].'[19] Sand reported related but quite distinct effects in a case of his own, where a sixty-three-year-old builder, suffering from 'premature senility', noted that although he 'has a good appetite', the patient had experienced a gradual decline in weight from 190 lbs to around 150 lbs; such case histories were presented by Sand (and Schmidt in turn) as part of the evidence for a need to effect a rejuvenation.[20] The use of case histories itself was reflective of a broader emphasis on individual narratives in rejuvenatory discourse. When recounted by practitioners such as Schmidt and Sand, they emphasised causation and progress, clearly linked to the relevant surgical intervention, whilst those which occupied texts aimed at a more general readership encompassed what Brian Hurwitz has termed 'the sentimental tale', designed to persuade and inspire as much as inform.[21]

The cases recorded by Norman Haire and reprinted by Schmidt demonstrate a further relationship between eating habits and rejuvenation procedures. For example, in the account of a 'novelist . . . A.B.' who was fifty-three years of age and who underwent a double-sided vasectomy, carried out by Haire on 19 March 1922 under spinal anaesthetic, the notes reveal that 'eating well' was a marker of general health and wellness following the operation, rather than as a specific indicator of rejuvenation.[22] In other cases, however, even Haire – a strong advocate of the benefits of the Steinach operation as a means of effecting rejuvenation – recognised the importance of 'the usual routine of dieting and massage for a few weeks' following seemingly effective surgical interventions.[23] As well as the gaining of weight, specific effects of successful Steinach operations, performed by Haire, resulted in in 'appetite and digestive powers' being 'improved'; one retired medical practitioner and 'man of letters' who underwent the operation on 19 March 1923 reported that

---

[18] Others included B. Kramer who was principally concerned not with endocrinology, but with nutrition. See Tisdall, 'A Note on the Kramer-Tisdall Method'.
[19] Schmidt, *Conquest of Old Age*, 108.   [20] Ibid., 109.
[21] Hurwitz, 'Narrative Constructs', 65.   [22] Schmidt, *Conquest of Old Age*, 115.
[23] Ibid., 116.

he had experienced 'increase in appetite and excellent digestive powers' within a year.[24]

Schmidt reported only selected cases from the hundred or so which he claimed to have overseen. Of these, in just over half he noted the appetite of the patient before and after treatment, and in almost all cases deployed weight gain as an indicator of successful rejuvenation. Several cases bear out the striking relationship between restoration of youthfulness and diet. For example, after being diagnosed with '[t]ypical male climacteric' and 'prostatic atrophy', a fifty-one-year-old factory owner underwent right vasoligature at the hand of Schmidt. The restoration of physical, mental and sexual powers was accompanied by a gain of around eight pounds in weight. However, most tellingly, when the patient suffered from influenza around eighteen months after the operation, '[i]n spite of the febrile illness ... with considerable falling-off in the appetite, his weight has been maintained.'[25]

For his part, Voronoff's earlier works eschewed any meaningful connection between habits of consumption and longevity. In his 1920 book *Vivre*, translated into English by his wife Evelyn Bostwick and published as *Life* the same year, Voronoff explicitly ruled out any such close relationship. Invoking the arguments first cast by Georges-Louis Leclerc, Comte de Buffon, in the eighteenth century, Voronoff noted that 'the duration of life does not depend on habit, custom, or quality of food.'[26] In this distinction, Voronoff found support from Leonard Williams who, in the 1927 Cavendish Lecture to the West London Medico-Chirurgical Society, argued for a strict separation between the action of vitamins and the endocrine system.[27]

This marked a somewhat dramatic reversal for Williams, who in a 1921 letter to *The Lancet* had personally endorsed periodic fasting for rejuvenation, a method which he had found yielded positive results in the case of diabetic patients.[28] Williams had already indicated his belief that the combination of a long large intestine and consumption of 'flesh-food' – features of physiology and diet deemed evolutionarily incompatible – were responsible for premature death and senescence.[29] However, whilst he then gradually softened his views on the importance of correct eating for rejuvenation, fasting remained a

---

[24] Schmidt, *Conquest of Old Age*, 116–18. Many, but not all, of these cases, of course, focussed equally or in greater detail on the restoration of sexual potency in male patients as an indicator of successful rejuvenation. This has been noted elsewhere, but the focus on sexuality has obscured the fact that rejuvenation was a process which involved numerous physiological indicators. See, for example: Sengoopta, *The Most Secret Quintessence*; Hirshbein, 'The Glandular Solution'.

[25] Schmidt, *Conquest of Old Age*, 128.

[26] Voronoff, *Life*, 5. For the original French edition, see: Serge Voronoff, *Vivre*.

[27] Williams, 'Senescence and Senility'.   [28] Williams, 'Fasting', 1245.

[29] Williams, 'Chronic Intestinal Stasis', 538; Williams and Lyon-Smith, 'Chronic Intestinal Stasis', 472.

popular means of promoting youthfulness despite the emergence of hormone surgeries as a more high-profile method.

Advocates of hormone-driven therapies had good reason for avoiding the recommendation of specific diets for rejuvenation. For every prospective patient who wished to use surgical intervention to avoid having to effect lifestyle changes, others who were perhaps more wary of the expense and uncertainty of testicular grafting had the opportunity to enjoy similar benefits through dietary modification or, some argued, simply taking a daily vitamin-rich tablet. Gradual loss of weight was implicated by Schmidt and other purveyors of the Steinach operation as indicative of an organism in need of rejuvenation. The restoration of a larger, youthful appetite – and accompanying gain of weight – was therefore taken as an indicator of successful rejuvenation. However, others claimed instead that, rather than being simply affected by endocrine balance, adopting a different dietary strategy could itself yield a rejuvenating effect on the body.

Prolonged Restricted Diet: Rational Fasting

> I have frequently repeated the experience [of three-day fasting], and always with the same result. The first day, craving; the second, resignation; the third, rejoicing and rejuvenescence.[30]

> After 50, the sensation of a full stomach should be avoided at all costs.[31]

The pre-war emphasis on moderation was intimately connected to late-Victorian anxieties about degeneration at the level of both the individual and the population, drawing inspiration in particular from late nineteenth-century treatises which addressed the crisis accompanying middle age.[32] Individual responsibility for maintaining health and vitality through diet was paramount; the food reformer and fierce anti-vivisectionist Charles E. Reinhardt argued in his 1910 book, *Diet and the Maximum Duration of Life*, 'the chief cause of the infirmities of old age ... is the process known as "auto-intoxication", or self-poisoning.'[33] Personal accountability was at the heart of Reinhardt's understanding of diet, which he saw as an extension of personal cleanliness, an interior and exterior bodily state which would 'naturally reach the mind and the morals'.[34] Reinhardt drew on the work of Elié Metchnikoff in his book which, priced at just a shilling, attracted a wide audience following positive

---

[30] Williams, 'Fasting', 1245.   [31] Lorand, 'Steinach's Rejuvenation Operation', 470.
[32] In his synthetic account of anxiety surrounding diet for the professional working man, Guy Beddoes noted the 'far reach of digestive derangement', which was thought to influence a wide range of physiological states. Beddoes, *Habit and Health*, vii.
[33] Reinhardt, *Diet*, 5.   [34] Ibid., 6.

comments in a large number of local newspapers, where he was described primarily as a 'well-known dietetic specialist'.[35]

Herman Weber's call to moderation – aired first in 1903 – continued to act as an important touching-stone for those commenting on how diet might extend lifespan in the immediate aftermath of World War One. A review of the fifth edition of his work, published in 1919, in *Nature* suggested that a 'clean life' such as that advocated by Weber would prevent 'the degeneration of the blood-vessels and other organs' and the absorption of toxins through the bowels. By drawing on cases where some family members had followed a regimen of moderate eating and drinking, combined with exercise in the fresh air, and some had not, Weber had seemingly provided 'evidence ... strong enough to support his claim'.[36] An emphasis on moderation was central to many other dietary schemes. The author Reddie Mallett, who published an extended treatise *Nature's Way*, outlining a means of attaining 'health without medicine' in 1930, attached special importance to diet. In his treatment of that subject in 1925, Mallett outlined a diet which 'may deserve the consideration of those who would follow in Nature's way'.[37] The noted American psychologist and educationalist, G. Stanley Hall (1846–1924), who in 1922 published a major treatise, *Senescence: The Last Half of Life*, was similarly praiseworthy of a relatively simple diet, particularly for the elderly. Citing John Madison Taylor (1855–1931) with approval, Hall argued that '[w]e must put aside, as we advance [in years], some articles of diet of which we are fond', basing his perspective on the mirroring between childhood and old age, both being 'toothless' states.[38]

As well as an emphasis on 'simple' diets, the effects of a prolonged, restricted diet were also of interest, and not just for those who sought to rejuvenate the organism. Francis G. Benedict and his colleagues at the Nutritional Laboratory of the Carnegie Institute of Washington spent much of World War One attempting to understand how the body responded to 'an entirely new and heretofore practically unrecognized nutritional level' which arose when food supplies were radically reduced through blockades.[39]

When it came to public audiences, however, advice tended to be simple. It is worth quoting at length from Jean Frumusan's 1923 work *Rejuvenation*, in

[35] 'Advice on Diet', *Globe*, 9 November 1910, 4; 'Literary Notices and Extracts. Books and Magazines', *Derbyshire Advertiser and Journal*, 21 October 1910, 18; 'Bookland', *Berwickshire News and General Advertiser*, 15 November 1910, 4.

[36] 'Nutrition and Longevity', 528.

[37] Reddie Mallett, *The Gospel of Feeding, from Childhood to Old Age*. London: Watts & Co., 1925, 39.

[38] Hall, *Senescence*, 232. For more on Taylor, a leading figure in American children's medicine, see Hinsdale, 'Memorial: John Madison Taylor', 41.

[39] Benedict, Miles, Roth and Smith, *Human Vitality and Efficiency*, 4.

which he outlined some of the key 'precepts for attaining to old age, or a little catechism of the healthy life'. He later expanded on these in far more detail in a more specific text, *The Cure of Obesity*. Frumusan's advice in *Rejuvenation* included directions to

give a substantial but light breakfast ... avoid artificial and exciting tonics ... Eat slowly and moderately, do not drink at meals, chew conscientiously and leave the table with a sensation of lightness, with the ability to eat more. ... Be carnivorous at one meal and vegetarian at the next. Once a month give the organism a rest by fasting for twenty-four or forty-eight hours, preceding the fast by a purgative. During the fast, drink large quantities of water or herb teas.[40]

This exhortation to a specific regimen of eating was interspersed with guidance on numerous other aspects of daily living, including sleep, exercise, environment, occupation, general disposition and the relationship between physical and intellectual work. Like many writers of the period, Frumusan equated early retirement with a loss of energy and vitality.[41] Indeed, Frumusan's appreciation for the myriad factors which might contribute to health and potential longevity drew in large part on the ongoing significance of the non-naturals (not identified by him as such, but clearly visible) in understanding and preserving whole-organism health. For example, in the case of 'Mme. P., aged 58', who arrived at Frumusan's clinic 'in such a state of physical ruin that life had become odious to her' and 'overwhelmed with fat', his proposed regimen included purges, dietary modification, a programme of therapeutic massage and exercise, and a course of 'galvanic and sinusoidal hydro-electric applications'.[42]

Published in English just a year later, Frumusan's manual for reducing – *The Cure of Obesity* – took a dramatically different approach. In it he addressed diet in isolation, divorcing it from almost all other factors, race excepting, which might affect longevity and health. Historical readings of *The Cure of Obesity* have focused exclusively on the divisions of habits of corpulence along racial lines; for example, Sander Gilman has noted that Frumusan characterised Jewish people as having a tendency towards obesity, without further comment.[43] Contemporary reviews of Frumusan's work in the mainstream medical press noted that, notwithstanding its 'liberality of the verbiage', *The Cure of Obesity* presented 'a radical but rational method of reducing' which might act to prolong life and health.[44] Those sympathetic to his aims and methods were more effusive. In an advertising brochure for Yerbama – the 'life preserving tea from Parana' – Frumusan was described as a '[l]eading

---

[40] Frumusan, *Rejuvenation*, 121.   [41] Ibid.   [42] Ibid., 123–24.
[43] Gilman, *Fat*, 105–07; Gilman, 'Fat as Disability', 51; Gilman, 'Thoughts on the Jewish Body', 5.
[44] Frumusan, *The Cure of Obesity*, 701.

authority on Rejuvenation ... a celebrated medico in Paris'.[45] The 'cult of reducing' – much noted in the existing literature – was indeed a prominent feature of the early twentieth century, drawing inspiration from significant treatises on this subject from the second half of the nineteenth century.[46]

Leonard Williams – supporter of Voronoff and a key British rejuvenation populariser – advocated a similar regimen to that of Frumusan. In both the medical and popular press Williams noted that his health was maintained through 'a short [three-day] fast occasionally', during which, on the first day he 'felt well', on the second 'very well', and the third, 'very well indeed'.[47]

Dietary guides were not only the preserve of medical practitioners, of course, and during the early 1920s manufacturers of a range of products went into print in order to establish the centrality of their wares to healthy diets. Amongst these was Heudebert Foods, based in Middlesex, well known for their 'diabetic bread', 'digestible crispbreads, biscottes and gressinettes' and other 'dietetic foods'.[48] In a series of extended 'dietetic summaries', Heudebert outlined theories of dietary disruption within specific organs, such as the stomach or intestine, before recommending hugely detailed diets. These included both their own products – pitched as a component in an otherwise mixed diet – as well as water-only, milk-based and vegetarian systems.[49]

The Heudebert products were calculated to appeal to a consumer market increasingly familiar with complex diets and natural management of illness and sub-optimal health. In the early twentieth century, the naturopathic 'movement' in Britain was little more than a collection of disparate therapeutic approaches to bodily disorder. As Jane M. Adams has noted, however, 'it was not until the interwar period that naturopaths began to assert a more coherent identity in Britain.'[50] The popularity of naturopathy was in many ways a reaction against an increasingly dominant technological modernity. Andrew Pitcairn-Knowles was emblematic of this shift. As a celebrated

---

[45] 'Yerbama the life-preserving tea from Parana', c.1930, Patent Medicines 19 (13a), 1, John Johnson Collection, Bodleian Library, Oxford (hereafter Johnson Collection); 'Does Yerbama Lengthen Life? By a Well-Known Writer', c.1930, Patent Medicines 19 (13b), 6, Johnson Collection.

[46] Simpson, *The Handbook of Dining*; Davies, *Foods for the Fat*. For discussions of obesity cures and the culture of reducing in the secondary literature, see Zweiniger-Bargielowska, *'The Culture of the Abdomen'*.

[47] 'Effects of Fasting. Craving, Resignation and Rejuvenescence', *Yorkshire Evening Post*, 10 December 1921, 4.

[48] '[Advertisement]', *Buckinghamshire Herald*, 23 June 1933, 8; 'The Heudebert Foods Co., Ltd.', *Burnley Express*, 9 February 1938, 1; 'Fine Groceries for Every Occasion', *Kent and Sussex Courier*, 5 January 1940, 5; 'Dietetics', *Dumfries and Galloway Standard*, 28 June 1941, 10.

[49] Heudebert Laboratories, *The Diet in Diseases of the Digestive Tract. Part 1*; Heudebert Laboratories, *The Diet in Diseases of the Digestive Tract. Part 2*.

[50] Adams, *Healing with Water*, 173.

journalistic photographer, he travelled extensively throughout Europe before founding the 'Riposo', a 'health hydro and dietetic establishment' in the English coastal resort of Hastings in 1911.[51] As a Fellow and advocate of the Nature Cure Association of Great Britain and Ireland (established in 1920), he staked his reputation in naturopathy on the methods of Emanuel and Johann Schroth, the father-and-son originators of a century-old hydro-therapeutic regime.[52]

Through the 'Schroth Regeneration Cure', according to Pitcairn-Knowles, 'tens of thousands have recovered their health, when they appeared to be approaching their graves.'[53] The treatment was based around 'the healing power of the dry diet', with 'infrequent short intervals for drinking', considering that 'water-logging' was the cause of much preventable disease.[54] A mixture of '"dry" days' and '"drink" days' involved almost exclusive consumption of bread products and wine, respectively, with 'two-third to a whole bottle of wine' indicated on days four and seven.[55] This was then followed by the nightly application of a 'full-body-pack', consisting of a wet sheet, 'next to the skin', covered in 'two large eiderdowns'. The patient was effectively 'sandwiched between the two eiderdowns', with hot water bottles applied to make the process more tolerable.[56] As well as being effective against rheumatism, insomnia, neuralgia, and 'all forms of blood poisoning', amongst many others, Pitcairn-Knowles heralded the Schroth method in treating age-related conditions such as arterio-sclerosis, varicose veins and the perennial challenge of 'auto-intoxication' of the digestive tract.[57]

Writing more extensively on the development of the 'Schroth Diet', Pitcairn-Knowles revealed further important aspects of how the regimen should be observed. First, the reliance on carbohydrates – 'starchy foods' – should not be carried beyond the confines of the treatment, and only pursued under expert supervision. Second, even the slightest introduction of meat during the treatment caused a reversion to ill health.[58] He also promoted the method and his own Riposo 'Nature Cure Resort' by issuing vegetarian recipe pamphlets, despite the fairly simple combination of breads and wine indicated

---

[51] Victoria and Albert Museum, 'Andrew Pitcairn-Knowles'.

[52] Pitcairn-Knowles, *Schroth Regeneration Cure*, 3.   [53] Ibid., 3.

[54] Pitcairn-Knowles, *Schroth Regeneration Cure*, 4. The Schroth Cure was heavily reliant on the separation of food from drink, a position echoed in much of the vegetarian literature of the period. See Hosali, *The Humane Diet Leaflets*, 4.

[55] Ibid., 5.   [56] Ibid.   [57] Ibid., 6–7.

[58] Pitcairn-Knowles, *The History and Development of the Schroth Cure*, 37. Pitcairn-Knowles also documented the treatment through photography, capturing in more arresting ways the physical experience of undergoing such treatment. See: Andrew Pitcairn-Knowles, 'The Schroth Cure – lying in a pack', c.1910, E.3623-2004, Victoria and Albert Museum; Andrew Pitcairn-Knowles, 'The Schroth Cure – The Monument Erected By Schroth's Cured Patients', c.1910, E.3620-2004, Victoria and Albert Museum.

in the regime.[59] Indeed, Pitcairn-Knowles also claimed that the treatment was effective in overcoming obesity, itself a significant object of concern in inter-war Britain.

Emphasis on the health benefits of reducing body weight was not merely a response to national anxieties about population fitness, however; it was also fundamentally rooted in changing attitudes towards the life course. For example, Frederick L. Hoffman, the German-born medical statistician who probed aspects of racial and occupational public health in relation to US healthcare insurance through his work with the Prudential Insurance Company, argued in 1928 that 'the increase in the average weight on the part of many persons past middle life is a serious menace to their future health and longevity.'[60] Like many, Hoffman argued that there were no 'inherent physical reasons why bodily weight should increase after thirty', noting instead that sedentary lifestyle practices and poor dietary habits were the root cause of such problems.[61]

If hormone surgeries were reliant on specialist medical oversight and reporting – albeit incorporating subjective patient experiences – the expertise of lay fasters was critical in establishing the efficacy of dietary restriction as a rejuvenation method in the public domain. A lengthy article on the practices of the 'veteran faster', Mr Tuohy, in the *Bedfordshire Times* in May 1927 noted that he had refined the fasting regime such that he regarded it as a far superior method to the 'grafting of glands'. The seventy-two-year-old Tuohy's claimed methods involved far more radical periods of abstention from food – up to forty-two days – but he also maintained a strict vegetarian diet at all other times, with a preference for uncooked food, which did not risk introducing 'impurities into the blood'.[62] Clement Jeffrey, author of *Human Power* and advocate of so-called natural living, also drew parallels with unnatural and ineffective endocrine treatments, arguing in a lecture at Mortimer Hall, London, in October 1927 that 'the only solid foundation of a happy, long and useful life was obedience to the laws of nature.'[63] The event was delivered

---

[59] Riposo Recipes, *Two Completely Meatless Meals*.

[60] Hoffman, *Some Problems of Longevity*, vi. For more on Hoffman, whose 1896 publication *The Race Traits and Tendencies of the American Negro* had argued quite explicitly that African Americans were far more prone to disease – a claim which he later retracted – see Sypher ed., *Frederick L. Hoffman*.

[61] Hoffman, *Some Problems of Longevity*, vi.

[62] 'Interview with Mr Tuohy, the Veteran Faster', *Bedfordshire Times and Independent*, 27 May 1921, 8.

[63] 'Rejuvenation. Right v. Wrong Methods', *Leamington Spa Courier*, 2 March 1928, 6. The lecture was widely reported in local periodicals throughout Britain. Strikingly, although Clement dismissed the possibility of using Steinach- or Voronoff-inspired treatments, the headline in the *Bellshill Speaker* read 'Putting Back the Hands of Time. Rejuvenation by Monkey Glands', demonstrating the extent to which glandular therapies had come to occupy a singular place in public rejuvenation discourse. See: 'Putting Back the Hands of Time. Rejuvenation by Monkey

in support of the Pearson Fresh Air Fund, established in 1892 to enable disadvantaged children to undertake outdoor activities, and Clement advised his audience to 'clean up the system by fasting and other methods, and ... become rejuvenated both in body and mind'.[64]

In his book *Old Age: Its Causes and Prevention* (1912), the American anti-ageing advocate, author and businessman Sanford Bennett proclaimed that a specific regime of exercise and diet had 'thrown off the conditions of age' and enabled him to 'become, physically, a young man again'.[65] Bennett's account was subtitled *The Story of an Old Body and Face Made Young*, highlighting his claim that modification of the diet and a strict regime of exercises – 'muscular contractions' – could result in a literal restoration of youth. Drawing on his earlier 1907 publication, *Exercising in Bed*, he railed against 'dangerous allopathic methods', instead raising a 'plea for Nature's methods of cure'.[66] The system of eating proposed by Bennett relied on a diverse range of authorities, from the writings of Luigi Cornaro (c.1467–1566), a Venetian nobleman who wrote treatises on the long life, to the more recent works of Arnold Lorand (1865–1943), physician at the Carslbad Spa and advocate of everyday rejuvenation. Lorand himself was cautious about the use of extensive fasting and the omission of food groups from the diet. As he argued, 'true vegetarians frequently present a pale, unhealthy and prematurely aged appearance.'[67]

Bennett's dietary method was essentially twofold: he advised periodic and total fasting, followed by a vegetarian diet characterised by 'well-cooked vegetables'.[68] Standard components such as fat were useful for achieving an 'increase of fatty tissues', yet even Bennett did not believe 'that life can be prolonged to extraordinary ages by any particular article of food'.[69] His own personal experience was critical in establishing his authority in matters of diet; *Old Age* abounded with explicit references to 'twenty-five years of experiment upon my own body' and the rejection of 'all medicines'.[70]

Sanford Bennett was one of the most high-profile advocates of rejuvenating methods in the twentieth century prior to World War One, and his exercises, promising rejuvenation at an old age, were hugely popular, particularly in the

Glands', *Bellshill Speaker*, 28 October 1927, 7–8; 'Do Monkey Glands Restore Youth?', *West London Observer*, 21 October 1927, 7; Clement, *Human Power*.
[64] 'Rejuvenation. Right v. Wrong Methods', *Leamington Spa Courier*, 2 March 1928, 6.
[65] Bennett, *Old Age*, 28.
[66] Bennett, *Old Age*, 30–31; Bennett, *Exercising in Bed*. I will return to Bennett and other practitioners of physical culture in Chapter 5.
[67] Arnold Lorand, *Health and Longevity through Rational Diet: Practical Hints in Regard to Food and the Usefulness or Harmful Effects of the Various Articles of Diet*. Philadelphia, PA: F. A. Davis, 1913, p. 398. Lorand's other works included a more general treatise on combating old age, *Old Age Deferred*, as well as *Life Shortening Habits and Rejuvenation*.
[68] Bennett, *Old Age*, 135.   [69] Ibid., 189.   [70] Ibid., 18 and 19.

United States, as he harnessed the powerful cultural cachet of the physical culture movement, then at its height.[71] Paradoxically, he revelled in his 'young boy appetite', yet at the same time castigated excessive consumption in noting that 'we all eat too much'.[72] Others, including the prominent physical culture advocate, Eugen Sandow, who had earned his fame in his native Germany as a bodybuilder, joined the call for dietary intervention in response to generalised anxieties about degeneration and obesity which accelerated from the 1880s.[73]

Sandow travelled extensively and, although his work was particularly influential in Britain, built up an international audience across Europe and North America by staging spectacular strongman shows and through his popular periodical, *Sandow's Magazine of Physical Culture* (1898–1907), which enjoyed notable yet brief success as the first bodybuilding magazine.[74] Sandow placed less 'emphasis on a healthful diet' than his great rival Bennett and shunned the use of any special foodstuffs. Despite this, in his 1897 exercise guidebook, *Strength and How to Obtain It*, he included a table listing the 'Nutritive Qualities of Foods' and stressed the importance of letting at least two hours elapse between eating and exercising; this despite asserting in the same publication that he had 'no belief in special diet'.[75] For someone who claimed that following a particular diet was largely irrelevant to the purpose of maintaining a youthful, vigorous body, Sandow acknowledged surprisingly specific practices of eating, including Fletcherism.[76] For example, he would

abjure anything intoxicating, confining myself mostly to beer and light wines. Tea and coffee I never suffer myself to touch. All I impose upon my appetites is that they shall be temperately indulged. I endeavour to have my meals at regular hours, and prefer that they shall be simple and easy of digestion. I always take care to chew my food, proper mastication being a *sine qua non* of health.[77]

Completing the Anglo-American trio of physical culture gurus who also attempted to assert their authority over what constituted a healthy diet designed to prolong youthfulness and vitality in the pre-vitamin era was Bernarr Macfadden. Macfadden, who established a publishing empire to promote his

---

[71] Martschukat, 'The Necessity for Better Bodies'; McKenzie, *Getting Physical*.
[72] Bennett, *Old Age*, 26 and 126.
[73] Zweiniger-Bargielowska, *The Culture of the Abdomen*, 242.
[74] Scott, 'Body-Building and Empire-Building'.
[75] Chapman, *Sandow the Magnificent*, 175; Sandow, *Strength and How to Obtain It*, 13, 35 and 90.
[76] Derived from Horace Fletcher, Fletcherism was a system of eating based on chewing food until it had become liquid and thereby easier to digest. For more on Fletcher, see Christen and Christen, 'Horace Fletcher (1849–1919)'.
[77] Adam ed., *Sandow on Physical Training*, 164–65.

ideas, drew on his personal experience of the links between a sedentary lifestyle and poor health to establish the magazine *Physical Culture* in 1899. Like Bennett, Macfadden extolled the virtues of a vegetarian diet and period fasting as a means of achieving rejuvenation.[78] Through his early publications Macfadden argued that '[t]here is but one way of creating a normal appetite and that is by fasting' and noted that, although vegetarianism was preferable, 'I am not one of those who holds that a high degree of health cannot also be acquired and retained with a mixed diet.'[79] By the early 1920s, in the context of emerging excitement about the nutritional potential of vitamins, Macfadden had reconfigured his arguments to provide a new rationalisation for his system. For example, whereas in his 1901 book *Strength from Eating* he had concentrated on factors such as the 'acid properties' of fruits which 'are valuable in assisting the digestive process' and, like Sandow, 'thorough mastication ... until it [food] is an actual liquid', later works drew on the language associated with vitamins.[80] Macfadden presented his updated arguments in *Eating for Health and Strength*, first published in 1921. In this text, he adopted scientific terminology to support his system, claiming that 'a single vitamine, which in quantity may be less than one thousand[th] of the weight of the food, is absolutely essential to life.'[81] Further, and more pertinently for Macfadden's aims as an entrepreneur,

Those of us who have studied the food question from a more practical, human standpoint had observed much evidence of the superiority of natural foods. The discovery of vitamines backs, with scientific fact and theory, these more practical human observations.[82]

Just as Macfadden's work was reconfigured through multiple editions, other publications, such as Otto Abramowski's simple and accessible pamphlet *Fruitarian Diet and Physical Rejuvenation* (1911), continued to be reprinted after World War Two. In the rapidly changing landscape of nutrition practices in the first half of the twentieth century, this manual for preserving health and youthfulness enjoyed remarkable longevity, even if its disciples did not experience similar effects. The text was published originally by the Order of the Golden Age. The Order was established in the mid-1890s by Sidney Hartnoll Beard and, through their various books and their periodical, *The Herald of the Golden Age*, sought to promote the cause of vegetarianism from a Christian perspective.

---

[78] Griffith, 'Apostles of Abstinence'. For more biographical details on the fascinating and colourful life of Macfadden, see: Ernst, *Weakness Is a Crime*; Adams, *Mr America*; Endres, 'The Feminism of Bernarr Macfadden'.

[79] Macfadden, *Strength from Eating*, 73.   [80] Ibid., 177 and 188.

[81] Macfadden, *Eating for Health*, 21.   [82] Ibid., 45–46.

Other authors, including Bramwell Booth (1856–1929), the second General of the Salvation Army, from 1912 until his death, after his father, William Booth (1829–1912), noted explicitly the links between vegetarianism and youth. As Bramwell Booth argued in his short pamphlet, reprinted from *The Herald of the Golden Age*, '[m]ost of the instances of great age are to be found among those who from their youth have lived principally, if not entirely, on vegetables and fruit.'[83] Beard himself argued strongly that this diet should be pursued as a matter of urgent moral duty.[84] When the Order relocated to South Africa in the late 1930s, the organisation quickly faded into obscurity, yet Abramowski's work continued to appear in print. The success of his pamphlet – still recommended in some quarters of the vegetarian movement – was something of an exception to the relatively short-lived fashions of the period, when dietary innovations competed for public attention and scientific credibility.

Whilst Abramowski's book dealt only tangentially with the subject of old age, F. W. D. Mitchell's *A Key to Health and Long Life* (1914, second edition 1922) argued explicitly that 'the most significant symptom of the approach of old age is the decline of the digestive powers.'[85] Mitchell had begun his medical training in Dublin in the 1880s but withdrew despite successfully completing examinations in anatomy and physiology, and by the early twentieth century occupied the post of Secretary of the Congested Districts Board in Ireland.[86] Having sketched out a pre-vitamin system of dietary management in his initial publication in 1914, Mitchell then drew on the public attention afforded to the significance of accessory food factors in a subsequent edition eight years later. In this, he reserved special praise for '"Vitamine", which escapes chemical analysis and seems to be almost synonymous with the quality known as "freshness"'. Having asserted that fresh foods contained an abundance of this substance, Mitchell advocated a diet which shunned 'salted or preserved foods' which could cause 'the blood [to become] weak and unhealthy'.[87] He echoed Bennett's call to ensure that foods were cooked appropriately, as overcooking might destroy the essential 'vitamin quality',

---

[83] Bramwell Booth, *The Advantages of Vegetarian Diet*. London: The Order of the Golden Age, c.1925, 2.

[84] Beard, *Is Flesh-eating Morally Defensible?*; Beard, *A Comprehensive Guide-Book*; Bates, *Anti-Vivisection and the Medical Profession*, 69–98.

[85] Mitchell, *A Key to Health and Long Life*, 163.

[86] 'Medical News', *British Medical Journal*, 29 October 1887, 973–75, 973; Royal Commission on Congestion in Ireland, *Appendices to the First Report*, 22. The Congested Districts Board of Ireland was established in 1891 by the then Chief Secretary for Ireland, Arthur Balfour, in an attempt to combat poverty and poor quality of life in West and North West Ireland. This has been seen largely as an extension of more active attempts to derail arguments for Home Rule. See Breathnach, *The Congested Districts Board of Ireland*.

[87] Mitchell, *A Key to Health and Long Life*, 2nd edition, 115.

favouring fresh fruit and salads over cooked food, and castigating in particular margarine, which he considered 'deficient in the vitamines'.[88]

As Mitchell was not a medical professional, he sought to bolster his credibility in a number of other ways. He drew heavily and explicitly in his own work on the writings of key authorities, including Cornaro, the celebrated English physician George Cheyne, Hermann Weber, Caleb Saleeby and Elié Metchnikoff, and also appealed to his own relationship with medicine by reprinting letters which he sent to the *Hospital Gazette* and *Medical Times*.[89] His intervention – aimed at a non-professional audience – did not go unnoticed by the medical press. A review of the 1922 edition in the *British Medical Journal*, for example, remained critical of Mitchell's arguments, yet also noted that 'if the public for whom it is more suited read and follow its directions the result will be all to the good.'[90]

Many of the materials cited by Mitchell were produced by high-profile members of the medical profession. Weber, for example, argued specifically that vitamine was 'destroyed by boiling', particularly in the case of milk, which was otherwise considered to be 'the most useful article of food ... the most perfect food'.[91] Weber had trained in Marburg and Bonn before settling in England to practice in 1854. He advocated environmental cures and health retreats in cases of consumption and turned his attention late in life to the relationship between diet and longevity, delivering his lecture on the subject to the Royal College of Physicians at the age of eighty.[92] Just as Bernarr Macfadden used emerging ideas about the role of vitamins in his later publications to provide new scientific justification for his earlier ideas, so too did later editions of Weber's book retrospectively integrate such information into his existing arguments. However, far from identifying vitamins as all-powerful, they were but a small, yet important, part of Weber's scheme of nutrition, which stressed above all the centrality of balance across the diet.[93] In this regard, he drew analogies with the animal kingdom in order to demonstrate one of the key tenets of his argument which went against many of the self-proclaimed dietary experts of this period: that abstaining from flesh in the

---

[88]   Ibid., 115–16. Macfadden made a similar argument, noting that '[t]he cooking process may destroy or reduce the available quantity of vitamines [in leafy green vegetables].' Macfadden, *Eating for Health*, 152.

[89]   These letters were included as appendices in both the 1914 and 1922 editions. Mitchell, *A Key to Health and Long Life*, 151–59.

[90]   'Notes on Books', *British Medical Journal*, 16 December 1922, 1179–80, 1179.

[91]   Weber, *On Longevity*, 87 and 89.

[92]   Weber and Weber, *Climatotherapy and Balneotherapy*. Frederick Parkes Weber, Hermann's son, was a prominent physician in his own right. See F. Parkes Weber, 'MD Thesis 1892 F P Weber: On the Association of Chronic Interstitial Nephritis with Pulmonary Tuberculosis', 1892, PP/FPW/B.337/1:Box 160, Wellcome Library.

[93]   Weber, *On Longevity*, 80–81.

diet was not self-evidently positive for overall health. The rationale behind this was, as the prominent English eugenicist Caleb Saleeby, an adviser to the Minister of Food during World War One, noted in his 1921 work *The Eugenic Prospect*, that 'the herbivore, eating the green leaf, does well; and the carnivore, eating the herbivore, does no worse.'[94] This, Saleeby and Weber maintained, was because the leaves were the true site of vitamin generation, and these remarkable substances simply made their way up the food chain in an uncomplicated fashion.

In earlier editions of his work, Weber placed great emphasis on the purity of milk as a foodstuff. For the purpose he drew largely on the assertion of one of the most significant figures in the longevity movement of the early twentieth century, Elié Metchnikoff (1845–1916). Writing before World War One, Metchnikoff almost singlehandedly initiated the idea that 'beneficial microorganisms should be introduced into the colon to fight the toxicity' produced by the digestive process.[95] This toxicity, he argued, which arose from decomposition, was the cause of not only intestinal complaints but also the ageing process.[96] To combat these destructive processes, Metchnikoff advocated the consumption of yoghurt, the natural bacterial content of which would modify the internal environment in such a way as to prevent the build-up of toxins to a dangerous level.[97] However, although the regular consumption of yoghurt was a unique feature of his approach to maintaining a healthy diet – and consequently remaining youthful – Metchnikoff also drew on similar practices of abstention and dietary restraint as those promoted by the likes of Weber and Saleeby. These included '[t]he avoidance of alcohol and the rigid exclusion from diet of foods that favour putrefaction, such as rich meats'. The ultimate goal of Metchnikoff's system of dietary modification was nothing less than extension of the average lifespan, and he cited the prominent role played by soured milk foods in a number of national contexts, from the 'Leben raib' (a soured milk prepared from the milk of buffaloes or goats) of Egypt to 'prostokwasha' (coagulated, soured, raw milk) consumed in Russia.[98] As he summarised, '[t]he fact that so many races make soured milk and use it copiously is an excellent testimony to its usefulness.'[99]

---

[94] Saleeby, *The Eugenic Prospect*, 183.   [95] Stoilova, 'The Bulgarianization of Yoghurt', 19.
[96] Later proponents of this view included William Arbuthnot Lane. See Lane, 'Chronic Intestinal Stasis'.
[97] Metchnikoff, *Prolongation of Life*. Some authors have argued that this approach was the defining precursor to modern practices associated with probiotics, notwithstanding earlier pregerm approaches to cultivating gut flora. See, for example: Mackowiak, 'Recycling Metchnikoff'; McFarland, 'From Yaks to Yogurt'; Tauber and Chernyak, *Metchnikoff and the Origins of Immunology*. John Harvey Kellogg was another high-profile advocate of the important role played by auto-intoxication from diet. See Kellogg, *Autointoxication or Intestinal Toxemia*.
[98] Metchnikoff, *Prolongation of Life*, 171–72.   [99] Ibid., 174.

Metchnikoff implicated germs of disease, albeit indirectly, in the ageing process, in addition to his much-publicised theory that the length of the colon was inversely proportional to expected, natural lifespan.[100] However he did so in a way which reinforced traditional narratives about the desirability of a simple diet, especially the avoidance of heavy foods and adherence to the 'rules of rational hygiene'.[101] Throughout, Metchnikoff argued that 'vegetable substances contain an acid principle which retards our mortal enemy putrefaction.'[102] These ideas were not displaced, but rather reinterpreted in the era of vitamins which followed World War One; a simple, raw diet of fresh, natural foods was now beneficial for preserving health and rejuvenating body and mind by virtue of its vitamin content. Although Frederick L. Hoffman did not mention vitamins once in his 180-page treatise on longevity, published in 1928, these fractional yet powerful constituents of foodstuffs attained a popular status as determinants of health.[103] We move now to consider what role contemporary commentators saw for vitamins in achieving a renewal or prolongation of youthfulness.

Vitamins and the Reconfiguration of the Food–Ageing Complex

> These mysterious substances were first called ... the 'Accessory food substances' ... which may without exaggeration be described as the essence of life.[104]

In 1919, at the same time as Herman Weber was promoting caution in cooking, for fear of damaging '*vitamine*, which is destroyed by boiling', the American biochemist E. V. McCollum published a text outlining how recent findings in the identity of vitamins might give cause to rethink what constituted a 'healthy' diet.[105] In *The Newer Knowledge of Nutrition*, McCollum, who had with Marguerite Davis isolated Vitamin A in 1913 and confirmed the identity of Vitamin B two years later, promoted 'the great protective foods' of 'dairy produce from cows fed on green leaves and the green leaf itself', which he regarded as 'a most essential part of the diet'.[106] This represented something of a significant shift from many of the mid- to late-nineteenth century texts on

---

[100] Vischer, *Old Age*, 98–99.   [101] Metchnikoff, *Prolongation of Life*, 183.
[102] Amos, *The Humane Diet Leaflets: 15*, 4.
[103] Similarly, the popular 1923 treatise on diet by John Harvey Kellogg shunned the language of vitamins, mobilising not biochemical but evolutionary and behavioural arguments in favour of a vegetarian diet, such as children's supposed natural reluctance to eat meat, and the fact that the ultimate carnivore – the dog – thrives on a diet with very little meat. Kellogg, *The Natural Diet of Man*, 258–59.
[104] Belfrage, *What's Best to Eat?*, 24.   [105] Weber, *On Longevity*, 89, original emphasis.
[106] McCollum, *The Newer Knowledge of Nutrition*; 'Nutrition and Longevity', *Nature* 104 (1920), 527–28.

diet and longevity, which had emphasised the importance of animal foods in older people. For example, the American physician and author of popular medical texts, John Gardner, claimed in the 1875 edition of his popular text on longevity that the natural preference of 'aged persons' for foods such as 'mutton, poultry, game, and often for gelatinous food, rather than beef, pork, lamb, or veal', was 'in accordance with physiology' and indicative of the error inherent in adopting a vegetarian diet.[107]

Instead, the discovery of vitamins appeared to 'confirm the vegetarian in his faith in fresh fruit and vegetables, and whole meal bread', as reported in the *Jarrow Express* as early as 1917.[108] McCollum was himself opposed to the word 'vitamine' and suggested instead a more complex system of nomenclature based on the water- or fat-soluble nature of the particular substance.[109] The considerable uncertainty and confusion surrounding the nomenclature of vitamines (which were also termed 'accessory food factors' and known by their individual names) persisted well into the late 1920s.[110] Whatever the favoured term, there was near-consensus amongst medical professionals and biologists alike that vitamins – as well as being implicated in the case of deficiency diseases such as beri-beri, scurvy and pellagra – played a critical role in maintaining normal metabolic function. A major 1919 report, commissioned by the UK-based Medical Research Council (MRC) and led by vitamin figurehead F. Gowland Hopkins, argued for the primacy of vitamins on the basis that 'if minute amounts of certain constituents are removed from natural foods, such foods wholly fail to support nutrition, and grave symptoms of actual disease may supervene.'[111]

The rise of "vitamania" was as much a socio-economic phenomenon as a medical one.[112] By the mid-1920s, the vitamin content of food, alongside its mineral and caloric composition and long-established categories of protein, fat and carbohydrate, was widely acknowledged to be a key factor in determining its nutritional value within both specialist and lay discourse. The implications for diet were obvious: the specific functions of different vitamins and the health requirements of the individual dictated the foods which they should eat. Following a decade in which rejuvenation of both individual and nation had become an object of societal fascination, these still-imperfectly-understood substances were endowed with extraordinary capacities to modify human physiology and intervene in the ageing process.

[107] Gardner, *Longevity*, 49.   [108] 'A Vital Element in Food', *Jarrow Express*, 13 April 1917, 5.
[109] McCollum and Kennedy, 'The Dietary Factors Operating'; McCollum and Pitz, 'The "Vitamine" Hypothesis'.
[110] 'Nomenclature of the Accessory Food Factors', *Nature* 68 (1928), 480–81.
[111] Medical Research Committee, *Report on the Present State of Knowledge Concerning Accessory Food Factors*, 1.
[112] For perspectives on vitamins, see: Apple, *Vitamania*; Carpenter, *The History of Scurvy*.

But how best to introduce vitamins into the diet? As Rima D. Apple has argued, in the United States the early debate was not 'who could sell vitamins', but 'who could judge vitamin supplementation'.[113] This was manifestly not the case in early twentieth-century Europe, where the food supply to tables was affected significantly as the proximity of conflict had a far more profound nutritional effect. In this context, vitamins functioned as an 'advertiser's dream', just as much linked with ageing as nutrition.[114]

Manufacturers attempted to capitalise on the appeal of vitamins to sell specific products, such as Fleischmann's Yeast, Quaker Oats and Welch's Grape Juice, many of which emphasised their place in a diet which promoted vigour and preserved health.[115] In the case of Fleischmann's Yeast, promotional material even claimed that it was naturally 'rich in hormone-like substances'.[116] However, others sought to integrate vitamins within a broader vision of rejuvenation. The Théiron School of Life, an organisation based (in Britain at least) initially in Bond Street, London, later in Henrietta Street and the less salubrious St. Martin's Lane, and which offered a correspondence course in 'how to remain young and achieve, how to develop a pleasing personality [and] how to overcome "old-age"', was one of a range of organisations which promoted rational healthy eating as part of a system which enabled adherents to reach these lofty goals.[117] The method, declared a whole-page advert in *The Observer* on 27 October 1935, was suitable especially for 'old young men' and 'faded young women'.[118] Although scant records of the Théiron School remain, newspaper advertisements and published courses aside, the practical guides, promotional materials and study questions for subscribers offer a fascinating insight into a little-recognised organisation which promised to 'give you back youth, beauty and vitality' with '[n]o operation, no danger'.[119] It seems that the enterprise originated in 1930 with the scientific endeavour and personal experience of a 'professeur Théiron' in Brussels, who drew on the transformative and controversial cellular immortality studies of Alexis Carrel to claim that, given the correct

---

[113] Apple, *Vitamania*, 84.
[114] Levenstein, *Revolution at the Table*, 152. Levenstein does not consider the characterisation of vitamins in relation to the aging process, and other authors only mention this briefly in passing. See, for example, Scrinis, *Nutritionism*, 188.
[115] Levenstein, *Revolution at the Table*, 153.   [116] Ibid., 197.
[117] Théiron School of Life, *Théiron Method*, title page; 'Youth, Personality and Achievement', *Yorkshire Post*, 15 May 1931, 1; 'I Would Not Accept £100 to Be without the Théiron Method', *Cheltenham Chronicle*, 1 July 1933, 9; 'Don't Grow Old', *Staffordshire Advertiser*, 8 April 1950, 6.
[118] 'Renewed Youth. Personality and Achievement. Body and Soul Under the Microscope', *The Observer*, 27 October 1935, 28.
[119] 'Personal', *Western Daily Press*, 21 May 1931, 6.

environmental conditions, life could be extended dramatically beyond its current limits.[120]

Diet was central to the approach of the Théiron Method and strongly connected with both the glandular system and ageing.[121] As one of the introductory sections on 'Scientific Feeding' explained,

[W]hen one considers that the glandular system determines one's personality, and that these glands require certain chemicals which are frequently absent from the diet, or eaten in a haphazard sort of way, there is no doubt that the character is more or less determined by what one eats.[122]

Much of this hinged on chemical elements as constituent parts of food, underpinned by claims to scientific authority:

The new science of bio-chemistry demonstrates that a man who takes insufficient oxygen into his system, develops a depressed and hopeless outlook in life ... A man who eats food containing an excess of carbon becomes incurably lazy, mentally stupid, and loses ambition. ... Those people who do not secure sufficient hydrogen take on the appearance of premature age.[123]

An impact on personality or health was identified for almost every conceivable chemical element, including nitrogen (responsible for 'magnetic' personality), phosphorous (intelligence), sulphur (excitability), sodium (restlessness), 'chlorin' (gloom), 'silicum' (baldness) and magnesium (sensitivity to heat). Whilst the student of the Théiron Method was introduced to these more traditional, 'mineral' components of food, special place was reserved for 'certain chemical combinations, which we have termed "vitamins," [which have] opened up an entirely new field of dietetics'.[124] The fact that these were, in the case of cereals, for example, located principally in 'the hull or outer covering' led the method to classify refined white bread as inferior, just as Hermann Weber, Benjamin Gayelord Hauser and others had done a decade earlier on almost exactly the same grounds.[125]

The Théiron Method was unequivocal in rejecting the consumption of 'flesh food', which was considered to be 'not for humans'.[126] However, the diet suggested was also described as being distinctive from vegetarianism, which led to 'lack of health and vitality ... sallow skin and other unwholesome

---

[120] 'Une Methode Intelligente de Vivre', *Le Petit Parisien*, 8 October 1930.

[121] Matthew Thomson, who provides a very brief reference to the Théiron School (with reference only to a later, more general textbook on practical psychology from 1936), suggests that this was an example of 'practical psychology', an approach which gained popularity particularly in the 1930s. However, that is to misrepresent the Théiron method, which relied as much on nutrition and exercise as what Thomson terms the use of 'subconscious mental powers'. See Thomson, *Psychological Subjects*, 47 fn. 186.

[122] Théiron School of Life, *Théiron Method*, 143.   [123] Ibid., 251.   [124] Ibid., 251.

[125] Ibid., 251; Weber, *On Longevity*, 98.   [126] Théiron School of Life, *Théiron Method*, 196.

symptoms'.[127] The rationale for this was that the Théiron School advocated eating only sun-ripened vegetables, as these contained the greatest proportion of vitamins A, B and D. Turnips, beetroots and other root vegetables were considered off-limits – adherents were advised to 'feed these vegetables to your cow' – whilst the dietary advice was also tailored according to complexion.[128] Happily for those of a fair disposition, in the case of ice cream, 'blondes can eat it and enjoy it without much harm to themselves', whilst '[b]runettes who feed upon ice-cream, and drink iced drinks ... interfere with their digestion, and bring about an unwholesome condition sooner or later.'[129] Even many of the external signs associated with ageing were attributed to dietary indiscretion: '[o]ne of the most important causes of greying hair is wrong diet.'[130]

As a means of promoting health, the modified vegetarian diet advocated by the Théiron School was also rooted in claims of a scientific nature. For example, the relatively short alimentary canal of humans compared to flesh-eating animals, the fact that most 'carnivorous animals are active at night', and the lack of teeth or claws 'with which to tear flesh' all provided justification for taking such an approach to diet.[131] In the competitive interwar landscape of both complementary and conflicting methods of rejuvenation, the ability to speak authoritatively on matters of human physiology and pathology was essential for success. Advocates of almost all products and procedures made some appeal to expertise in this regard, and both new and existing approaches now claimed to be rooted in emerging forms of scientific knowledge.

It is difficult to say with any certainty exactly what impact the Théiron method had on the everyday practices of rejuvenation through diet and exercise. However, two things are certain. First, as discussed, in the expensively produced and lavishly illustrated publications emanating from the School, vitamins played a key role in anchoring theories of rejuvenation and youthfulness. Second, the School itself came to the attention of one of the most prominent commentators on rejuvenation from the period, Maurice Ernest, with promotional materials appearing in his papers, highlighting at least some recognition for its activities.[132]

At the same time, it was not alone as an organisation which promoted everyday lifestyle changes which, if implemented, promised to rejuvenate followers. Another such method was the Batt-Baird Himalayan Vitality System, promoted by physicians Jill Cossley-Batt and Irvin Baird. Together, American husband-and-wife explorers Cossley-Batt and Baird were part of a British–American expedition to the Himalayas in 1931–32, which uncovered what the *New York Times* described as 'a tribe living in isolated conditions to

[127] Ibid., 255.   [128] Ibid.   [129] Ibid., 260.   [130] Ibid., 529.   [131] Ibid., 196.
[132] Evans, 'The Problem of Death', 19.

great age and free of disease and the pressures of civilization'.[133] Within the year, the Scottish-born Cossley-Batt and Baird had published a book 'full of vital information regarding the keeping of the "body beautiful and healthy"', which aimed to 'eliminate all the poisons and acids of Deterioration' through 'different Food Combinations'.[134]

Responding self-consciously to the aftermath of the Great Depression in which 'peoples have become enveloped in the maelstrom of events, causing them to drift to and fro', Baird and Cossley-Batt outlined a system based 'on the proper combinations if foods and their reaction on the body'.[135] As well as esoteric aspects of diet, such as regular 'Himalayan oil', they argued, in common with many would-be dietary authorities that, '[t]o keep yourself youth looking [sic], [you should] avoid cooked fruits and vegetables. To cook these wonderful gifts of nature, means to destroy, to devitalise, and de-mineralise them.'[136] Specific chemical constituents of food – just as in the case of the Théiron method – were afforded specific properties in relation to the body. 'Fluorin [sic]', for example, '[p]reserves youth, and is a protector against infections, bone disease, and fear', whilst iron was characterised as '[t]he master-chemical which keeps the life-force in harmony in the body . . . [giving] warmth, magnetism, mental endurance, creative ability, success, ambition, and vitality.'[137]

At the same time, Cossley-Batt and Baird were somewhat unusual in highlighting the social pressures which led to a demand for rejuvenation:

To-day. . . the necessity for keeping one's body youthful is imperative. In face of fierce competition, we are compelled by the driving force of economics to draw more on our mental and physical energy. . . . Happily enough, there are many men and women who are beginning to realise that some steps must be taken to restore their former beauty, if they are to regain their energy and youthfulness, and remove those obnoxious wrinkles.[138]

Eating habits were central to their system, with a focus on vitamins and mineral substances. Although vitamin content was heralded by some as the supreme indicator of nutrition value and the definitive explanation for why some diets appeared to confer prolonged youthfulness and health, it was just as significant in creating spaces for the re-rationalisation of diet as it was in instituting new practices. For example, the Australian medical practitioner Otto Abramowski, physician at the Mildura District Hospital in north-west Victoria, wrote in his widely publicised eating manual, *Fruitarian Diet and Physical Rejuvenation* (1916), that '[c]ooked food is *dead* food. A diet full of

---

[133] 'Irvin Baird Dead; Explorer was 63; Himalayan Tribe Found by Former Correspondent', *New York Times*, 31 January 1964, 27.
[134] Baird and Cossley-Batt, *Elixir of Life*, ix.   [135] Ibid., xi.   [136] Ibid., 24.
[137] Ibid., 34–35.   [138] Ibid., 55.

dead material forces the body to great exertion in order to extract the few living particles.'[139] Subsequent editions concretised such dietary practices in the action of vitamins, which were now invoked as the key elements of '*natural food and natural drink*'.[140]

The vitamin content of food, and its preservation, was often connected with retention or restoration of bodily vitality. The British physician Haydn Brown (1864–1936) had previously argued that the modern scourge of sleeplessness rendered technological developments entirely superfluous (how could we make the most of the electric telegraph if its effects were to induce insomnia?).[141] However, in vitamins, Brown considered that medical science might have unlocked the key to understanding the preservation of vitality, not to mention a means of retaining bodily integrity in older age. In his 1924 text, *Vitality and Diet*, he dedicated an entire chapter to vitamins, which he described as 'the essential food of vitality'.[142]

Institutionally, the MRC had earlier commented in detail on the biochemistry of vitamins in their 1919 report on the topic. Throughout the early 1920s they continued to regard research into the actions of vitamins as an area of significant priority, establishing a dedicated Nutrition Committee in 1922.[143] However, by the early 1930s, a follow-up study confirmed that the major medical research body in Britain had become an advocate for the centrality of vitamins in health throughout the life course. By the time that a de facto third edition of their original 1919 publication appeared in 1932 as *Vitamins: A Survey of Present Knowledge*, the language of 'accessory food factors' had disappeared, whilst a more robust claim that a deficiency of vitamins in diet during youth led to an increased likelihood of developing various age-related diseases in later life was inserted.[144] The report was authored by a Committee jointly appointed by the MRC and Lister Institute for Preventive Medicine, including Frederick Gowland Hopkins and Edward Mellanby. Their roles in the 1932 report, however, were reversed, with Hopkins – serving at the time as President of the Royal Society and having recently received a Nobel Prize – taking a far less prominent role, and Mellanby acting as Chair.[145]

In addition to the established deficiency diseases of pellagra, rickets and beri-beri, the report considered a far wider range of conditions, some of which were explicitly connected with certain demographics. For example, osteomalacia – the softening of bones, occurring frequently because of a

[139] Abramowski, *Fruitarian Diet and Physical Rejuvenation*, 9.
[140] Abramowski, *Fruitarian Diet* (1946), 9.   [141] Brown, *Sleep and Sleeplessness*.
[142] Brown, *Vitality and Diet*, 73–132.
[143] 'Nutrition', 1922–1923, FD 1/5298, National Archives, Kew. For more on this emphasis of the MRC, see Oddy, *From Plain Fare to Fusion Food*, 115–17.
[144] Medical Research Council, *Vitamins*.   [145] Ibid., 2.

deficiency of vitamin D – during times of hunger affected principally 'middle-aged and old people of either sex'.[146]

Whilst the original 1919 report had attracted attention primarily within circles of professional scientists and (selected) medical practitioners, the 1932 iteration drew responses in the mainstream newspaper press, with commentaries appearing in *The Daily Telegraph* as well as numerous regional outlets.[147] The inclusion of extensive tables detailing the nutritional values of foods was, in some ways, indicative of the competing claims advanced about specific foodstuffs and the increasing rejection of individual foods as the harbingers of rejuvenation. At around the same time, for example, James Oliver, Consulting Physician to the Hospital for Women, London, and Consulting Gynaecologist to the King George Hospital in Ilford, Essex, argued in *The Medical Press* that 'the wonder-working powers of vitamins … instructs us not so much as to what we should eat, but informs us rather why we eat what we do.'[148]

Whilst organisations like the Théiron School and individuals such as Andrew Pitcairn-Knowles were promoting the youth-making properties of certain approaches to diet, the apparent ability to produce refined (or, it was even claimed by some, synthesized) vitamins – known invariably as 'extracts' – saw the reconfiguring of the commercial landscape of dietary supplements. Critically, by the advent of World War Two, vitamins had come to occupy a place of pre-eminence within rejuvenation discourse. For example, reflecting a marginalisation of endocrine solutions, Benjamin Gaylord Hauser, the prominent American naturopath and self-help author, claimed that '[n]ot through the monkey jungle, but through less spectacular paths shall we find the road to prolonged youth. … It is in the vitamins that you must seek the antidote to the accumulated poisons of the years.'[149] In a major later intervention on the subject, *Look Younger, Live Longer* (1955), Hauser neatly encapsulated the tensions between the partially distinct aims of attaining youthful appearance and promoting longevity whilst he continued to promote a healthy and balanced diet as a sure-fire way to achieve both longer life and beauty.[150]

---

[146] Ibid., 227 and 240.

[147] 'The Vital Vitamin. Deficient Diet in Youth. Cause of Illness in Later Years', *The Daily Telegraph*, 28 July 1932, 6; 'Vitamins to Keep You Fit', *Leeds Mercury*, 28 July 1932, 6; 'Dietetic Value of Vitamins. The Proper Feeding of Infants', *Western Daily Press*, 28 July 1932, 6.

[148] Oliver, 'Food and the Natural Limited of Man's Life', 293.

[149] Hauser, 'Prolong Youth … But Without the Surgery'. In: *Old Age etc. (Third Series)*, 1919–1955, PP/FPW/B.7/3/1, Wellcome Library.

[150] Hauser, *Look Younger*.

Extracts and Preparations: YEAST IS LIFE!

Diet is an important factor in the maintenance of reasonable longevity, and by this it must not be inferred that the individual should become a 'neurotic fad'.[151]

By the 1930s, the medical profession and retail pharmacists alike were decrying food 'faddism' with an almost singular voice in both Britain and, most prominently, the United States. As J. A. Nixon, Physician to the Bristol Royal Infirmary and Professor of Medicine at the University of Bristol, noted in the Long Fox Memorial Lecture on 28 October 1930, '[t]he spread of a smattering of knowledge combined with prejudice, speculation and credulity has given rise to an amazing amount of food faddism and inspired hosts of food cranks.'[152] The professional anxiety about quasi-cults emerging around particular foods, substances or modes of eating was set against the backdrop of attempts to perfect the so-called rational diet in order to achieve rejuvenation, promote longevity and safeguard health. The changing understandings of the importance of dietary components also underpinned the marketing of a range of new diet-related products. These ranged from Kutnow's Powder which promised to provide 'certain alkaline solvents to assist the functioning of the digestive tract', enabling the user to 'start toward rejuvenation', to later examples of tablets containing yeast and chlorophyll 'for rejuvenation and vital energy'.[153]

Eric J. Trimmer's work on the history of rejuvenation has dismissed many of these products as 'therapeutically worthless', peddled by quacks.[154] However, the supplements constituted a significant and lasting market. In the years immediately prior to World War One, the promotional claims drew largely on the humoral tradition of bodily structure and the nineteenth-century tradition of patent medicines and nostrums, such as liver and kidney pills, blood-purifying tonics and elixirs. In the United States, the introduction of Pure Food and Drug Act in 1906 began the process of removing from the marketplace some of these, targeting products such as Dr Kilmer's Female Remedy, Lydia E. Pinkham's Vegetable Compound and the incomparably named Moyer's Oil of Gladness.[155] This piece of legislation sat at the confluence of consumer,

---

[151] 'Current Medical Topics', *Retail Chemist*, September 1935, 232.
[152] Nixon, 'The Long Fox Memorial Lecture', 257.
[153] 'A Natural Aid to Bodily Vigour', *The Tatler*, 9 March 1921, xvii; 'You Want Vital Energy?', *The Scotsman*, 29 April 1938, 69.
[154] Trimmer, *Rejuvenation*, 70–71.
[155] 'Impression and bite trays; patent model', c.1870, Smithsonian National Museum of American History, 2012.0165.699; 'Dr Kilmer's Female Remedy', c.1890, National Museum of American History, 2000.0137.088; 'Lydia E. Pinkham's Vegetable Compound', c.1910, National Museum of American History, 293320.1616.

industry and scientific desires to bolster confidence in both domestic and international markets.[156] However, it would be misleading to see it as a genuinely watershed moment; the persistence of similar products – many of which claimed to rejuvenate and restore body and mind – not just beyond 1906 but well into the interwar period demonstrates their continuing significance and resilience in the face of efforts to regulate the US healthcare market.

In Britain, attempts to ensure 'purity' in food and drug products had important antecedents in the form of late nineteenth-century public health legislation, such as the Adulteration of Food and Drugs Acts (1860, 1872) and the Milk and Dairies Act (1914). However, legislation comparable to that introduced in the United States did not come until much later with the Food and Drugs Act (1938), which was the first to introduce penalties for false or misleading labelling.[157] In this context, therefore, it is especially instructive to consider the British case, where a *laissez-faire* approach to national regulation of foodstuffs and their promotion created a marketplace within which supposedly rejuvenating food products and dietary supplements could be advertised with relatively little regulatory oversight.

Yeast, a substance long since claimed to promote health, was amongst the most prominent substances in extracts and supplements. Its supposedly high vitamin content conferred on it remarkable agency in the maintenance of youthfulness. Manufacturers such as Irving's – who produced Yeast-Vite tablets – made bold claims about their wares (see Figure 3.1). In the case of Irving's, they hailed their product as '[t]he greatest medical discovery of the century' which could produce beneficial results in a huge range of complaints, from headaches and constipation to fevers and anaemia. Tellingly, however, their advertisements also promised that '[a]ll users ... will note the extraordinary rejuvenating powers. In many cases even wrinkles and crowsfeet disappear and the buoyancy of youth is prevalent.'[158] Later Yeast-Vite advertisements went even further, claiming a specific 'timetable' for positive effects on health. Within fifteen minutes, for example, consumers could expect 'nerve pains' to give way to 'glorious relief' and 'deliverance' from headaches. In the longer term, rheumatism, constipation and impure blood would be alleviated within thirty-eight hours.[159]

---

[156] Barkan, 'Industry Invites Regulation'.

[157] Phillips and French, 'Adulteration and Food Law'. For more on the relationship between this legislation and cosmetics, see Chapter 6.

[158] 'Yeast is Life! Irving's Yeast-Vite Tablets a Lightning Pick-me-up', *Leeds Mercury*, 19 October 1925, 6. Chapter 6 will consider in more detail the specific dietary advice given as part of the promotional activities around skin care products; the focus here is from the perspective of dietary supplements, but there was a strong appreciation of the value for the skin of a proper diet, however that might be defined.

[159] 'Yeast-Vite and YOUR health register', *Aberdeen Press and Journal*, 19 October 1929, 5.

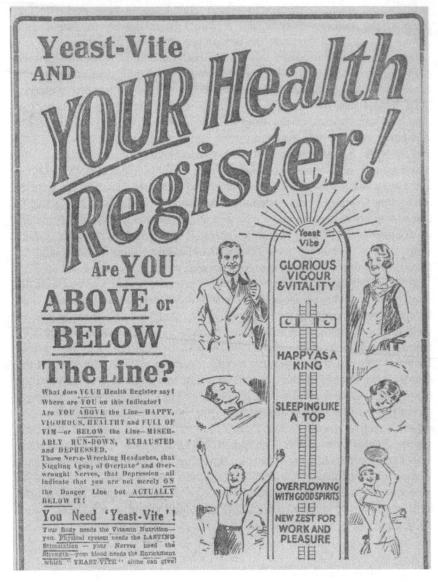

Figure 3.1 An advertisement for Yeast-Vite demonstrating its supposed effects, promoting models of both male and female health, happiness and, crucially, productivity.
('Yeast-Vite and YOUR health register', *Aberdeen Press and Journal*, 19 October 1929, 5.)

As well as the focus on the ability of dietary supplements to reverse both the sensations and the appearance of ageing and promote vitality, less-than-subtle references to sexual performance also permeated the claims made about vitamin supplements. Advertisements for Sea-Vitoid tablets, produced by Hygienic Food Products Ltd., located in Holborn Street, London, made just such an assertion; these 'new Vitamin-Seaweed tonic tablets ... have a most marked effect on sluggish organs of the body' as well as promoting 'increased growth of the hair'.[160] Such promotional claims were placed strategically with extracts from other newspapers and scientific periodicals which noted that Vitamin A was one of 'the two great life-lengtheners among foods', the other being oysters as a result of their high iodine content.[161]

In addition to the explicit claims of rejuvenation made by manufacturers of certain products, more subtle reference to the power of vitamins in foodstuffs also focused on linked personal qualities. For example, the advertising material for Mason's 'O.K.' sauce, claimed that it 'stabilises the blood, thereby increasing energy and vitality' owing to the significant content of fruits *'richest in vitamins'*, such as lemons, grapes and oranges.[162] Rejuvenation was therefore intimately bound up with earlier debates about both maximising bodily energy and creating purity of the blood, with natural sources such as fruits and marine organisms frequently described by manufacturers as containing especially high levels of active substances.

Despite this proliferation, resistance to the introduction of supplements and 'bottled vitamin concentrates' came from a variety of sources, including figures both within and beyond the medical profession. H. C. Corry Mann, for example, claimed in a lecture to the World Dairy Congress in London on 29 June 1928, that 'one of the most extensively advertised vitamin preparations has ... been singularly futile in my hands.' Instead, he urged that 'fresh food, prepared and distributed under modern conditions of cleanliness' would provide a far more suitable means of supplying vitamins, as well as minerals such as calcium, into the diet.[163] Corry Mann's explicit reference to the superior hygienic practices of the age reflected a fascination with what technological intervention could do for public health.[164]

By the end of the interwar period, products which had previously claimed to treat more generalised nervous disorders and almost all aspects of sub-optimal

---

[160] 'New Life from the Deep! SEA-VITOID Tablets', *Birmingham Gazette*, 22 February 1927, 6; 'New Life from the Deep! SEA-VITOID Tablets', *Birmingham Gazette*, 4 May 1927, 10.

[161] 'Sea Breeze in an Oyster. Iodine in Every Swallow. Life-Lengthener', *Daily Herald*, 4 April 1927, 3.

[162] 'Vitamins and Daily Food', *Gloucestershire Echo*, 8 May 1925, 4, original emphasis.

[163] 'Vitamins. A Doctor's Warning against Synthetic Products. A Handicap', *Devon and Exeter Gazette*, 30 June 1928, 4.

[164] For more on this, see Smith, *Clean*.

health were now marketed by manufacturers as guardians of youthfulness, vitality and energy. Many of these drew on the supposed universal power of vitamins, linking deficiency to the premature onset of old age. One such product was Vitamina, the 'secret of new youth at any age', which was developed by the 'French savant' and disciple of Professor Berthlot, Dr Paulin.[165]

Marketing materials emphasised Paulin's scientific credentials alongside the designation of Vitamina as 'not a drug but [a] natural food of the highest order', which

introduces Vitamins and Mineral Salts into the Blood Stream in the correct proportions found in Nature ... rendering the blood beautifully clean and fluid. This improved Fluidity at once enables the Heart to circulate it, without effort, into the furthermost tissues and automatically build Strong Nerves and Radiant Health.[166]

In Britain, two products of the late interwar period which also emphasised their natural origins were Vikelp and Oystrax. The former – 'a concentrated extract of a Pacific Ocean plant' – was claimed by its manufacturers to be 'the richest known source of 9 of the 12 minerals essential to health and well-being' as well as containing critical 'vitamins and food iodine' considered equally valuable.[167] Advertisements for Vikelp in the late 1930s embodied a sense of national hygiene in the face of World War Two. 'A fit Britain is a strong Britain', proclaimed a promotional spread in the *Daily Herald* in October 1939; 'at a time like this you must give courage to those around you', and if the reader felt unable to do so, then it was considered 'ten to one you suffer from mineral deficiency', with the body missing 'essential minerals and vitamins'.[168]

Vikelp represented more than this, however. Rather than acting alone, manufacturers argued that it exerted its rejuvenating effect through the glandular system. Advertisements encouraged consumers to '[r]efuel your glands with Vikelp's [m]inerals and [v]itamins' to bring 'new health, vigour, strength, calm nerves, rich red blood'.[169] Within the chemist trade, internal promotion focused on Vikelp's suitability for 'thin rundown nervous people'; these '[h]ealth and body building tablets' were filled with '[s]ea minerals in readily assimilable [*sic*] form'.[170]

Oystrax, a similar product which contained 'raw oyster stimulants, vitamins [and] general invigorators', especially 'Vitamin E, the "gland-toning"

[165] '[Advertisement]', *Daily Herald*, 2 May 1939, 13. Berthelot was one of the most prominent chemists of the late nineteenth century, and by the 1890s he claimed that chemistry would eventually enable the synthesis of all foodstuffs, replacing natural products just as the new science of electricity would ultimately render gas obsolete.
[166] '[Advertisement]', *The People*, 6 August 1939, 13.
[167] '[Advertisement]', *Daily Herald*, 13 October 1939, 9.
[168] '[Advertisement]', *Daily Herald*, 13 October 1939, 9.
[169] '[Advertisement]', *Daily Herald*, 25 August 1939, 11.
[170] 'Vikelp Tablets', *Merchandise Bulletin*, 10 May 1937, 5196.

Vitamin', claimed that both men and women past the age of forty could 'feel as young as ever'.[171] First advertised in 1937 through local newspapers in Britain, both Vikelp and Oystrax continued to be marketed as restorers of vigour until the early 1950s, reflecting a general anxiety around World War Two about the energy and fitness of the British populace.[172] Indicating that there was a particular target audience in mind, the promotional materials for Oystrax explicitly referenced the circumstances of 'MEN, WOMEN, PAST 40', who might be able to 'feel young as ever' through a simple course of tablets containing 'raw oyster stimulants, vitamins, general invigorators'.[173] These products promised a restoration of youthfulness and vitality, making accessible to a wider audience the rejuvenatory possibilities of 'glandular re-fuelling treatments'.[174]

Manufacturers rarely claimed that their rejuvenating products had entirely consistent or instant effects; some deliberately avoided making such positive statements, most likely to avoid inflating consumer expectations. However, the advertising materials for Oystrax proclaimed that 'you can become full of life, energy and vitality IN 10 MINUTES' through the extremely high content of 'Vitamins A, B, C, D and E' as well as 'a new triple-strength Iron ... [to] re-build, re-vitalize and re-juvenate you *permanently* [sic]'.[175]

As well as the active vitamins, minerals and more nebulous 'life elements' cited in advertisements, a further common denominator to many of these products was their reliance on raw materials derived from nature, and the sea in particular. For example, another supplement from the stables of the Hygienic Food Products company, Seaweena, claimed to promote 'health from seaweed!' as a 'wonderful vitalizer, refreshing rejuvenator, [and] powerful vitamin tonic'.[176] Indeed, seaweed and extracts from other marine organisms came to embody the powerful rejuvenating capacity of nature, paralleling a rise in naturopathic methods endorsed by key advocates of rejuvenation, such as Arnold Lorand and Andrew Pitcairn-Knowles.[177] Even manufacturers such as Hancock & Co., who produced pamphlets promoting products containing

---

[171] '[Advertisement]', *Liverpool Evening Express*, 21 March 1939, 2; '[Advertisement]', *Yorkshire Evening Post*, 5 November 1937, 8; '[Advertisement]', *Manchester Evening News*, 28 August 1939, 7; '[Advertisement]', *Sheffield Evening Telegraph*, 18 May 1939, 2.

[172] For the latest advertisement in the British press, see '[Advertisement]', *Aberdeen Evening Express*, 15 June 1954, 14.

[173] '[Advertisement]', *Portsmouth Evening News*, 31 August 1939, 7.

[174] '[Advertisement]', *Daily Mirror*, 21 July 1939, 20.

[175] 'Rundown People Needs Vitamins plus Iron plus a Stimulant', *Cambridge Daily News*, 23 January 1939, 1.

[176] 'Seaweena', *Western Daily Press*, 21 October 1926, 11.

[177] For more on the history of seaweed specifically as a medical and food product, see Mouristen, *Seaweeds*. For more general accounts of the context of naturopathy from the late nineteenth century onwards, see: Cayleff, *Nature's Path*; Whorton, *Nature Cures*; Brown, 'Nineteenth-Century American Health Reformers'.

glandular extracts, platinum, palladium and cerebral-lecithin, also noted the inclusion of 'active vitamins' in products designed to promote longevity and prevent 'senile decay'.[178] Their promotional literature – dating from around 1930 but continuing through the 1940s – noted several products derived from natural sources, including 'anti-rheumatic bath salts' which contained 'Canary Islands sea-weed', a 'Japanese sea-wrack slim figure bath treatment' and the singular 'Arabian orange poppy ankle reducing cream'.[179]

One of the most enduring products in this period, Phyllosan, also appealed to a high content of chlorophyll as reason for efficacy. Described in some of the earliest newspaper coverage as 'a new extract in tablet form of watercress, spinach and other green plants' which might be a 'rival to lime juice in preventing scurvy', it persisted in the marketplace for almost fifty years.[180] Like many products which became successful in the public sphere, Phyllosan started life in the clinical environment; in this case that was at 'several London hospitals, where patients have been rejuvenated by a course of treatment'.[181] In common with many personal accounts of rejuvenation, Phyllosan was lauded for its ability to produce 'rejuvenation without operation'. In promotional literature a curious mix of humoral theories of bodily regeneration co-existed with chemical symbols explaining how Phyllosan was able to exert such a remarkable effect on the body:

Phyllosan is certainly the greatest specific yet discovered for enriching the blood . . . and eliminating the *physical signs of advancing years*. By its remarkable chemical structure, Phyllosan possess the properties of restoring to normal all physical and vital forces . . . The composition is represented scientifically in the formula (C16, H18, N2O).[182]

Amongst the beneficial effects were an improvement 'in general health . . . an increase in appetite, energy and the joy of life'.[183] Aimed squarely at those over the age of forty – a long-running advertising campaign which ran for well over a decade claimed that it would 'fortify the over-forties' – Phyllosan was arguably the most successful everyday rejuvenation product of the period.[184]

---

[178] Hancock & Co., *Foreign Prescriptions*, 7.

[179] Hancock & Co., *Foreign Prescriptions*, 17, 27 and 28. Subsequent issues of this forty-eight-page leaflet of different preparations appeared as 'Combating the Ravages of Time' and 'Rejuvenation' in the early 1940s, claiming to alleviate 'the pressure of years' through 'vitaminised gland treatments'. See: 'The Pressure of Years' *St Andrew's Citizen*, 19 December 1942, 2; 'Personal', *Milngavie and Bearsden Herald*, 19 December 1942, 1; 'Personal', *Berwick Advertiser*, 7 January 1943, 2.

[180] 'Rival to Lime Juice: Plant Extract for Curing Scurvy', *The Scotsman*, 13 December 1923, 10.

[181] Ibid., 10.   [182] 'Rejuvenation Without Operation', *Yorkshire Post*, 5 June 1924, 4.

[183] '[Advertisement]', *Daily Record*, 8 February 1939, 5.

[184] For early and late examples of the advertising campaign, see: 'Are you over forty?' [Advertisement], *Berwickshire News*, 18 December 1945, p. 1; 'Phyllosan' [Advertisement], *Aberdeen Evening Express*, 9 February 1955, 15. The 'fortifies the over-forties' campaign was instigated in 1945, but Phyllosan was marketed at this demographic from its origins in the 1920s.

Allied to this, the emergence of Sanatogen – first as a 'Nerve-Tonic Food' supplying 'organic phosphorus and protein', later in a variety of forms – as an analogue to Phyllosan emphasised the openness of the market for preparations. Sanatogen, produced by the Loughborough-based Genatosan Ltd., included testimonials from both doctors and patients, even though it was a product available freely over the counter.[185]

The ubiquity and public visibility of these extracts and rejuvenating supplements, continuing in the post-war period, forces us to challenge the dominant historical narrative that public discourse surrounding rejuvenation in the interwar period was largely rooted in hormones and the endocrine system. Rather, the ageing body's supposed decreasing ability to extract nutritive value from food provided a powerful rationale for age-specific optimum diets, many of which were calculated to restore or preserve youth.

Legacy and Conclusion

In March 1941, Linus Pauling delivered a lecture at the Hotel Pennsylvania in New York. During the event, those who sat closest to Pauling noted that he seemed listless and his face was swollen. A few days later he was assessed at the Hospital of the Rockefeller Institute and diagnosed with Bright's disease.[186] As part of his treatment, overseen by the noted nephrologist Thomas Addis, Pauling followed a carefully managed diet, including significant vitamin supplements.[187] By the late 1960s, Pauling's engagement with the use of vitamins in managing disease and health had changed, however; he had become a vocal advocate of what was termed 'megavitamin therapy'. Based on his experience, Pauling argued that huge quantities of, in this case, vitamin C had the capacity to preserve health and, critically, extend lifespan. So strong was his belief in the power of vitamin C that, in 1986, Pauling published a book proposing a method of longevity, *How to Live Longer and Feel Better*, exhorting readers to ingest large quantities of a wide range of vitamins.[188]

---

[185] Genatosan Ltd., *The Good Life*. A more complete consideration of Sanatogen and Phyllosan, both of which arguably came to prominence in postwar Britain, is beyond the scope of this particular study, but it is perhaps sufficient to note that these iconic products of the 1950s and 1960s were not developed in the context of either World War Two or the NHS. Rather, they were a product of the 1890s and the interwar period, respectively, inspired by a generalised interest in avoiding degeneration and maintaining the health and functionality of the human organism throughout the life course. Sanatogen itself moved from occupying a position as a 'nerve tonic' for those who were 'startled at the least sound' to a whole-body rejuvenator. 'I was startled at the least sound', *Everybody's Magazine*, 38:5, 5 May (1918), 111.

[186] Peitzman, *Dropsy, Dialysis, Transplant*, 72–73.

[187] Linus Pauling, 'My Love Affair with Vitamin C', 27 January 1992, Ava Helen and Linus Pauling Papers, Oregon State University Library, MMBBKT.

[188] Pauling, *How to Live Longer*.

One might think that this indicated a commitment on the part of Pauling to a biologically determined understanding of ageing, yet his belief in the value of vitamin-orientated therapies did no such thing. As he later wrote,

If we think that people are older than their years or younger than their years – physiologically – what does that mean. The way to tell how old a person is to look at him, I've discovered. There is no way of taking a sample of blood and putting it in an apparatus and having it reveal a physiological age of 33.7 years, or anything like that. Nobody knows how to determine physiological age.[189]

Pauling has been characterised as an outlier, yet he was far from alone in promoting extraordinary health claims for vitamins. The self-help market burgeoned with advice on vitamin-orientated dietary practices for both health and longevity.[190]

The ongoing post-war search for a diet guaranteed to cause rejuvenation of the whole organism was not restricted to individual properties of food, such as vitamins.[191] The 'moderation' advice of earlier periods, typified in the early twentieth century by interventions on the subject by Herman Weber and others, was reconfigured into caloric restriction, which now stands as one of the most effective method for postponing senescence in animal models.[192] In 2003, for example, a review of the available scientific literature found strong evidence that caloric restriction extended lifespan 'in a variety of species, including rats, mice, fish, flies, worms, and yeast'.[193] More recent studies have explored the application of this method to higher animals, especially primates.[194] Our understanding of the links between diet and longevity, as well as health and disease, remains incomplete, whilst contemporary debate over the constitution of a 'healthy diet' continues to mirror the interwar public and professional discourse on the subject.

Vitamins had become an additional dietary factor to consider when attempting to effect rejuvenation. In 1960, for example, the Health Publishing Corporation, based in Hackensack, New Jersey, issued several books extolling the health benefits of 'natural raw juices', yet also claimed, through their periodical *Health Saver*, that '893 prematurely aging patients at the Hillman

---

[189] Pauling, 'My Love Affair with Vitamin C', 1.

[190] See, for example, numerous works by Leonard Mervyn: Mervyn, *Vitamin C*; Mervyn, *The B Vitamins*; Mervyn, *Vitamins A, D, K*.

[191] As an archetypal example of physician-driven dietary advice from the post-war period, see Cantor, *Dr Cantor's Longevity Diet*.

[192] Conniff, 'The Hunger Gains'; Wilson, 'Calorie Restriction Diet'. See Weber, *On Longevity*, 119.

[193] Heilbronn and Ravussin, 'Calorie Restriction and Aging', 361.

[194] See, for example: Mattison et al., 'Impact of Caloric Restriction'; Mattison et al., 'Caloric Restriction Improves Health'.

Clinic in Birmingham, Alabama were completely rejuvenated' after a 'diet rich in protein, vitamins and minerals, and added dried brewer's yeast and liver extract'. Critically, '[t]he above food supplements are in all health food stores', demonstrating the increased ubiquity of previously specialised dietary supplements in the food marketplace in the United States.[195]

The themes of interwar dietary rejuvenation were therefore not limited temporally. There was strong and significant continuity of dietary approaches to promoting youthfulness beyond 1945, and the caloric restriction promoted under the guise of 'rational fasting' continues to underpin important aspects of contemporary research into life extension. Historians have linked different dietary habits with almost all major sociocultural factors; however, the reciprocal relationship between eating and ageing – the food–ageing complex – has largely been obscured by a focus on broader connections between eating and health, with food much recognised as operating in the space between everyday consumption and health.[196] By focusing on ageing as a primary object of concern, we see that dietary habits and rationales did not exist in isolation from other forms of rejuvenatory practice. Most writers on the subject drew inspiration from other spheres of biomedical thought, whether implicating food in the healthy functioning of the endocrine system or combining their dietary regimens with physical activity. Diet was, of course, linked to specific organs and organ systems in ways which intersected with prevailing social anxieties, but the interwar imperative to restore vitality to the whole organism largely displaced such close connections.[197] Food permeated the body in its entirety; its active constituents, like vitamins, reached far beyond the digestive tract, the stasis of which had been implicated in premature ageing, decay and death by Elié Metchnikoff.

The extent to which actual practices of eating were transformed along these lines in this period is uncertain. Even within the constituency of medical professionals and lay experts who agreed that changes in diet could prolong youthfulness there was substantial divergence of opinion. What is clear is that the advent of vitamin science precipitated a re-justification of existing approaches to food preparation and consumption, and underpinned a boom in vitamin- and mineral-rich supplements, advertised directly to consumers across the full range of newspapers and periodicals. Other products such as cod liver oil were now desirable not (only) because of general nourishing 'fat-forming' properties – commonly trumpeted in late nineteenth-century

---

[195] 'Is This the Secret of Rejuvenation?', *Health Saver* 3:2 (1960), 61.
[196] Haushofer, 'Between Food and Medicine'; Whorton, *Inner Hygiene*; Bauch, *A Geography of Digestion*; Finlay, 'Early Marketing of the Theory of Nutrition'; Brock, *Justus Von Liebig*, especially 215–38.
[197] Miller, *A Modern History of the Stomach.*

advertising – but (also) because of its high Vitamin D content.[198] That cod liver oil in particular had come to represent a class of food or supplement whose benefits were predicated on vitamin content is amply demonstrated by advertising campaigns for vitamin-rich Radio Malt which heralded its superiority to fish oils.[199]

Notwithstanding these new products, the interwar discourse surrounding rejuvenation, ageing and their links to diet was deeply rooted in pre-war attitudes towards food and its relationship with physical degeneration. The discovery of vitamins simply represented a new way of justifying particular diets, whilst food faddisms, such as the yoghurt diet advocated by Metchnikoff, came in for increasing criticism in both the medical and lay press as numerous so-called balanced diets claimed to be effective, especially 'in middle life, to "wash out" the impurities of the body'.[200] The connection between other rejuvenation methods, especially hormone treatments, and appetite also served to reinforce the close relationship between food and ageing, made more concrete in the public realm by the twin attention afforded to rejuvenation and vitamins.[201]

In the sense that rejuvenation was both a prolongation of youthfulness and an extension of life, very few rationalised food consumption as solely connected to rejuvenation. In contrast to hormone treatments and procedures, the maintenance of a suitable diet was also responsible for improved health, with rejuvenation one of many consequences of observing such a regime. Within this, multiple approaches, from vegetarianism to the consumption of raw foods and fasting, vied for supremacy by invoking both claims about digestive process and the fantastical powers of vitamins. The ambition to reduce, much noted in the secondary literature, masks a more complex picture in which the truly rejuvenated individual was often cast as being able to sustain greater food consumption and gain, not lose, weight.

Dietary intervention encompassed both natural and synthetic means of warding off the signs of old age. In the following chapter we see how the

[198] 'You Versus Winter', *Falkirk Herald*, 27 October 1928, 3; 'Wisdom of Feasting: Christmas Festivities a Barrier Against Illness', *Sheffield Daily Telegraph*, 6 January 1927, 5; 'Avoid Imitations', *The Scotsman*, 6 February 1904, 1; 'Louis de Jongh, M.D. Light-brown Cod Liver Oil', *Illustrated London News*, 18 September 1897, 25.

[199] 'New Vitamin Food Supersedes Cod Liver Oil', *The Scotsman*, 8 March 1927, 5.

[200] Webster, *Beauty and Health*, 17.

[201] Although abstinence was a core pillar of the health regimens of many who sought to encourage diets which promoted the maintenance of youthfulness, it was generally – though not exclusively – exonerated from any meaningful role in causing premature ageing or, in its absence, promoting youthfulness. A full and complete consideration of alcohol, and its attendant links with temperance, moderation and morality, is beyond the scope of the present study, but it is worth noting that Hermann Weber, for example, claimed that the popular doctrine 'wine is the milk of old people' was highly misleading, and that 'alcohol, excepting in great moderation, is even more dangerous to the aged than to the younger people.' Weber, *On Longevity*, 162–63.

strong nineteenth-century tradition of technically based amateur electrotherapy continued through the interwar period, fuelled by increased public fascination with the prospect of restoring youthfulness and postponing senescence as well as a reconfiguration of electrical technologies into a far wider range of electrical products. One might have expected the use of electricity – as well as its kindred technologies of diathermy and violet ray treatments – to fall sharply out of favour by the 1920s as chemical models of bodily control came to dominate. However, this was manifestly not the case, as a reconfiguration of electrical machines and increasing public comfort with and trust of electricity created a second wave of engagement with domestic devices.

4   Electrotherapy, 1925–1932

In 1906, *The Weekly Welcome* ran an advert for the Pulvermacher Battery Belt. Touting electricity as 'the only natural remedy for all weak men and women', the belt required the user to 'have constant application [for] several hours at a time ... [which could not be done] in doctors' offices'.[1] The Pulvermacher company – originally called the J. L. Pulvermacher Galvanic Establishment – had been manufacturing and promoting their belts and batteries since the 1840s, asserting that galvanism was 'nature's chief restorer of impaired vital energy'.[2] By the turn of the twentieth century these electrical devices had become ubiquitous, with extensive newspaper advertising for domestic products and electrotherapy embedded within mainstream clinical practice. Increasingly, manufacturers claimed for their products the ability not just to combat loss of energy and poor overall health but to enhance the personal aesthetic and interact favourably with other forms of lifestyle management.[3]

The potential for electricity to transform domestic, work and public life was a source of intense fascination for consumers in the late nineteenth and early twentieth centuries. As several historians have noted, the craze for electric belts and other products designed to produce rejuvenating effects in the privacy of the home, particularly in men, grew steadily through the latter part of the nineteenth century, coinciding with the use of similar treatments by a newly professionalised community of electrotherapy practitioners.[4] Meanwhile, the introduction of domestic electrical technologies along highly gendered lines reconfigured the relationship between women, men and these supposedly assistive devices in the home.[5] Public and domestic spaces became

---

[1] '[Advertisement]', *The Weekly Welcome*, 29 August 1906, iv, with thanks to the Thackray Medical Museum.

[2] 'Electricity Is Life', *Bedford Record*, 30 June 1877, 7.

[3] The J. L. Pulvermacher Company, for example, claimed in promotional materials for their 'Hydro-Electric Voltaic Chains', distributed in the United States, that 'strict attention to diet, exercise, bathing, pure air, etc., should be observed in all cases.' Pulvermacher, *J. L. Pulvermacher's Patent Portable Hydro-Electric Voltaic Chains*, 4.

[4] Senior, 'Rationalising Electrotherapy'; Lori Loeb, 'Consumerism and Commercial Electrotherapy'; de la Peña, *The Body Electric*; Morus, *Shocking Bodies*.

[5] Gooday, *Domesticating Electricity*.

experimental as electricity was applied in new and uncertain ways. By the early twentieth century non-specialist consumers were increasingly able to secure direct access to electrical therapeutic devices which had previously been the preserve of medical and pseudo-medical practitioners, bringing electrical forces into contact with bodies far removed from the medical gaze.

Despite this flourishing market, John Senior has argued that by the advent of the 1920s amateur electrotherapy in Britain had largely become defunct.[6] This perspective has recently been refined by Anna Wexler, who identifies a significant difference between the 'medical battery' – characterised as a 'shock-producing electrotherapy device' – and later incarnations of domestic electrotherapeutic devices, which included 'vibrating machines, high-frequency devices like the Violet Ray, and so-called oxygen delivery systems like the Electropoise'.[7] Focussing predominantly on the United States, Wexler also argues that, during the 1920s and 1930s, 'there was always an underlying implication that [electrical] rejuvenation would target a sick or tired body, not a healthy one.'[8] Nevertheless, we still know very little about how these technologies were configured with respect to ageing, even though many of the manufacturers and promoters of these devices made claims about their efficacy in cases of premature old age.

In this chapter I argue that, in the period between the claimed demise of domestic electrotherapy and the emergence of electro-convulsive therapy in the late 1930s, electrotherapy devices were reconfigured from simple batteries into a range of equipment, much of which promised not only to preserve health but to ward off the effects of the ageing process and restore youthfulness. These included rejuvenating face masks which employed the technique of diathermy, electrical massage and exercise devices, and violet ray apparatus, many predicated on elaborate theories of bodily function and in which technical developments spanned public and professional domains.[9] There was a lively, controversial and diverse culture of electrical treatment in the interwar period; the marketplace was the preserve of not just esoteric individuals peddling their wares, but high-profile global entities such as the Ediswan Company and beauty magnates including Elizabeth Arden and Helena Rubinstein. All this took place against a backdrop of the greater explanatory power afforded to hormones and vitamins and their physiological function.

---

[6] Senior, 'Rationalising Electrotherapy'.

[7] Wexler, 'The Medical Battery in the United States', 190.

[8] Wexler, 'Recurrent Themes', 193.

[9] On occasion these technologies acted indirectly to enhance other means of restoring youthfulness. For example, the internal Boots Company magazine *The Bee* noted in June 1931 that, 'by using the ultra-violet ray test, they [product developers at Boots] are able to select only oils of unimpeachable quality [for use in various beauty products].' 'One Glance. . .and he knows!' *The Bee*, June 1931, 249–50, 249.

With hormonal changes and dietary balance increasingly implicated as the causes or effects of the natural ageing process, it is doubly surprising to find electrical accounts of rejuvenation retaining such popularity.

The Electrical Body

A rich tradition of galvanic and faradic therapy, practised in Britain during the nineteenth century, was a highly significant part of both mainstream medicine and the domestic device market.[10] Towards the end of the Victorian period organisations such as the Zander Electropathic Institute courted controversy by producing and marketing electric belts and other devices which claimed to effect dramatic physiological change in both men and women. Such claims – that 'electricity is life' – drew on the ascendant power of neurology which, through the development of theories of cerebral localisation advanced by the likes of Paul Broca and David Ferrier, purported to explain numerous bodily mechanisms through the combined motor, sensory and processing functions of the central nervous system.[11]

Electric batteries, belts, corsets and even so-called flesh brushes, almost all employing similar modes of action, were the mainstay of domestic, amateur electrotherapy during the latter stages of the nineteenth century, joined by increasingly large and stable electrical devices, deployed under medical super-vision in the clinic.[12] Subsequent developments and refinements in electrical technologies resulted in a transformed landscape by the immediate aftermath of World War One. Reflecting on the reasons behind the 'numerous' changes in the practices of electrotherapy over the preceding decade, H. Lewis Jones – a prominent member of the British Electrotherapeutic Society – argued in 1902 that '[t]he general introduction of electric lighting supplies had not only helped greatly to extend the practice of medical electricity, but had also provided the profession with a new and valuable agent in the sinusoidal current.'[13] By 1905, the inclusion of several additional innovations, such as

---

[10] Iwan Morus has explored the development of electrotherapy in Victorian Britain. The practice sat at the intersection between commercial and professional interests, and drew on changing ideas from numerous emerging scientific and medical disciplines from physics to neurology. Morus, *Shocking Bodies*.

[11] For more on the work of Broca and Ferrier, see: Finn, 'The West Riding Lunatic Asylum'; Greenblatt, 'Huglings Jackson's First Encounter'; Harrington, *Medicine, Mind, and the Double Brain*; Oppenheim, *Shattered Nerves*. Principal amongst the texts which established the nervous system – underpinned and interrogated by electrical force – as a powerful physiological mode of control was Ferrier's 1876 publication, *The Functions of the Brain*.

[12] 'Dr Scott's Electric Flesh Brush', c. 1881, Electrotherapy and Vibrators Ephemera, Box 1, EPH47.17 Wellcome Library; Pall Mall Electric Association, 'Dr. Scott's electric corset: health, strength, comfort, elegance: a great boon to delicate ladies: a beautiful invention', c. 1882, Electrotherapy and Vibrators Ephemera, Box 1, EPH475.15, Wellcome Library.

[13] 'British Electro-Therapeutic Society', 519.

high-frequency apparatus, at a major exhibition of electrotherapeutic instruments suggested that highly technical, larger devices were possessed of the capacity to transform medical practice, even as theories of hormone-mediated, chemical physiology were coming to predominate.[14] Indeed, the identification of acetylcholine in 1913 by the British pharmacologist Henry Dale suggested that even the supposedly all-powerful network of electrical signals governing physical action, thought and health, had its basis in chemical interactions. As Dale himself noted in a letter to T. R. Elliott – a key figure at University College Hospital – in late 1913, 'Here is a good candidate for the role of a hormone related to the rest of the autonomic nervous system.'[15] When acetylcholine was further confirmed as an active and powerful neurotransmitter by Otto Loewi experimentally in 1921, the gradual erosion of electrical supremacy might have been supposed to be complete.[16]

However, electrotherapy as a broad therapeutic field had established a diverse and seemingly effective presence within professional medicine in Britain, with electrical departments at most major hospitals, dedicated institutes, and an extensive manufacturing and promotional network which continued to refine and develop new devices. For example, the 1919 catalogue of apparatus for various forms of electrotherapy, issued by Watson & Sons Ltd., spoke volumes about the extensive nature of electric devices available for professional use. Mirroring textbooks in both presentation and, to some degree, content, this was much more than a simple price list.[17] Included alongside images of a large range of devices were technical descriptions of the construction, modes of application and likely therapeutic outcomes, highlighting the extent to which the hardware of electrotherapy was intimately bound up with theoretical perceptions of both normal and pathological bodily function. Such approaches also resonated with the long-standing body-as-machine metaphor – in this case, a machine underpinned by electrical force.

---

[14] The British Electrotherapeutic Society was relatively short-lived, established in 1901 before merging with the Royal Medical and Chirurgical Society of London (later the Royal Society of Medicine, from 1909) just six years later. 'Council Minute Book', 1901–1907, BES/A/1, Archives of British Electrotherapeutic Society, Royal Society of Medicine, London; 'Apparatus at the Annual Exhibition of the British Electrotherapeutic Society', *Medical Electrology and Radiology* 6 (1905), 62.

[15] Henry Dale to T. R. Elliott, 11 December 1913, Wellcome Library, GC42/15. For more on the Elliott–Dale interactions, see: Max R. Bennett, *History of the Synapse*. Amsterdam: Harwood Academic, 2001.

[16] Loewi, 'Über humorale Übertragbarkeit der Herznervenwirkung'. Dale and Loewi – lifelong friends – were jointly awarded the 1936 Nobel Prize in Physiology or Medicine, recognising their achievements. See Feldberg, 'Henry Hallett Dale. 1875–1968'. Dale himself wrote an extended obituary for Loewi: Dale, 'Otto Loewi. 1873–1961'.

[17] For more on the critical paratextual content of medical trade catalogues, see Jones, *The Medical Trade Catalogue*.

The language and imagery of electricity within bodies was perhaps just as critical. In his practical rejuvenation guide, *Never Grow Old*, published in 1920, the Parisian physician Louis Henri Goizet, argued that 'since the vital adducent current ceaselessly brings new material to replace the material destroyed for the needs of combustion ... one cannot see any reason for the death of the human body by wear and tear.'[18] For Goizet, 'the vital current [of the body] is the living man himself, animated by an incessant general movement which is the result of each partial movement of the cells.'[19] Adhering to such an interpretation of bodily function allowed Goizet to side with almost all mainstream medical practitioners in rejecting so-called faddism – adherence to highly specific dietary regimes – yet still endorse his own system of rejuvenation, a 'method of superficial tractile [*sic*] rubbings', which would enable adherents 'to be young up to one hundred years of age'.[20] The use of electrical metaphors and claimed modes of action within the body were common, and were mobilised by advocates of methods of rejuvenation based on means other than through the application of electricity to the body. Commenting on an earlier, more slender text also penned by Goizet, the *New York Times* noted in 1913 that the author 'at an advanced age preserves almost boyish vigor and alertness ... [and] says that his youthfulness is entirely due to his discovery'.[21]

Tellingly, during his tenure as a member of the prestigious Faculty of Medicine in Paris some years previously, Goizet had published an extensive text in support of the Charles Brown-Séquard. In the preface to this volume, published in around 1891 as *La vie prolongée au moyen de la méthode Brown-Séquard*, Goizet claimed:

As far as we know, the Séquardian vaccine is not only an aphrosidiac; it is a regenerator, a force ... It does not cure any disease, but as most human affections stem from general or partial debility of the organism, it restores vigour and the evil disappears of itself.[22]

Goizet offered a defence of the method, covering its application in a wide range of conditions, and concluded after almost 350 pages that 'the discovery of Brown-Séquard is one of the greatest blessings with which our century has bestowed upon humanity.'[23] After such a robust endorsement of

---

[18] Goizet, *Never Grow Old*, 39.   [19] Ibid., 48.   [20] Ibid., 191.

[21] 'How to Live 100 Years. Aged French Doctor Says He Keeps Young by Massage', *New York Times*, 3 August 1913, 3.

[22] Goizet, *La vie prolongée*, 6. My translation of the original text: 'Qu'on le sache bien, le vaccin séqurdien n'est pas seulement un aphrosidiaque, c'est un régénérateur, c'est une force ... Il ne guérit aucune maladie, mais comme la plupart des affections qui éprouvent l'humanité proviennent de la débilité générale ou partielle de l'organisme, rendant à celui-ci sa vigeur, le mal disparait de lui-même.'

[23] Goizet, *La vie prolongée*, 349. My translation of the original text: 'la découverte de Brown-Séquard d'être un des bienfaits les plus grands dont notre siècle ait doté l'humanité.'

organotherapy, it is not surprising to find the Goizet confirming his continued faith in rejuvenation almost three decades later. However, it is telling that even in an era where natural heirs of Brown-Séquard, such as the hormone-wielding Steinach and Voronoff, were at the forefront of rejuvenation discourse in both public and professional domains, Goizet formulated an elaborate system of massage as his rejuvenation method of choice. His articulation of life as a product of 'a vast atomic current created by the motions of the planets and the suns of the universe' suggests that recent discoveries in atomic structure, not endocrinology, were of far greater influence.[24]

A near-contemporary of Goizet was Bernard Hollander. Born in Vienna in 1864, he moved to London at the age of nineteen to study physiology at King's College Hospital under the tutelage of David Ferrier. Having spent a period back in Vienna practising psychiatry, Hollander returned to London and became a naturalised British subject in 1899.[25] In keeping with many of the leading neurologists of the mid- to late nineteenth century, he was greatly inspired by phrenological principles and sought to reinstate a role for a scientifically respectable phrenology in psychiatric practice and therapeutic surgery.[26] To this end, Hollander published his first treatise on the subject – *Scientific Phrenology* – in 1902, and established the Ethological Society, with its attendant journal, the *Ethological Journal*, two years later in 1904.[27] In this capacity he promoted what has been described as an 'odd mix of phrenology, heredity, and eugenics', though the combination of these disciplines in the early twentieth century was rather more a part of the intellectual mainstream than might be supposed.[28]

For our purposes, Hollander's key intervention in theories of electrotherapy came in 1920 when he invoked electricity as a primary physiological and therapeutic power. In his well-received two-volume treatise on the localisation of character traits, *In Search of the Soul*, Hollander argued that

Electricity is known as a great force in physical nature … Why should it be thought impossible that a[n electrical] nerve force can emanate under certain conditions from the operator and can control his subject?[29]

---

[24] 'How to Live 100 Years', 3.   [25] 'Dr Bernard Hollander', 316.

[26] Hollander, *The Mental Symptoms of Brain Disease*. Rhodri Hayward has characterised Hollander as a neurologist, though it is somewhat misleading to describe him in this way. See Hayward, *The Transformation of the Psyche*, ch. 4, fn. 63.

[27] Hollander, *Scientific Phrenology*. Hollander also continued to promote the significance of cerebral localisation within phrenological circles. See, for example 'Dr Hollander on Localisation of Mental Faculty', 402–03.

[28] Romani, *National Character and Public*, 260.

[29] Hollander, *In Search of the Soul*, 303. Reviewing the book in the *Journal of Neurology and Psychopathology*, Hubert J. Norman noted that 'Hollander, without dogmatism, has carefully endeavoured to work out the hidden springs of character.' Norman, 'In Search of the Soul', 97.

The power of electricity in nature, and in particular its 'stimulating and rejuvenating action', was widely recognised, not least by Andrew Balfour, Director-in-Chief of the Wellcome Bureau of Scientific Research, in his 1923 article in *The Lancet* on how bodies might be prepared to adapt to hot, humid climates.[30] The application of electricity, Balfour argued, would serve to prime or adapt the body to these kinds of environments; it was a benign, protective force which could be applied safely to enhance the physiological capacity and resilience of the human organism.

For his part, Hollander had by the early 1930s modified and expanded his specific views on the nature of electricity in relation to the human body into a fully fledged system of rejuvenation. Much like the promotional strategies which surrounded the personal electrical products of the nineteenth century, Hollander argued that '[w]ith increasing years – generally after sixty-five – there is a gradual diminution in vital energy, and a slowing of the various functions of the body', rejecting the biological inevitability of old age.[31] Critically, Hollander claimed that, in addition to the abuse of the body through drinking, overeating and immoral habits, '[a]t the close of life the energies become less and less, the movements become less frequent, and less energetic, atrophy begins, and death is the end.'[32]

Underpinning the natural bodily energy identified by Hollander was electricity. In a chapter entitled 'What Is Life?' he mobilised the ideas of the physiologist George Washington Crile, whose work in surgical preparation and the emotions had been a source of inspiration, whom Hollander quoted with reverence: '[a]ccording to Professor Crile, the famous American authority, "The processes which distinguish the living from the non-living are due to electrical forces within the protoplasm, which endow it with the essential processes of irritation, assimilation, and reproduction".'[33] For Hollander,

[t]here can be no doubt that a force resembling electricity, if not identical with it, is constantly generated in the body[;] ... it is now generally recognised that all vital processes have their associated electrical currents. In fact, all matter, both living and lifeless, is but electricity. The whole living body may be compared to an electric battery.[34]

---

[30] Balfour, 'Problems of Acclimatisation', 85. Balfour was a specialist in tropical medicine who had acted as sanitary advisor to the Sudanese government and had in 1923 been appointed as Director of the London School of Hygiene and Tropical Medicine. 'Sir Arthur Balfour', 245–46.

[31] Hollander, *Old Age Deferred*, 1.   [32] Ibid., 14.

[33] George Washington Crile, quoted in Hollander, *Old Age Deferred*, 37–38. For more on Crile, including a comprehensive list of obituaries, see Royal College of Surgeons of England, 'Crile, George Washington (1864–1943)'.

[34] Hollander, *Old Age Deferred*, 38.

In addition to Crile, Hollander drew on associated researchers from across the world, all of whom gravitated around electrical explanations of bodily health and control.[35] Fundamentally, he argued, 'electricity is generated in the lungs with every inspiration, and is conveyed by the blood-stream to every cell in the body, the brain receiving the larger supply, and representing the seat of the highest potentials.'[36]

In ascribing such agency to electricity, Hollander was far from alone. In his 1924 textbook, *Practical Electrotherapeutics and Diathermy*, written explicitly 'to furnish students, surgeons and general practitioners with the basis for a practical understanding of the application of electric power ... in the treatment of their patients', G. Betton Massey argued that recent discoveries in the electrical nature of matter, driven by 'J. J. Thompson, Rutherford, and other English physicists', provided an empirically confirmed basis to electrotherapy.[37] Indeed, the conditions which Betton Massey identified as being particular amenable to treatment by various forms of electrotherapy, especially diathermy, were, as we shall see, arguably just as variable and extensive as those referenced by purveyors of direct-to-consumer rejuvenation devices. Even those who advocated New Thought as a means of promoting self-directed internal healing, such as Grace Stuart, described internal bodily functions in electrical terms. Stuart's 1925 rejuvenation manual, *Gland Treatment*, captured in both its title and its methods the focus on the endocrine system, yet reserved special place for the 'electric currents running from these glands' throughout the body; the control of these currents, she argued, had enabled her to have 'attained greater results ... than any patient of the greatest scientist or surgeon'.[38]

The influence of these 'electric currents of health, strength, youth and beauty' over the body were at the heart of a number of diverse theories of rejuvenation, many of which were developed specifically to underpin commercial activities targeting lay consumers.[39] A striking example appeared just one year later when the British brewer's chemist Otto Overbeck (1860–1937) entered the electrotherapy market with electric body comb, known as the Overbeck Rejuvenator.[40] This was one of the most

---

[35] Amongst these were Wladimir Wishnjakoff, Piper, Einthoven, W. A. Jolly, Adrian, Ecripsy, Jagadis Chandra Bose, Schweninger, Berger, Jacobson, Cazzamali, and Sauerbruch.

[36] Hollander, *Old Age Deferred*, 42.

[37] Massey, *Practical Electrotherapeutics and Diathermy*, v and 2.

[38] Stuart, *Gland Treatment*, 12–13 and 28.   [39] Stuart, *Gland Treatment*, 29.

[40] As well as the controversy surrounding the Rejuvenator, which attracted considerable interest from the medical establishment in both Britain and Australia, Overbeck himself remains a controversial figure. In Grimsby, where he was the scientific director of Hewitt Brothers Brewery, he was a patron to a large number of children's organisations, such as the Dolphin Swimming Club. In early 1929 he was charged with eighteenth alleged sexual crimes, including indecent assault and gross indecency, before being acquitted on all counts. For full records of

high-profile, yet conventional, electrotherapy devices of the interwar period and illustrates how far non-medical entrepreneurs were able to enter the rejuvenation marketplace.[41] The eponymous inventor was not a physician, rather a successful entrepreneur who was able to exploit his position as an outsider, unbounded by the codes of practice under which medical professionals operated.[42] Despite his lack of formal medical training, Overbeck mobilised numerous forms of authority to reinforce the impression that customers who purchased the Rejuvenator were under a form of medical care-at-a-distance. The 1938 directions for use of the Supreme Model of his instrument, for example, referred to the 'many patients' who had written to Overbeck enquiring about the device.[43] This acted alongside his extensive use of other promotional strategies – testimonials, patents, his own claims to be a 'well-known British scientist' – to create an impression of trustworthiness through adverts and pamphlets.[44]

It is unclear exactly how Overbeck developed the Rejuvenator, but he claimed that the original idea stemmed from 'early primitive apparatus consisting of a bundle of brass wires connected to a cheap pocket-lamp battery'.[45] He owned numerous volumes on household medicine, including the popular treatise *Virtue's Household Physician* (1907), but his personal library is hardly sufficient to explain his commercial venture in electrotherapy.[46] What is certain, however, is that Overbeck made strenuous efforts to differentiate his own therapy from that based on the endocrine system. A full-page advertising campaign in the popular weekly periodical

the proceedings at Derby Assizes Court, which were covered extensively in the local press, see: 'Grimsby Scientist for Trial', *Yorkshire Post and Leeds Intelligencer*, 11 January 1929, 10; 'Grimsby F.R.G.S. in the Dock', *Derby Daily Telegraph*, 27 February 1929, 1; 'Scholar Tried by Jury', *Derby Daily Telegraph*, 28 February 1929, 1; 'Allegations Against Scientist', *Derbyshire Advertiser*, 1 March 1929, 29; 'Scientist Discharged', *Derbyshire Advertiser*, 8 March 1929, 29.

[41] I have addressed elsewhere some of these issues in a previous publication which charted the significance of Overbeck's efforts to establish his own professional credibility: Stark, 'Recharge My Exhausted Batteries'.

[42] For more on the development of professional medical responses to processes of patenting and profit-making, see Jones, 'A Barrier to Medical Treatment?'

[43] Overbeck's Rejuvenator Ltd., *Overbeck's Rejuvenator: Supreme Model*, 26

[44] Stark, 'Recharge My Exhausted Batteries'; 'Scientist Rises from the Couch of Old-Age Invalidism to Take Up an Active Life', *The Farmer and Settler*, 8 September 1938, 3.

[45] 'Hope for the Aged. Electricity to Make Old Folk Young. Grimsby Man's Theories', *The Telegraph*, 20 February 1925, n.p.

[46] Copies in Overbeck's personal collection include: Herbert Buffum, *Virtues' Household Physician*. London: Virtue Book Company, 1905, Overbeck's, National Trust, NT 3041278; H. De Vere Stacpoole, *The Doctor: A Study in Life*. London: T. Fisher Unwin, 1914, Overbeck's, National Trust, NT 3041282. Other relevant objects in his collection included the "Readson" High Frequency apparatus, a violet ray device, an 'Improved Magneto-Electric Machine, for Nervous Diseases', and a Q-Ray Electro Radio-Active Dry Compress, all held at Overbeck's, National Trust, uncatalogued.

Tit-Bits touted the 'prospect of life-long youth and freedom from ill-health without gland-grafting or other operation'.[47]

In support of his business venture, Overbeck penned a treatise on medical electricity and its relationship with human health. Originally titled *A New Electronic Theory of Life and Rejuvenation*, the first edition appeared in 1925, and made explicit references to his method and device.[48] This went through multiple editions, by the third of which Overbeck had removed all mentions of the Rejuvenator. In a hand-annotated copy he struck through references to the Rejuvenator, abandoning the more explicit self-promotion of his own devices in favour of establishing his independent scientific credibility.[49] By the advent of the fourth edition, published in 1932, the Rejuvenator was again front-and-centre, a manifestation of 'Overbeck's scientific methods' for the application of electricity to the body, which depended on the fundamental nature of electrical energy in all matter.[50] Within this framework, Overbeck was in fact doing little more than recapitulating arguments made at least seventy years by the J. L. Pulvermacher Company which, in a 1853 promotional brochure for the Hydro-Electric Voltaic Chain, claimed:

when a person is in perfect health . . . the Electricity of the system is in perfect harmony, and equally diffused, no particular part or organ possessing a larger amount than another, and the nerves, which spread like a net-work over and through the whole body, act as conductors for the nervous fluid, or Electricity.[51]

In 1928, concerned that unsuspecting consumers might be doing more harm than good, the British Medical Association commissioned Harold Bright, an electrical engineer, to carry out an independent assessment of the Overbeck Rejuvenator to determine its effects. Bright concluded the current created by the device was around one microampere, in his view far too low to make any impression – either positive or negative – on the user. He also noted that, although higher currents could be achieved using different attachments (up to around 100 microamperes), the oily residues of the body seemed to act as an insulator, whilst the teeth of the patented body comb (see Figure 4.1) were too large to allow effective contact with the scalp.[52] As well as this electrical evaluation, which focused mainly on safety, practitioners at the Royal Free Hospital also tested the Rejuvenator on a number of patients. The report of these tests indicated that in most cases there was no observable improvement;

---

[47] 'Better Health for All and Longer Life', *Tit-Bits*, 3 November 1928, 268.
[48] *Overbeck's New Electronic Theory*.
[49] Ibid . Annotated copy held at Overbeck's, National Trust, uncatalogued.
[50] Ibid., 4th edn, 91 and 132, held at Overbeck's, National Trust, NT 3041280.
[51] Pulvermacher, *J. L. Pulvermacher's Patent Portable*, 7.
[52] 'The Overbeck Rejuvenator', SA/BMA/C.458: Box 124, Wellcome Library.

Aug. 9, 1927.   1,638,407

O. G. C. L. J. OVERBECK

ELECTRIC BODY COMB

Filed April 30, 1925

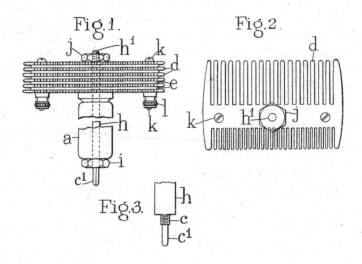

Inventor

Otto G. C. L. J. Overbeck

by Knight Bro
          attorneys

Figure 4.1 Patent images showing Otto Overbeck's US patent for an electric body comb. His other patents were also for the same part of the device, demonstrating the extent to which he attempted to persuade users of its novelty and efficacy despite only a small part of The Rejuvenator being patented, and multiple times over. Otto Overbeck, 'Electric Body Comb', US Patent 1,638, 407, 9 August 1927.

the only suggested benefit – the promotion of hair growth – was ultimately attributed to either the placebo effect of 'other factors'.[53]

Whilst the Rejuvenator may not have attracted public criticism from the medical profession as a whole – an expected state of affairs given the anxiety of the BMA as potential legitimators of spurious medical devices – individuals did not share such reticence. In an explicit attack on promoters of multiple forms of rejuvenation, A. V. Hill, during the third Stephen Paget Memorial Lecture, delivered before the Research Defence Society on 12 June 1929, argued that there 'is no self-styled prophet, no soothsayer or fortune-teller, no food faddist, no purveyor of patent medicines or electrical "rejuvenators," who cannot, given a little plausibility, secure a following.'[54] As the only person associated with an electrical device known as a 'rejuvenator', it is hard not to draw the conclusion that Overbeck himself was indeed the intended target. Hill, furthermore, was no side-line commentator. As the joint recipient of the 1922 Nobel Prize with Otto Fritz Meyerhof, and successor to Ernest Starling as the Professor of Physiology at University College London, Hill had demonstrated the production of heat during muscle contractions, marking a key contribution to the emerging research field of biophysics.[55]

The instructions for using the Rejuvenator were both complex and vague. According to the simplified 'Time Card' of application, neuralgia, for example, should be treated for 'a few seconds to 4 minutes', whilst the head should be treated in all cases before attending to 'the affected part' of the body.[56] However, we do have more details about how the Rejuvenator should be used. In February 1932, Overbeck wrote to his sister-in-law Mrs Brett, including a Rejuvenator for use by her son and his nephew, Maurice. In his letter, Overbeck noted that '[t]he book will give you full instructions', but also that the treatment should be applied 'on getting up & going to bed & better still if after dinner also – on the head – 3 minutes with each comb before changing over.'[57] In an undated follow-up letter, addressed simply to 'my dear Professor [Maurice]', Overbeck noted: '[b]y all means keep the machine going after you have quite recovered & for some time, to prevent sliding back. With it you will soon become stronger than all the other boys; and far more intelligent from using it on your head.'[58]

By the early 1930s, the promotional materials for the Rejuvenator had attracted enough notoriety in Australia, a key market for Overbeck, that the device became a matter for discussion within Parliament. On 29 November

[53] Ibid.   [54] Hill, 'Enemies of Knowledge', 1386.
[55] Hill was elected as a Fellow of the Royal Society at the age of just thirty-two. Katz, 'Archibald Vivian Hill'.
[56] 'Time Card', n.d., Overbeck's, National Trust, uncatalogued.
[57] Otto Overbeck to Mrs Brett, n.d. February 1932, Overbeck's, National Trust, uncatalogued.
[58] Otto Overbeck to Professor [Maurice Brett], n.d. February 1932, Overbeck's, National Trust, uncatalogued.

1934, the Member of Parliament for Kalgoorlie in Western Australia, Albert Green, posed three questions to the Minister of Health and former Prime Minister William "Billy" Hughes. Green asked, first, whether the promotional material for the Rejuvenator, 'which is described as "The Elixir of Life" machine', had come to his notice; second, if Hughes was aware that 'some returned soldiers, who are bad nervous cases due to war service', were a particular target for such promotion; and third, 'to ascertain whether this method is of real medical value, or whether on the other hand, it is wholly without any merit whatever'.[59] In response, Hughes indicated his awareness of the issue and confirmed an investigation into the efficacy of the Rejuvenator. Reporting back less than a month later on 12 December 1934, Hughes noted that, 'in the opinion of the Health Department this apparatus is not to be regarded as a reliable method of treatment, and advice has been given to the Trade and Customs Department that the article may be regarded as coming within the list of prohibited articles in respect of which the ignorant or innocent purchaser should be protected against himself.'[60]

Although the ruling effectively banned the Rejuvenator from the Australian market, Overbeck's promotional efforts in Britain and elsewhere continued unabated. There was also a lively trade in second-hand instruments throughout the late 1930s into the mid-1940s, shown through a large number of classified advertisements offering Rejuvenators for sale, often in conjunction with other related devices, such as the Raydo electric hair brush and infra-red home appliances.[61] This culminated in the publication of another book by Overbeck, *The New Light*, in which he described an 'electronic philosophy of the universe'.[62] Here, in a rambling commentary on the role of electricity as an attractive force in physiology and medicine, and in society in the form of a 'Deistic potentiality', Overbeck described the human body as '37 odd trillion cells glued together, filled with juices carrying electronic currents, and depending for their life upon the continuation of those particular styles of current'.[63] For Overbeck, '[w]hen Darwin spoke of the "survival of the fittest," he was unconsciously enunciating this electronic theory.'[64]

New Kinds of Medical Electricity: Diathermy and the Violet Ray

Although supplying the body directly with electricity, suffusing the tissues with lost energy in the process, continued well into the twentieth century, other

---

[59] 'House of Representatives', 699.   [60] 'House of Representatives', 1081.
[61] '[Classified Advertisement]', *The Times*, 10 March 1944, 1; '[Classified Advertisement]', *The Times*, 1 September 1945, 1; '[Classified Advertisement]', *The Times*, 7 November 1936, 3; '[Classified Advertisement]', *The Times*, 25 September 1937, 2; '[Classified Advertisement]', *The Times*, 6 November 1937, 2; '[Classified Advertisement]', *The Times*, 12 February 1938, 2.
[62] Overbeck, *The New Light*, front cover.   [63] Ibid., viii and 75.   [64] Ibid., 76.

manifestations of electrotherapy also gained traction in the public sphere. The transformation of more conventional electrotherapy into these new forms served two key purposes. The first was to provide alternative and strikingly modern forms of treatment for a range of conditions. The second was to propagate the use of medical electricity more generally. The introduction of modified and enhanced forms of electrotherapy was one reason why, from the perspective of public medical consumers, electricity remained a viable and effective means of alleviating the signs of ageing.

Two principal manifestations of this new medical electricity came to prominence in the interwar period for the purposes of rejuvenation – violet ray therapy (also known as high-frequency treatment) and diathermy. Both found expression in varying degrees in the clinic and the home and were tested on a huge range of ailments and illnesses. By 1931, for example, E. P. Cumberbatch, speaking to the Medical Society of London, noted that 'there was hardly a region of the body to which diathermy had not been applied.'[65] Diathermy and violet ray treatments straddled the boundaries between professional medical practice, beauty therapy and domestic self-treatment.

Violet Rays: Testing Patients' Limits

The foundational technical work in developing new forms of electrotherapy was carried out almost simultaneously by physician Jacques Arsene d'Arsonval and engineer Nikola Tesla in the 1890s.[66] Each produced larger-scale apparatus capable of producing high-frequency outputs for therapeutic purposes, and in a climate where electrotherapy was part of mainstream, conventional medical practice, the prospect of applying this new and powerful force to the human body was tantalising.[67] Technical limitations of the original apparatus restricted early violet ray devices to clinical use; these were frequently large, expensive, and required significant practical expertise to operate effectively.[68] Manifestations of high-frequency electrotherapy suitable for use in the domestic context was another step still; medical texts from the first decade of the twentieth century remained broadly speculative about the likely impact of these devices in a range of diseases and conditions. In his 1903 treatise, for example, Chisholm Williams, who had qualified as a Member of the Royal College of Surgeons and Licentiate of the Society of Apothecaries before embarking on a successful career as an electrotherapist at the West

---

[65] 'The Medical and Surgical Uses of Diathermy', 181.
[66] For the most recent authoritative account of Tesla's work in this area, see Morus, *Nikola Tesla*.
[67] Culotta, 'Arsonval, Arsène D'.
[68] Tesla, 'High Frequency Oscillators'. Tesla himself identified the possibility of applying this method to the body, noting that the therapeutic uses might be varied. Rhees, 'Electricity – "The Greatest of All Doctors"'.

London Hospital, argued that high-frequency current was 'a general therapeutic agent ... able to produce a general electrification of the cells of the
whole body'.[69] The early apparatus advocated by Williams was diverse and
included whole-body electrical cages (see Figure 4.2) in which the patient
stood and was 'saturated by being placed in the field of the currents', as well as
an insulated, electrified 'couch ... whilst he holds in his hands metal electrodes'.[70] Conditions such as cancer, haemorrhoids, diabetes, obesity, dyspep-
sia, rheumatism and pulmonary tuberculosis were all singled out by Williams;
for each he outlined the principles underlying the mode of action of the violet
rays, and also included examples of successful treatments which he had
overseen.[71] Critically, Williams noted, out of his twenty-three cases of
neurasthenia, '[e]ight were about the "climacteric"', illustrating both the inher-
ently gendered and implicitly age-related nature of neurasthenia as a
condition.[72]

As well as the more general applications promoted by Williams and others,
specific investigations in the first decade of the twentieth century focussed on
the effect of violet rays on the appearance of both pathological and non-
pathological signs associated with ageing. In 1906, for example, the New
York dermatologist George M. Mackee published a paper in the *New York
Medical Journal* exploring how 'the high frequency spark' might be
deployed in cases of premature hair loss.[73] By the 1920s, high-frequency
treatment represented a new and exciting reformulation of traditional
electrotherapy, having come to prominence before World War One. The
bulk of the medical literature from this period considered the violet ray as
a novel and effective treatment of various conditions, including rickets and
tuberculosis, and especially in the case of cutaneous diseases and in
dentistry.[74]

In addition, simplifications in design and operation, as well as increasing
cultures of mass production, enabled the violet ray to become a highly prized
aesthetic device. The 'ideal home treatment' provided by the Sterling Violet
Ray High Frequency Generator, for example, was supposedly capable of
'giving the skin a healthy, glowing appearance' as well as 'alleviating brain

---

[69] Williams, *High-Frequency Currents*, 5.   [70] Ibid., 132 and 134.   [71] Ibid., 157.
[72] Ibid., 166.
[73] MacKeen, 'The High Frequency Spark', 180. Premature baldness, of course, had already
attracted considerable attention amongst late nineteenth-century medical practitioners and
commentators. See, for example: 'The Causes and Treatment of Premature Baldness', *Medical
News*, 21 January 1893, 82; 'Lactic Acid as a Remedy for Baldness', *New York Medical
Journal*, 21 October 1899, 595. See also, for an overview, Segrave, *Baldness*.
[74] Eberhart, *A Working Manual*. 'The Violet Ray', 153; Tisdall, 'The Etiology of Rickets; Fisher,
'Experiments on the Bactericidal Action'; Troup, 'Individual Overdose; 'Treatment of Industrial Rheumatism'.

130 HIGH-FREQUENCY CURRENTS

2. Auto-conduction by the Solenoid.

The noteworthy feature of this method is that the patient is not in actual metallic contact with the solenoid. The solenoid is made like

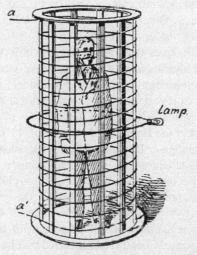

FIG. 53.—UPRIGHT AUTO-CONDUCTION CAGE.

a cage, and large enough to envelope the patient, who either stands up inside it or lies on a couch, as shown in Fig. 39. Smaller cages may be used for arm, leg, etc.

Figure 4.2 An outline of a large-scale, clinical electrotherapy device.
Source: Chisholm Williams, *High-Frequency Currents in the Treatment of Some Diseases*. New York: Rebman Company, 1903, 130

fag [and] exhaustion', according to advertisements from 1920.[75] Such promotional materials suggested a technology already fully mastered, yet patents for
violet ray apparatus dating from the early 1920s reveal that even basic features
of domestic devices were still unsettled. For example, on 31 January 1923, the
German-born Benno F. Jancke, employed by the American company Eastern
Laboratories, was able to file documents relating to an almost-complete therapeutic violet ray device 'capable of ready and economic manufacture, and
hence capable of sale at a popular price'.[76] Given that the earliest patents of
Otto Overbeck, recognised the following year, protected just one small component of his device, this strongly suggests that domestic violet ray devices
remained in their (commercial) infancy when compared with more 'traditional'
forms of electrotherapy. Other technical developments of the period included
more robust handles, necessary to protect the delicate glass applicators
according to representatives from the Master Electric Company, one of the
most prominent and long-standing manufacturers of violet ray apparatus.[77]

Other useful comparisons across conventional and ultra-violet ray
electrotherapy devices reveal that similar professional and political anxieties
attended their use, particularly beyond the confines of the clinic. In written
answers to questions in the House of Commons on 17 May 1926, the Labour
Member of Parliament Harry Day, representing the constituency of Southwark
Central, drew the attention of the then–Minister of Health, Neville
Chamberlain, 'to the increasing use of the ultra-violet ray by masseurs,
barbers, and other unqualified persons'. Further, Day continued, 'in view of
the danger produced by over-dosage in certain cases, if he will consider action
with a view to the registration of all persons who utilise this method of
treatment?'[78] In response, Chamberlain asserted that he had not received any
evidence of such dangers, a reply which drew surprise from members of the
medical profession, such as the London-based practitioner M. Weinbren, who
had recognised the potentially damaging effects of excessive ultra-violet
treatment.[79]

These exchanges were indicative not only of the ambiguous medico-
aesthetic status of the violet ray but also of the challenges presented by
nomenclature. When Day returned to the issue in 1927 – describing the 'violet

---

[75] 'Health. The Sterling Violet Ray High Frequency Generator', *The Bystander*, 1 September
1920, viii.
[76] Jancke, 'Violet-Ray Generator', 1. This came notwithstanding a much earlier patent from
1904 in which Charles F. W. Horn, acting independently, had protected one of the first high-
frequency devices 'which may be conveniently employed in the application of the ultra-violet
rays to the cure of diseases'. Horn, 'Ultra-Violet-Ray Electrode', 1.
[77] Muller and Lorenze, 'Holder for Terminals of Violet-Ray Apparatus'.
[78] 'Written Answers (Commons) of Monday, 17th May, 1926'.
[79] Weinbren, 'The Public,' 80–81.

ray lamp being a potential danger in the hands of an amateur and inexpert' and requesting Chamberlain to introduce legislation to control its use – he was questioned by Sir Harry Brittain on whether he had 'not failed to differentiate between the violet and ultraviolet rays, which are quite different things'.[80] Brittain's question was especially pertinent since the near-concurrent development of UV lamp therapy and violet ray devices – the former a variation of phototherapy, the latter electrotherapy, but both frequently implicated in the treatment of similar conditions – suggests that the ambiguity might have engendered confusion on the part of at least some potential lay consumers. Indeed, even manufacturers such as Watson & Sons, who produced both violet ray and ultra-violet devices amongst numerous electrotherapy products, noted that 'High-Frequency or Violet-Ray Treatment should ... not be confused with Ultra-Violet or Artificial Sunlight Treatment.'[81] Newspapers frequently used both violet ray and ultra-violet ray treatment interchangeably, adding to and reflecting this uncertainty.[82]

Partly in response to anxieties about non-specialists mishandling the technology, formal training in the use of high-frequency electrotherapy, as well as diathermy, was well established by the outset of the 1930s. Writing in 1930, W. Claughton Douglass compiled a textbook specifically for candidates for the Chartered Society of Massage and Medical Gymnastics Diploma in Diathermy and High Frequency.[83] In this manual, Claughton Douglass, the Medical Director of the Comely Bank Electotherapeutic Clinic and one of the examiners for the Diploma, outlined some of the key principles underlying both electromagnetism in general and the application of such forces to the body. His description of the mode of action of violet ray devices gives a striking indication of the sensory experience of both patient and practitioner:

The current of the high frequency apparatus having been switched on, the vacuum electrode glows with a violet coloration (if air filled). As the current is strengthened, blue streaky sparks flow with a crackling noise from the external surface of the glass; ... the electrode should be quickly applied to the skin ... while the current is increased in strength until it has reached the limits of toleration of the patient. ... Sparks will pass with a crackling noise between the electrode and the skin of the patient, and the skin itself will become hot and produce erythema.[84]

---

[80] 'Commons Sitting of Thursday, 17th March, 1927'.
[81] *The "Sunic" High-Frequency Apparatus for Violet-Ray Treatment*, c.1924, Wellcome Library, WN26 1924-27W33c, n.p.
[82] 'Violet-Ray Treatment', *Birmingham Daily Gazette*, 26 October 1932, 4; 'Mysterious Violet-Ray Effect' *The Bioscope*, 19 February 1930, 97; 'Sun Parlours Planned in New Derby Mental Hospital', *Derby Evening Telegraph*, 16 June 1937, 7.
[83] Douglass, *The Elements*, v.   [84] Ibid., 69.

He went on:

If the electrode is raised, a violent torrent of sparks will pass and cause intense stimulation of the skin, with a rapidly produced erythema, which, unless the electrode is promptly replaced on the skin ... will go on to form burns. This severe stimulation is sometimes desired.[85]

Such treatment was recommended in cases of neuritis, persistent headache, sleeplessness and other 'nervous cases', and to promote wound healing and relieve pain from ulcers.[86] Nor was Claughton Douglass himself neutral with respect to the merits of individual devices; he endorsed specific apparatus for the purpose of diathermic treatment, including the "Sunic" Diathermy Apparatus of Watson & Sons and the "Intertherm" device produced by Stanley Cox Ltd.[87]

The "Sunic" High Frequency Apparatus for Violet-Ray Treatment – part of a broader range of "Sunic" appliances – was a flagship product for Watson & Sons, a mainstream medical device firm. These were large-scale cabinets generally designed for use in specialist medical establishments. The hand-held Ajax Violet Ray Generator promoted actively during the late 1930s was a different proposition altogether, with treatment 'carried out in the comfort of one's home'.[88]

The mature violet ray therapy which characterised the 1930s reflected the expanded context of such treatments. The manufacturer of Rogers Vitalator, Ideal Home Electrical Appliances, deployed messages calculated to appeal to an audience of lay consumers, both men and women. Promotional materials, including a dense thirty-two-page brochure, claimed superior outcomes and easier application when compared with diathermy, and outlined a broad range of health benefits including 'better flow of blood, ... stimulation of the process of assimilation, ... deeper and easier breathing, ... [and] increase in the discharge of urine'.[89] According to the brochure, the Vitalator was key to 'general good health, ... beauty and sport', cementing a link between outward and inward bodily health.[90] Amongst the ailments which were amenable to treatment were stomach and intestinal disorders of various kinds, thrush, mumps, chest pain, paralysis, convulsions, hysteria and even joint dislocation, all of which could be treated with a huge array of forty different electrodes.[91]

Some violet ray devices were designed to be used in the home, whilst others appealed to physical therapists who intended to expand the range of treatments which they offered. 'Mr Sparks' of St. Helen's, for example, described himself in newspaper advertisements as a purveyor of 'massage, medical electricity,

[85] Ibid.   [86] Ibid., 71.   [87] Ibid., 104 and 108–09.
[88] 'Violet Rays', *Daily Mirror*, 5 April 1938, 4.
[89] Ideal Home Electrical Appliances, *Health*, 3.   [90] Ibid., 4.   [91] Ibid., 7–10.

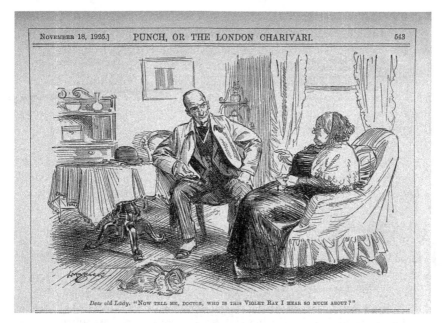

Dear old Lady. "NOW TELL ME, DOCTOR, WHO IS THIS VIOLET RAY I HEAR SO MUCH ABOUT?"

Figure 4.3 Violet Ray was also the stage name of a popular singer during the 1920s.
Source: 'An old lady asking her doctor about "Violet Ray" referring to high-frequency rays. Reproduction of a drawing after H.M. Brock, 1925', reproduced by permission of the Wellcome Collection CC BY

high-frequency (violet-ray), infrared and radiant heat lamp' treatments, whilst the Arbroath clinic of masseur J. M. O'Neil boasted even broader options, including 'sun-ray treatment, violet-ray, ultra ray. Electric blanket – electric nail-planing [and] electric bath.'[92] Treatment with the violet ray became a staple of the beauty parlour and the physical therapist; the 'Wise People's Beauty Parlour' in Lincoln advertised in February 1933 that a course of six violet ray therapy sessions was available at a cost of ten shillings, men being treated in a 'special cubicle where privacy is assured'.[93] The provision of private facilities for male clients highlights the recognition that, in sharp contrast to more typical rejuvenating offerings such as dying grey hair, the application of the violet ray was typically a more personal, revealing encounter, especially for those whose treatment necessitating exposing their bodies.

---

[92] 'Massage', *The Reporter*, 19 May 1939, 16; 'For Sun-Ray Treatment', *Arbroath Herald*, 2 September 1936, 8.
[93] 'Lincoln's Latest Beauty Parlour', *Lincolnshire Echo*, 2 February 1933, 3.

Organisations such as Bower Electric Ltd., London, promised to 'cultivate youth and beauty with violet rays ... in your own home', highlighting the 'glowing feeling of pleasant warmth' produced by the treatment, as well as the status of the device which was '[u]sed by Hospitals, Specialists and by most Bond Street Beauty Salons'.[94] As well as conventional beauty parlours, dedicated premises for violet ray therapy were also an occasional site in major urban centres. The Ultra-Violet Ray Clinic in Sheffield, for example, was staffed by both 'male and female' attendants and offered multiple different forms of electrical treatment.[95]

Reflecting the diversity of violet ray instruments, by the early 1940s, patents relating to high-frequency electrotherapy had become increasingly focussed on minor improvements to existing designs, even as patentors themselves made sweeping claims about the relationship between electricity and disease. In his 1942 British patent for a minor electrical component which would 'increase the efficiency of ultra short [sic] wave treatment and apparatus by the employment in connection therewith of flat-topped electrical impulses', New Yorker Arthur Siegfried Milinowski Jr argued that, '[i]n the case of bacteria, their virulence varies with their electrical charge, while in the case of body cells, it seems probable that departure from normal [electrical] conditions will result in pathological conditions.'[96] For the violet ray, therefore, patents functioned as legitimate sites for scientific knowledge-making, as well as legal documents laying claim to technical innovations.[97] The repurposing of violet rays across new areas of health continued alongside ongoing use in the home.

Diathermy: Professional Practice and the Vienna Youth Mask

Whilst the pain threshold was a significant consideration for the application of violet ray treatment, patient experience was also a central factor in the application of diathermy, another manifestation of higher-frequency current, but which aimed to penetrate the body and create warmth within. For example, according to Claude Saberton, a radiologist practising in Harrogate, and former Medical Officer in the Electrical Department in the Royal Victoria and West Hampshire Hospital, '[t]he sensation of warmth first felt in the wrists gradually

---

[94] 'Cultivate Youth and Beauty with Violet Rays', *The Tatler*, 23 April 1924, 73.
[95] 'The Ultra-Violet Ray Clinic', *Sheffield Independent*, 28 November 1936, 11; 'The Ultra-Violet Ray Clinic', *Sheffield Independent*, 30 November 1935, 9.
[96] Milinowski, 'Electrotherapy', 1–2. In some ways, Milinowski's claims for the efficacy and effectiveness of electrotherapy went beyond even those of Otto Overbeck, implicating electrotherapy as a means of combating infectious agents such as bacteria in addition to diseases arising from electrical imbalance within the body.
[97] This expands the uses articulated by Gooday and Arapostathis in their work. See Gooday and Arapostathis, *Patently Contestable*.

increases and slowly spreads up the forearms towards the elbow; the wrists, however, always feel the warmest, and the sensation of heat gradually diminishes as the diameter of the forearm increases.'[98] Such reflections, which framed the limits of treatment which depended to a large extent on balancing therapeutic effectiveness with patient tolerance, were entirely typical of texts for both training and experienced physicians.[99]

The supposedly deeper penetration of diathermy treatment both reduced the risk of superficial injury and led to improved clinical results.[100] This greater control led, by the mid-1930s, to diathermy devices being commonplace in high-profile beauty salons, as well as being reintegrated into professional medical practice as adjuncts to existing forms of electrotherapy. For example, Stanley Cox Ltd., a large medical device firm principally orientated towards supplies for hospitals and clinics and based on Shaftesbury Avenue, promoted the Intertherm Diathermy Apparatus, which combined 'Diathermy with any other current used in Electro-Therapy'.[101] With evocative references to 'surging Faradism' and 'the warming action' of diathermy, the device promised improved results in a range of age-related conditions such as impaired nutritional absorption and rheumatism.[102] Similarly, The Medical Supply Association advertised a huge array of electro-medical apparatus for main current, as well as those for diathermy and short-wave treatments. Their 1934 brochure boasted four devices which combined 'Diathermy current in conjunction with Galvanic, Faradic or other current'.[103] These ranged from the relatively modest and simple Smart Bristow Faradic Coil, priced as low as £6.12.6, to the Limpet Rectifier with additional electrodes, priced at ten or twelve guineas, to the much larger floor-standing Universal Radiotherm Apparatus at £199.[104]

New products designed for domestic consumption continued to appeal to professional use as a marker of prestige and trustworthiness, reflecting the ongoing, parallel practice of electrotherapy in the mainstream medical domain. The manufacturers of Readson's Duo-Ray Apparatus, for example, claimed in adverts targeted at a lay audience that the device was 'used in the main hospitals in London, including the London, the Royal Free, King's College, and Guy's Hospital', all of which had well-established electrical

---

[98] Saberton, *Diathermy in Medical and Surgical Practice*, 25.
[99] Schliephake, *Short Wave Therapy.*   [100] Beaufort, *Diathermy*, 96.
[101] The company did not engage in any direct-to-consumer marketing during this period, though a limited number of their electrotherapy devices did appear in classified adverts and auction lists during the 1930s, indicating a possible informal market for such products beyond the confines of the medical profession. 'Messrs Jarvis & Co.', *West Sussex County Times and Standard*, 21 April 1933, 4; 'Classified Advertisements', *Daily Herald*, 9 June 1937, 14.
[102] Stanley Cox Ltd., 'The "Eclipse" Radiant Heat Hand Lamp', c.1935, EPH475, Electrotherapy & vibrators ephemera Box 1, Wellcome Library.
[103] Medical Supply Association, *New Electro-medical Apparatus*, 12.   [104] Ibid., 3, 5 and 14.

departments.[105] Professional bodies beyond physicians also sought to regulate the application of medical electricity. During the period from November 1929 to March 1932, the Chartered Society of Physiotherapy recorded at least 686 practitioners who were registered to practise 'light and electro-therapy without examination'.[106] This represented a dramatic increase from earlier numbers; during the whole period from July 1919 to December 1925, for example, only twenty-one such individuals were recognised by the society; in contrast, during the month of February 1932 alone, forty-five names were added to the register.[107]

Indeed, as well as established hospitals and institutions, many organisations dedicated to the practice of rejuvenating therapies afforded huge prominence to electrical treatments. The Alfred Eichholz Clinic, opened by the Prince of Wales in July 1934 at premises in Great Portland Street, London, boasted an illustrious Medical Advisory Board, chaired by Lord Moynihan and including Sir Humphrey Rolleston and then-President of the Medical Society of London, Sir John Thomson-Walker.[108] Named in honour of the late Alfred Eichholz, a Manchester-born medical practitioner and former chief medical inspector for the Board of Education, the clinic offered a dizzying array of electrical treatment – 'diathermy, faradism, galvanism, high frequency, infra red long and short rays, radiant heat, sinusoidal current, [and] ultra violet rays' – in addition to multiple forms of massage and baths.[109] Tellingly, the clinic was designed with input from electrical engineers as well as physicians, highlighting the multiple forms of technical expertise deemed necessary to successful treatment. The clinic had a further, distinctive feature, however. Following Alfred Eichholz's own close involvement with the National Institute for the Blind, particularly during his short retirement, the clinic was specially adapted for masseurs and masseuses trained at the School of Massage for the Blind.[110]

Technical dimensions of diathermy continued to occupy medical practitioners, particularly those associated with the Section of Physical Therapy, a branch of the Royal Society of Medicine. In both 1934 and 1936, the Section played host to major discussions on short-wave diathermy, yielding insights into its status within mainstream medicine. In the latter of the two meetings, as

---

[105] 'Readson's Duo-Ray Apparatus', *Merchandise Bulletin*, 26 April 1937, 5171.
[106] 'Medical electricity, medical gymnastics, light and electrotherapy', 1915–1932, Records of the Chartered Society of Physiotherapy, Wellcome Library, SACSP/D/2/10.
[107] 'Applications Passed by Council for Enrolment Without Examination in Light & Electrotherapy', February 1932, Records of the Chartered Society of Physiotherapy, Wellcome Library, SACSP/D/2/16, 3.
[108] *Alfred Eichholz Clinic.*   [109] *Alfred Eichholz Clinic*, title page.
[110] For more details on Eichholz's involvement with the National Institute for the Blind, see 'Alfred Eichholz'.

reported in the *Proceedings of the Royal Society of Medicine*, Dr Justina
Wilson noted that, '[i]n human tissues with their intricate arrangement of
capacities, resistances, and conducting paths, it is impossible for diathermy
to produce a homogeneous distribution of warmth.'[111]

Arguably the most high-profile diathermy device of the period – the Vienna
Youth Mask (see Figure 4.4) – was also produced by one of the most
recognisable names in the burgeoning global beauty industry: Elizabeth
Arden.[112] This appeared on the British market in the spring of 1927, and a
later commentary on 'The Highway of Fashion' in the high-end women's
magazine *The Tatler* offered an unfettered endorsement of the device, which
'really does firm and rejuvenate the facial tissues'.[113] Although the author of
this article, the regular beauty columnist M. E. Brooke, did not mention the
mechanism by which the mask achieved these remarkable effects, she did
highlight one of the most distinctive selling points: the mask was 'made of the
client's face' at the first session and was therefore tailored to their personal
aesthetic requirements.[114] Just three months later Brooke provided a second
endorsement of the Vienna Youth Mask, again eschewing any reference to
mode of action, but describing the treatment as in full accord with 'the laws of
science and hygiene'.[115] Arden's credentials were scarcely in doubt – her
flagship London salon was often characterised as the place where contemporary beauty was defined – yet the Vienna Youth Mask retained an aura of
mystery, drawing on interwar Vienna as a site of both experimental scientific
adventure and aesthetic good taste.[116]

According to a 1935 retrospective on the device, Arden herself claimed that
she had 'thought it up ten years ago, in Vienna, when she heard Professor
Steinach talk about diathermy – the application of heat to tissues in the body by
means of electrical current – and the benefits derived from it by soldiers whose
muscles and nerves had been injured in the World War'.[117] Arden's extrapolation of diathermy from the ovaries to the face was entirely in keeping with
the mode of others who looked to the endocrinologists for sources
of rejuvenation inspiration. Despite this, the term 'diathermy' did not appear
in any of her British promotional materials, even if the language of these
advertisements hinted at an underlying electrical force at work in the body
through references which Arden made to the cells of the body feeling

---

[111] 'Section of Physical Medicine. Discussion on Short-Wave Therapy', *Proceedings of the Royal Society of Medicine* 30 (1936), 211–20, 215.
[112] The focus here is on Arden's engagement with forms of electrical rejuvenation. For a fuller account of Arden and her company's commercial activities in skin care, see Chapter 6.
[113] M. E. Brooke, 'The Highway of Fashion', *The Tatler*, 21 December 1927, 568.   [114] Ibid.
[115] M. E. Brooke, 'The Quest of the Beautiful', *The Tatler*, 14 March 1928, 56.
[116] Marjorie, 'The Woman's Sphere', *The Sphere*, 12 May 1928, 290.
[117] M. C. Harriman, 'Glamour, Inc.' *The New Yorker*, 4 April 1935, 24–30, 24.

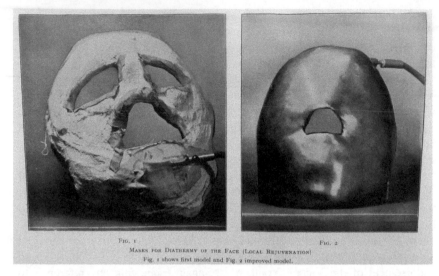

Fig. 1   Fig. 2
MASKS FOR DIATHERMY OF THE FACE (LOCAL REJUVENATION)
Fig. 1 shows first model and Fig. 2 improved model.

Figure 4.4 Peter Schmidt included images of various rejuvenation devices,
including the Vienna Youth Mask, which deployed similar techniques to
those used in the female Steinach Operation.
Source: Peter Schmidt, *The Conquest of Old Age: Methods to Effect Rejuvenation
and to Increase Functional Activity*. London: George Routledge & Son, 1931,
plate XXXIX

'tinglingly alive'.[118] Similarly, the exclusion of Steinach's name – he became
'a certain famous Professor of the University of Vienna' – set Arden apart from
her more endocrinologically inclined rival Helena Rubinstein who, as we will
see later, embraced hormone-infused skin creams.[119]

Whilst guidance on the use of diathermy by medical practitioners emphasised the limits imposed on treatment by patients' tolerance for discomfort,
Arden marketed the use of the Vienna Youth Mask as a luxurious and
pleasurable experience. At the same time, her promotional material emphasised the responsibility of women to use all the latest contrivances to avoid the
signs of ageing, noting that, '[i]n this enlightened age there is no excuse for
tired eyes and sagging skin.'[120] Paradoxically, she claimed that the Vienna
Youth Mask was both a technical innovation and achieved 'rejuvenation by
deep, *natural* stimulation'.[121] The device, Arden continued, 'pours into the

[118] 'The Answer to "What Is Youth?"', *The Sketch*, 1 May 1929, 243; 'The Answer to "What Is
Youth?"', *Britannia & Eve*, 1 June 1929, 123.
[119] 'The Answer to "What Is Youth?"', *The Tatler*, 12 June 1929, 515.
[120] 'Your Beauty Is at Your Fingertips', *The Sketch*, 25 September 1929, 636.
[121] 'Make a Plan for Beauty', *The Sketch*, 23 March 1932, 529.

inner tissue that electric energy which keeps one young', acting as an aid to, not a replacement for, conventional skin care regimes.[122]

Arden placed the Vienna Youth Mask not just in the context of contemporary scientific understanding of the body and its functioning, but in a far longer tradition of the search for prolonged youth. Promotional material evoked the mythical search by Spanish explorer Juan Ponce de León (1474–1521), who supposedly 'traversed half the globe, centuries ago, to find the Fountain of Youth'.[123] Tellingly, by the time this advertisement appeared in May 1933, references to 'the expert eyes' of a 'diathermic nurse' add a sense of scientific trustworthiness to Arden's practices.[124] Such 'expert direction', as other Arden advertisements claimed, was essential to achieving desired results 'in this zestful atmosphere where each passing hour brings a new measure of loveliness.'[125]

Electrical Devices for Youth

As well as therapies which could be generated by applying various forms of electricity directly to the body, rejuvenation could also seemingly be achieved by deploying other means which depended on electricity as a source of power. These included electrical combs, light therapy devices and mechanical contraptions which aimed to enhance exercise or reduce body fat. The Savage Health Motor, for example, hailed in advertisements to be the 'golf-course, riding-academy and gym all in one', was the product of the Savage Arms Corporation, established in 1894, and better known for its rifles and handguns.[126] The action of the device was calculated to strengthen 'the muscles and vital organs' through 'systematic stimulation of circulation', with equal benefits possible for both men and women.[127]

These devices – underpinned by electricity – sought either to replicate the beneficial effects of the natural world or to act as a substitute for lifestyle factors responsible for promoting longer life and health. In late summer 1910, the *Derby Daily Telegraph* reported on a recently published article in *The Lancet*.[128] Reflecting on the role of sunlight in the maintenance of overall health, the leading article noted that '[a] face burnt brown by the sun would seem ... to

---

[122] 'Are You Glad to See Yourself?', *The Tatler*, 19 November 1930, 357.

[123] 'Elizabeth Arden's Five-Point Plan', *The Tatler*, 3 May 1933, 211.

[124] Ibid., p. 211; 'Elizabeth Arden's Five-Point Plan', *The Tatler*, 24 May 1933, 339; 'Elizabeth Arden's Five-Point Plan', *The Tatler*, 10 January 1934, 79.

[125] 'Make a Plan for Beauty', 529.

[126] 'Health and Beauty at Little Cost! Savage Health Motor, Exerciser and Reducer'. Utica, NY: Savage Arms Corporation, c. 1930, Electrotherapy and Vibrators Ephemera Box 1, EPH+27:5, Wellcome Library, n.p.

[127] Ibid.

[128] '"You Do Look Well". A Medical View of the Sun-Burnt Face', *Derby Daily Telegraph*, 19 August 1910, 2.

be a sensible object of a holiday ... because the circumstances which conspired to produce the brown complexion have other factors favourable to an all-round healthy state.'[129] The significance of sunlight – whether natural or artificial – for health was widely recognised in the first decades of the twentieth century. However, the relative merits of these two were debated extensively by medical practitioners, those on the fringes of medical practice and lay experts.

The reconfiguration and expansion of different forms of electrotherapy during the interwar period also propagated new endeavours in rejuvenating electrotherapy. For example, Ernst Kromayer, the German dermatologist, explored modifications to the earlier Finsen Lamp which had been developed principally to treat diseases of the skin, such as lupus vulgaris. Unlike many other purveyors of electrically powered rejuvenating devices, Kromayer was a classical dermatologist in the mould of Nils Finsen; Kromayer's eponymous lamp, like that of Finsen, was primarily used for treating diseases of the skin rather than restoring lost youthfulness.[130] However, Kromayer engaged closely with signs of ageing, viewing these instead through the lens of disease. This was most visible in his discussion of plicae cutis – wrinkles – in a 1930 text on *The Cosmetic Treatment of Skin Complaints*. Considering what he described as the 'pathology' of wrinkles, Kromayer argued that 'the wrinkles in the face, which are cosmetically so abhorrent, cannot be effectively removed by means of the beauty-ointments, lotions, fomentations, massage, and electricity which are extolled in such glowing terms.'[131]

Francis Howard Humphris, who in the late 1930s co-authored a major text on emanotherapy with rejuvenation enthusiast Leonard Williams, was a prominent advocate for the rejuvenating properties of ultra-violet radiation.[132] In his 1929 treatise on *Artificial Sunlight and its Therapeutic Uses*, Humphris quoted a case overseen by Arnold Lorand in which 'an anaemic, very weak man', treated with an 'air-cooled mercury vapour lamp' for a period of just three weeks 'presented an aspect of blooming health with rosy cheeks'.[133] For all the purported benefits of this approach, however, Humphris also stressed 'that ultra-violet light treatment should only be given under, and by the orders of, a practitioner, and patients should be most specifically warned against indiscriminate so-called "sun baths".'[134]

As well as bespoke devices, new to the marketplace, all of which claimed to exert rejuvenating effects on the body in a more wholesale manner, electricity

[129] 'The Sun-Burnt Face'.
[130] For more on Finsen, see Jamieson, 'More Than Meets the Eye'. A larger-scale analysis of phototherapy by Tania Woloshyn has highlighted the critical role of visual materials – not least images of successful cases of treatment – in the legitimation of various forms of light therapy. Woloshyn, *Soaking up the Rays*.
[131] Kromayer, *The Cosmetic Treatment*, 97.   [132] Humphris and Williams, *Emanotherapy*.
[133] Humphris, *Artificial Sunlight*, 196–97.   [134] Ibid., 279.

also enabled the reimagining of simple everyday practices. The 'Letrik' electric comb is a key example. Produced by the Letrik Company, based in London, and specifically established for the purpose, the promotional material promised to 'make new hair grow from "dead"', restoring 'hair back to its youthful beauty'.[135] Similarly, White's 'Electric Comb', according to advertisements, was the essential device which 'really makes hair grow, stops greyness, brings back the colour, and waves the hair'.[136] In addition to the claims about creating a hair style as well as modifying the colour and texture of the hair, the creation of a new 'handbag size' indicates that this promoted primarily to women.[137] Other manifestations of the device, such as the Evans Electric Comb, deployed similar claims – within a single advert the headings 'stops falling hair now', 'baldness banished by Evans' and 'greyness goes for good' – suggesting common terms of reference for electrically powered combs, all with specific effects which included both the reversal and rectification of signs of ageing as well as aesthetic consequences.[138] The mode of action of these electric combs was firmly located in the ability of electricity to penetrate into the roots of the hair. As one advertising campaign for White's Electric Comb noted, it was effective in 'reviving the roots – waking them up – bringing them to life. Roots of hair that have become dormant are revitalised.'[139]

Works of fiction in the early twentieth century continued the well-established tradition of imagining the application of electricity as a life-giving force. Writing almost one hundred years after its pivotal appearance in *Frankenstein*, the British schoolteacher-turned-author Herbert Gubbins (1887–1950) deployed electricity as the most fundamental force in his science fiction work, *The Elixir of Life*.[140] Published in 1914, the novel imagined humanity in the year 2905, suffused with technical novelties yet with the

---

[135] 'You'll Have Wavy Hair – Same Day, New Hair – Same Week', *Daily Herald*, 28 October 1930, 13.

[136] 'See the Special Window Display', *Worthing Gazette*, 13 August 1930, p. 11; 'See the Special Window Display', *Grantham Journal*, 21 June 1930, 4; 'See the Special Window Display', *Yorkshire Evening Post*, 18 June 1930, p. 5; 'Going Grey?', *Bucks Examiner*, 31 January 1930, 6;

[137] 'Whites Electric Comb', *Bexhill-on-Sea Observer*, 14 June 1930, 5.

[138] 'New Hair in a Week', *The People*, 20 July 1930, 15; 'New Hair in a Week', *The People*, 31 August 1930, 6;

[139] 'White's Electric Comb', *The People*, 2 March 1930, 15.

[140] For a recent reflection on the centrality of electricity and 'the spark of being' in *Frankenstein*, and its continuing significance, see Fairclough, '*Frankenstein* and the "Spark of Being"'. Fairclough, in fact, argues that Shelley originally focussed on an 'obscure "chemical" experiment' as the source of animation, rather than 'galvanic shocks.' Fairclough, '*Frankenstein* and the "Spark of Being"', 399. Ulf Houe has advanced a similar view, that 'there is no mention of electricity at the moment of creation. There are "instruments of life" and there is a "spark of being," but no lightning, no Galvanic fluid.' See Houe, 'Frankenstein without Electricity', 95.

global population rendered illiterate in consequence. In his preface, Gubbins identified two paradoxical roles for electricity in the early twentieth century. The first was in underpinning 'an age of inventions with a negative nomenclature', emphasising the undesirable removal or lack induced by the expansion of electrical force, as in the case of wireless telegraphy or horseless carriage.[141] The second lay in the potential of electricity to add and recreate, in this case, lost youth to bodies faded by time.

Writing under the heading 'Prolonging Life', again in the preface, Gubbins outlined the recent scientific discoveries which underpinned his narrative. He claimed that, '[o]nly a short time ago two doctors in Paris proved that electricity would prolong life', leading those who were treated with 'an electric bath' to 'become young that they might extend the span of existence', invoking the recent discoveries of Marie Curie, Röntgen and Crookes.[142] In the future imagined by Gubbins, 'health-giving electrical appliances have removed the necessity of exercise to preserve, or drugs to restore health.'[143] Ultimately the promised 'electrical baptism', supposed to offer 'a guarantee of prolonged life' by removing 'every impurity encumbering and blocking up arteries and organs' proved to be a false dawn. On the final page of the novel, newspaper headlines proclaim, 'THE FINDING OF THE PHILOSOPHERS STONE' and 'THE ELIXIR OF LIFE FOUND', with the key protagonist, scientist Sir Thomas Browne, having failed in his plan to awake, rejuvenated, in the far future, yet still emerging as the inventor of a genuinely rejuvenating substance, a hybrid between electricity and radium: electrum.[144]

Legacy and Conclusion

On 19 June 1953, the Glasgow-based *Evening News* included a lengthy article outlining what was claimed to be an increasingly close relationship between beauty and heath. Amongst the supposedly 'new methods and treatments' which yielded beneficial effects on both appearance and 'lumbago, fibrositis, rheumatism, arthritis and kindred complaints', pride of place was reserved for the Rouathermic bath ('from the Continent') and 'the Traxator from Denmark which slims, tones and improves the blood circulation'.[145] Both were entirely dependent on electrical force but in quite different ways. The former supposedly acted to expose the body directly to a form of electrical energy, whilst

---

[141] Gubbins, *The Elixir*, n.p.
[142] Gubbins, *The Elixir*, Preface, n.p. Gubbins also described radium – 'the world's latest and most mysterious substance' – as exhibiting life-prolonging properties. Ibid., 33.
[143] Gubbins, *The Elixir*, 74.
[144] Ibid., 251 and 254. For a concise summary of the novel, see Bleiler and Bleiler, *Science Fiction*, 313–14.
[145] 'Beauty Is Now a Question of Health', *Evening News*, 19 June 1953, 86.

the latter drew on electric power to underpin a mechanical device to act on the body.

Electrical devices such as these, designed for home use, proliferated in the postwar period. Almost identical principles to those underpinning the simple electrotherapy devices of the 1920s have become part of mainstream pain relief, particularly in childbirth, through the development of transcutaneous electrical nerve stimulation (TENS) machines.[146] Similarly, the emergence of electroconvulsive therapy as a distinctive and high-profile manifestation of electrotherapy in the domain of psychiatry did not dampen the appetite for domestic products which claimed to promote everyday health and longevity.

In his book *Animal Electricity*, Robert B. Campenot identifies the key stages which underpinned the concretisation of 'body and brain' as 'electric machines'.[147] Campenot's account, with electricity and especially bodily electrical at its heart, necessarily excludes competing models, such as the chemical, which created a pluralistic understanding of how bodies worked. When we explore the lively electrotherapy marketplace of the 1920s and 1930s, driven by modernity, as a continuation of that described for the Victorian period by Iwan Rhys Morus, it creates an intriguing tension.[148] How and why did amateur electrotherapy persist in an age seemingly dominated by chemical explanations of bodily function? There are three principal factors, specific to electrotherapy, which underpinned such ongoing popularity. The first was the well-established institutional basis of electrotherapy which, by the turn of the twentieth century, extended through almost all major British hospitals, as well as the offices of individual physicians and dedicated electrical clinics. This was augmented by the extensive commercial networks which had emerged to support and shape the extension of electrical treatments. The second, broader reason was the emerging popularity and notoriety of rejuvenation more generally, to some extent rehabilitating the health-giving electrical devices of the Victorian period. Third, the seemingly successful application of transformed electrical tools, such as the violet ray, diathermic devices and electric lights, underpinned expanded and reformulated claims of efficacy. Whilst conventional electrotherapy devices did persist, therefore, the

---

[146] The language surrounding the efficacy of TENS therapy bears a striking resemblance to the justification for its use in the rejuvenation devices of the interwar period. For example, the NHS guidance on TENS notes that 'small electrical impulses are delivered to the affected area of your body ... [These] can reduce the pain signals going to the spinal cord and brain, which may help relieve pain and relax muscles.' NHS, 'TENS'.

[147] Campenot, *Animal Electricity*.

[148] Morus has argued that the body was 'the primary medium through which electricity was assimilated into Victorian culture', with electrical entrepreneurs successfully claiming not just to demonstrate electricity as spectacle but to harness and 'discipline' its actions. Morus, *Shocking Bodies*, 185.

rejuvenating devices of the interwar period shifted to accommodate these emerging technologies, adapted for domestic use.

There was almost no perceptible difference between the framing of the scope, theoretical basis and therapeutic efficacy of electrotherapy in a professional domain, as characterised by Claughton Douglass, and that suggested by proponents of rejuvenation devices marketed directly to lay consumers. At the same time, the celebration of discoveries in atomic structure and the pivotal role of the electron within atomic models appeared to confirm electricity as the most fundamental force of matter, even within chemical bodies.[149] This was built chiefly on the back of the popularisation of the power of the electron in the late nineteenth century and the subsequent claims of atomic structure advanced by J. J. Thompson and Ernest Rutherford in the early twentieth century. Electricity therefore retained a pre-eminence within scientific and popular discourse, and continued to underpin the reconfigurations of electrotherapy which both shaped and responded to public perceptions about how this powerful agent could be mobilised to combat the onset of signs of ageing.

The commercial content of books such as Otto Overbeck's *A New Electronic Theory of Life* was far from unique. Almost all textbooks and manuals for lay and professional medical audiences also endorsed and recommended specific products, effectively advocating certain configurations of equipment and the firms which manufactured them. In consequence, we can read Overbeck's efforts as an extrapolation of the pre-existing commercial-medical complex rather than a radical and unprincipled venture (notwithstanding the fact that other aspects of his promotional strategy certainly fell into this category).[150]

Whilst the marketing material of some electrical devices for use in the home claimed to mimic the effects of exercise through their reducing action and toning effect, the interwar period also saw significant changes in the deployment of physical culture. New forms of exercise – both those which enabled

---

[149] A key original paper was G. Johnstone Stoney's from 1894 in which he both popularised the term 'electron' and described the atom as an 'atom of electricity'. The fact that electrical forces now seemed to sit at the heart of matter provided strong justification for supposing that even the action of hormones was actually dependent on electrical forces. Stoney, 'Of the "Electron"'. The continuation of this electro-centric view of the physical world and human body also had strong cultural resonance with earlier ideas about the relative importance of the blood and electrical energy in the circulation. As the promotional materials of 'Dr Carter Moffat's Feather Weight Electric Body Belt' noted in the early 1890s, 'the blood is the life, but electricity is the life of the blood.' Carter Moffat, 'Electricity in Failing Health', London: London Health Electrical Institute, c. 1892, Clothing Ephemera, Box 1, EPH131:8, Wellcome Library, n.p.

[150] For more on the medical-commercial relationship in the late nineteenth and early twentieth centuries, see: Jones, *The Medical Trade Catalogue in Britain*; Jones, 'A Barrier to Medical Treatment'; Ueyama, *Health in the Marketplace*.

individuals to pursue regimes at home as part of a daily rejuvenating routine and very public, communal displays of (predominantly female) youthful, athletic prowess – offered a counterpoint to the electrical devices discussed in this chapter. We turn now to consider how exercise became a cornerstone of attempts to avoid the onset of the signs associated with older age, celebrating the natural capacity of the human body to be disciplined without either medical or technical intervention.

5   Exercise, 1930–1939

> Old age is simply a 'pose,' says Sir James Cantlie. When a man is young
> he requires no stimulus to take exercise of some form or another ... but
> when he reaches fifty years of age or thereby the spontaneity for exercise
> gradually dies away.[1]

James Cantlie (1851–1926) is now perhaps best known for his promotion of
first aid and expertise in tropical medicine, exemplified by his involvement in
military emergency medicine and as inaugural surgeon and lecturer in tropical
medicine at the London School of Tropical Medicine when it opened its doors
in 1899.[2] There is, however, an additional aspect to his work as a medical
practitioner which has gone largely unnoticed: the somewhat esoteric programme of exercise known as James Cantlie's Physical Jerks. Although this
system was just one trend in a period of numerous competing exercise regimes,
George Orwell chose to take inspiration from Cantlie's system: members of the
Outer Party in *Nineteen Eighty-Four* were required to carry out daily Physical
jerks, monitored by telescreens.[3] Failure to participate correctly in the Physical
jerks resulted in admonishment by Big Brother.[4] Similarly, Lily Pike's less
well-known 1924 play *The Rejuvenation of Grandpa* attributed the revitalisation of the titular character to a series of exercises termed physical jerks; the
play itself was 'suggested to the author by the accounts of the physical drill
classes of Sir James Cantlie'.[5] In the final scene, physical jerks are claimed by
the rejuvenated older man in question to produce 'old men and women made
young again'.[6]

Cantlie, 'the eminent Harley Street specialist' and 'keen supporter of a
movement to have a British System of Physical Training introduced', was

---

[1] 'Brochure of The British Institute of Physical Training (Instituted 1889)'. Aberdeen: The
Rosemount Press, 1925, Sir James Cantlie (1851–1926) Papers, Wellcome Library, MS.7941/
12, 3.

[2] Mark Harrison, 'Cantlie, Sir James (1851–1926)'.   [3] Orwell, *Nineteen Eighty-Four*.

[4] Ibid. In chapter 3 Winston is castigated by name through his telescreen after becoming
distracted.

[5] 'The Rejuvenation of Grandpa', October 1924, MS7941/11, Wellcome Library.

[6] 'Rejuvenation of Grandpa', 16.

138

adamant that '*Exercise! Exercise! Exercise!*' was the key to avoid becoming 'old at fifty'.[7] Alongside correct fuelling of the body – exemplified by dietary and electrical feeding as discussed in previous chapters – proponents of exercise regimes in the interwar period argued that training appropriate to both age and gender could prolong the youthful portion of life. By the late 1930s, numerous new groups offering particular kinds of physical advice and training were operating, many – but not all – making claims about the rejuvenating effect of exercise as well as its health benefits. Moving beyond established narratives concerning the increasing importance and social role of physical education for both young and old, this chapter explores how and why different forms of exercise came to be seen as the key to youthfulness, who rose to promote these, and how the life course of both men and women was further complicated by exercise regimes which claimed to restore lost vitality.[8]

In her recent book, *Exercise in the Female Lifecycle in Britain*, Eilidh Macrae charts the development of physical education for women through the middle part of the twentieth century. For Macrae, the primacy of the role of motherhood for women was a defining factor in shaping the nature of female physical education.[9] However, whilst this argument indicates that the pace of social change in the aftermath of World War Two was uneven in terms of gender, Macrae's acknowledged focus is on relatively early life, covering 'adolescence, marriage, pregnancy and motherhood'; this leaves our understanding of 'the process of negotiation between the ageing body and the sporting self' as incomplete, representing a very typical marginalisation of the elderly body as a key feature of the physicality of the life course in a period when ensuring maximum bodily productivity was a pressing national and familial concern.[10] Focussing closely, but not exclusively, on the period immediately preceding World War Two, this chapter interrogates the increasingly complex relationship between ageing and exercise in its myriad forms, from moralising physical culture to drill-style mass exercise for women. Whilst many of these initiatives were aimed at (and popularised by) a younger generation of athletic exemplars, the fact that much of the promotional material – including advertisements, publications and films – drew on the imagery of the young should not obscure from us the fact that older and prematurely aged people were also exhorted to engage in life-prolonging, rejuvenating exercise.

The public visibility of bodies has been interpreted as a key feature of physical culture, largely from a Foucauldian perspective in which the primacy

---

[7] Cruden, *The British Institute of Physical Training*, 13–14, in Sir James Cantlie (1851–1926) Papers, Wellcome Library, MS.7941/12, original emphasis.

[8] For the case of physical education in the United States, see Verbrugge, *Active Bodies*.

[9] Macrae, *Exercise in the Female Lifecycle*,   [10] Ibid., 221–22.

of medical observation of the body was reflective of a new and, implicitly, disturbing power relationship between professional and public.[11] Yet, through all of this extensive and well-established literature – which recognises that bodies were at the heart of physical culture at both the individual and collective level – there is little consideration given to the *ageing* body. This is doubly surprising given the characterisation of the interwar period as 'the morbid years', beset with anxieties about the 'moral miasma' of mass industrialisation and racial decline, even in the relatively liberal context of Britain.[12] We begin, therefore, with selected moments within the broad movement of physical culture, before turning our attention to forms of communal exercise, particularly through The Women's League of Health and Beauty, established in 1930, and finally considering the role of physical therapy such as massage and facial exercises in maintaining a youthful face and complexion. Throughout, the chapter sets these high-profile initiatives against the backdrop of everyday practices as captured by diarists through mass observation from 1937. Such accounts demonstrate that for some – men and women of all ages – rejuvenating exercises, such as the physical 'jerks' of Cantlie and others, became an indispensable part of daily routine.

A Confluence of the Non-Naturals: Physical Culture for Agelessness

> Jump out of bed immediately, and in full light, with unclothed body, perform the internal toilet of the organism by half an hour of physical culture, in regular rhythm, with slow inspiratory and expiratory movements.[13]

On 12 September 1918, David Lloyd George delivered a speech in Manchester against the backdrop of imminent allied victory in World War One, albeit at immense national cost.[14] The title of his address was 'Looking Forward', and Lloyd George struck an optimistic yet cautionary tone in his address. He identified the 'health and fitness of its people' as one of the most important areas of British society which should be monitored and improved in order to meet 'any emergencies of either war or peace'. Referencing the highest and lowest military service grades used by the army up to 1917, Lloyd George remarked that '[y]ou cannot maintain an A1 Empire with a C3 population.'[15] The regeneration and revitalisation of race – an expression of eugenic ideals in the interwar period – was therefore intimately bound up with issues of national security. The preservation of youthful strength and energy

---

[11] See, for example: Armstrong, *Political Anatomy of the Body*; Vertinsky, 'The Social Construction of the Gendered Body'; Kirk, 'Foucault and the Limits of Corporeal Regulation'.

[12] Overy, *The Morbid Age*, 70.   [13] Frumusan, *Rejuvenation*, 121.

[14] Monger, *Patriotism and Propaganda*, 199.   [15] *Lloyd George's Message*, 9–10.

represented an important strategy for maintaining economic productivity and protecting the realm.

With this goal in view, there was scarcely an aspect of physical and mental health which, in the eyes of its proponents during the interwar period, could not be enhanced or remedied by adherence to a regime rooted in physical culture. The so-called diseases of affluence in the late nineteenth century gave rise to a new imperative for maintaining levels of physical activity both within and outside the workplace.[16] In order to counter the technology-driven tendency for men (especially) to undertake sedentary occupations, forms of exercise and lifestyle modification were increasingly seen as a natural, essential modification to daily habits in order to prevent a worrying regression of the race.[17]

As I have argued elsewhere, the architects of physical culture in the early twentieth century made telling interventions far beyond exercise, advising on diet, work, leisure, sleep, sexual habits and lifestyle more broadly.[18] In the United States, two of the chief prophets of this approach were Sanford Bennett and Bernarr Macfadden, who we encountered in Chapter 3 in their capacities as self-styled experts in bodily management and performance. In Britain, Eugen Sandow established a similar reputation which made him one of the pre-eminent figures in the physical culture movement in the first decade of the twentieth century, whilst the Danish author and advocate of home gymnastic exercises, Jørgen Peter Müller (1866–1938, often known in his English publications as J. P. Muller), gained popularity in Britain through his English-language texts and dedicated Institute.[19] Collectively, these men were part of a broader trend in the representation of male bodies as repositories of unlocked physical potential, a trend extended in film and which came to permeate much later advertising strategies for everyday products which lay claim to improving health, such as margarine.[20]

In 1904, Muller published *Mit System* (*My System*), in which he outlined a fifteen-minute workout regime, to be performed daily. This, so Muller claimed, had transformed him from 'a delicate boy into one of the most successful all-round amateur sportsmen and athletes on the Continent'.[21] In common with Bennett, Macfadden and Sandow, Muller's own physical development from a

[16] McKenzie, *Getting Physical*; Martschukat, "The Necessity for Better Bodies".

[17] See, for example, the now classic collection of essays edited by J. A. Mangan and James Walvin, *Manliness and Morality*. In this volume, especially relevant are contributions by Roberta Park on biological thought and athleticism, and Allen Warren's account of the role of the scouting movement on concepts of masculinity and manliness.

[18] Stark, "Replace Them by Salad and Vegetables".

[19] Watt, 'Cultural Exchange, Appropriation and Physical Culture', 1922.

[20] Hand, 'Marketing Health Education', 481; Kirkham and Thumim eds, *You Tarzan*.

[21] Muller, *My System: 15 Minutes*, 4.

sickly child into a powerfully built man was central to legitimising his claim to speak with authority on matters of physical culture. The first English translation of the original Danish publication appeared just a year later, and in 1912 Muller moved to London and established the Muller Institute in Piccadilly, where clients could receive 'specialised instructions in Lieut. Muller's Methods of Physical Exercise, both personally and through the post.'[22] *My System* generated significant press attention, and was described in some quarters as an already 'famous' text, despite appearing in Danish only the preceding year.[23]

Muller's method was relatively simple – a series of eighteen exercises, set in the context of wider bodily management, which included those features so typical of physical culture, including 'suitable diet', 'sensible underclothing' (a perennial obsession of Muller), and 'moderate indoor temperature'.[24] The exercises were assured to transform the body 'from a fidgety, hypochondriacal master to an efficient and obedient servant', and included elaborate stretches, postures and balances (see Figure 5.1), designed to improve the hygienic action of the skin, circulation and digestion.[25] The male body was cast here as a lithe, functional unit, and the presence of a ubiquitous cricket jumper gave the distinct impression that the individual could retain a sense of gentlemanly dignity even when adopting such esoteric poses. The images convey a clear sense of suppleness, as well as strength and were accompanied by detailed descriptions and responded to one of Muller's central driving assumptions: that '[t]he vital force of the body does not reside in the arms.'[26]

To promote his regime (and, of course, his books), Muller quickly embarked a tour of Europe, giving quasi-performances and talks. On 9 April 1906, at the invitation of 'a number of gentlemen', he gave 'a demonstration of his celebrated system' at the Music Hall in Shrewsbury, presided over by the local mayor.[27] This was part of a packed schedule of similar engagements which he carried out during that month, such as those delivered in Exeter Hall (5 April), at the German Gymnastic Society in London (6 April) and at the Military

---

[22] Ibid., title page, original emphasis.

[23] 'For Country Readers', *Penny Illustrated*, 30 December 1905, 6; 'Fifteen Minutes Work a for Health's Sake', *Jedburgh Gazette*, 27 January 1906, 3; 'A New Book on Physical Exercises' *Dundee Courier*, 10 March 1906, 6.

[24] Muller, *My System: 15 Minutes*, 6.

[25] The language of Joseph Pilates's major publications on exercise and bodily health from the mid-1930s represents a striking continuity with that of Muller. For example, in the introduction to an updated edition of his classic 1945 text, *Return to Life*, Pilates, then aged 77, noted that the '[t]elephones, automobiles, and economic pressure all combine to create physical letdown', alleviated only by giving 'constant thought to the improvement of our bodies.' Pilates and Miller, *Return to Life*, 3–4.

[26] J. P. Muller, *My System: Fifteen Minutes' Work*, xiv.

[27] 'Physical Development', *Wellington Journal*, 31 March 1906, 7; 'By Invitation of the Committee', *Shrewsbury Chronicle*, 30 March 1906, 5.

EXERCISE No. 2.

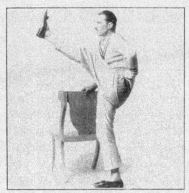

Fig. 11.

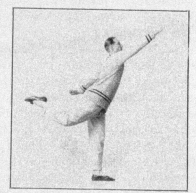

Fig. 12.

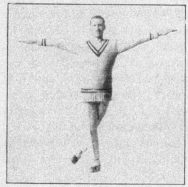

Fig. 13.

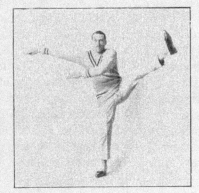

Fig. 14.

These photos and several of the others are of the Author's
eldest son, Ib, at the age of 22, 34 and 37 years

Figure 5.1 Muller's family were typically included as demonstrators of the
stretches, in a manner later mirrored by mother and daughter, Mary and
Prunella Bagot Stack, in the context of the Women's League of Health
and Beauty.
Source: J. P. Muller, *My System: 15 Minutes' Exercise a Day for Health's Sake.*
London: Athletic Publications Ltd., c.1925, 67

Gymnasium in Aldershot (11 April).[28] Faithful to his approach at all times, Muller was insistent that he would only 'give his performance throughout with open windows', with organisers at pains to note that 'the audience, who will not be engaged in active exercise, will not be subjected to any inconvenience in the way of draughts.'[29]

Although Muller was careful to position himself as the epitome of physical prowess, he also attempted to reach beyond a middle-aged male audience, including images of his own children performing various exercises and noting frequently throughout that particular instructions might apply 'both to ladies and gentlemen' or that variations might be preferable; in the case of Exercise No. 11, for example, '[f]or women it is better not to take the hands away as they rise.'[30] Despite this, Muller did not envision his system as equally well suited to women and men, noting in the preface to *My System for Ladies*, a follow-up text from 1911, that '"My System" ... was not especially intended for ladies.'[31] This modified system, which joined a similar adaptation for children, highlighted the extent to which Muller viewed male and female bodies as fundamentally different in both their structure and function, and in their maintenance.[32]

In their publications Muller, Bennett, Macfadden and Sandow all appealed not only to their strength and health, following periods of childhood weakness, but also to their ability to maintain a desirable physical state longer into later life. However, others addressed the relationship between age and exercise in more explicit terms. The journalist and prolific author Walter M. Gallichan, for example, noted in his 1929 guide *Youthful Old Age* that in old age 'the muscles stiffen more quickly after exertion.'[33] Gallichan was a controversial figure with a tendency for ostentatious prose who published a number of novels and wrote at great lengths against the women's movement.[34] He also theorised extensively on the subject of sex education and became a fervent supporter of eugenics, views clearly evident in his musings on the subject of old age and rejuvenation.[35] Notwithstanding Gallichan's outspoken views, his perspectives on the role of exercise in maintaining youthfulness into old age drew on a

---

[28] 'Mr J. P. Muller and "My System"' *Shrewsbury Chronicle*, 6 April 1906, 5.   [29] Ibid.

[30] Muller, *My System: Fifteen Minutes Work*, 124–25.

[31] Muller, *My System for Ladies*, 13. As we shall see later in the chapter, Muller's System – only later classified as a form of physical 'jerks' – remained popular for some decades, practised ritualistically in British homes as part of both morning and evening routines.

[32] Muller, *My System for Children*.   [33] Gallichan, *Youthful Old Age*, 9.

[34] For a brief biography of Gallichan, see: Hooper, 'Hartley, Catherine Gasquoine (1866/7–1928)'. See, for examples of Gallichan's work in these areas: Gallichan, *The Conflict*; Gallichan, *A Soul from the Pit*; Gallichan, *Modern Woman*; Gallichan, *The Critical Age of Woman*; Gallichan, *Youth and Maidenhood*.

[35] Gallichan, *The Art of Courtship*; Gallichan, *The Great Unmarried*. On eugenics, see Gallichan, *The Sterilization of the Unfit*.

range of popular ideas. He held that 'neglect of regular suitable outdoor exercise' was second only to 'auto-intoxication' as a cause of infirm old age.[36] Gallichan noted that although '[d]iet is of supreme importance in the avoidance of constipation ... [e]xercise comes next', echoing Elié Metchnikoff's pronouncements of the early twentieth century that intestinal stasis was the principal cause of old age infirmity.[37] As well as being the chief cause of cancer, Gallichan implicated constipation in 'depression of spirits, gloomy apprehension, lassitude of the brain, irritability, irascibility, and malaise of the mind'.[38]

Sedentary occupations in office work were prone to produce what Gallichan termed 'bowel derangement and displacement', evidenced by the seeming absence of constipation during holidays.[39] Critically, however, although Gallichan was concerned with preventative exercise measures in those of working age, he also noted that 'The necessity for exercises lasts till the closing days of human life, and the aged should be urged to take the kind of exercise suited to their years and their strength.'[40] Gallichan was explicit about the level of exertion appropriate to each stage of life, and reserved the bulk of his attention – as might be expected given his attitudes towards women – for men. For example, '[i]n early manhood and middle-age, the amount of daily physical exercise should be the equivalent of walking nine miles ... An old man should walk about five miles every day, and a woman at least three or four.'[41] The context and purpose of the exercise were equally as important as its nature and duration. For the elderly in particular, physical activity was at its most valuable when carried out as part of a relationship with nature and the natural world. Gardening, walking in the countryside and 'any other form of nature study' were considered superior – '[d]igging is a fine exercise' – while Gallichan reserved judgement on the merits of '"physical culturists" who proclaim that no one need grow old'.[42] He was especially scathing of James Cantlie's physical jerks, dubbed 'a rather drastic process for old joints and muscles'.[43]

In both Britain and the United States, the response to Gallichan was typical of that reserved for perceived interlopers on matters of health. For example, writing in the *American Journal of Public Health*, the Director of the State Hygiene Laboratory and Professor of Bacteriology at the University of Wisconsin, Madison, M. P. Ravenel, noted that the profession was 'tired of books written by non-medical men who think that some fad or another has saved their lives and preserved their health'.[44] Ravenel lamented the 'cocksure tone' and

---

[36] Gallichan, *Youthful Old Age*, 15. For more on auto-intoxication and diet, see Chapter 3.
[37] Gallichan, *Youthful Old Age*, 76.   [38] Ibid., 80.   [39] Ibid., 78.   [40] Ibid., 79.
[41] Ibid., 132.   [42] Ibid., 131–33.   [43] Ibid., 134.
[44] Ravenel, 'Why Not Grow Young?', 840.

dismissed Gallichan as nothing more than 'a disciple of Sir Arbuthnot Lane'.[45] This assessment was far from universal. Albert G. Nicholls, editor of the *Canadian Medical Association Journal* from 1930 to 1942, welcomed Gallichan's contribution on the subject of longevity. Nicholls noted that the book 'sets forth in a sane and helpful, and for us a very, convincing, manner his views as to right living', departing from the 'fads and "isms," cranks, "uplifters," and false prophets' so characteristic of the genre.[46]

The height of public fascination with hormonal rejuvenation produced a robust response from advocates of a more 'natural' approach to maintaining youthfulness. Arthur Abplanalp, the Swiss physical culture practitioner who wrote columns for *The Sketch* and personal fitness guides such as *In Perfect Shape All Your Life*, was one of a number of commentators who adopted the language of rejuvenation in order to draw on its cultural cachet.[47] He was formerly an instructor at the Sandow Institute, where he earned the nickname 'the Terrible Swiss', before establishing his own institution in London in 1921, promoting the benefits a rigorous and uncompromising form of physical culture throughout the life course.[48] Writing for a predominantly middle-class audience in periodicals during the mid-1920s, Abplanalp emphasised the importance of 'strictly hygienic physical exercises in promoting health and vitality', particularly for older men, in 'counteracting the many injurious influences of our over-civilised age'.[49] These made use of his 'exercising apparatus suitable for reducing corpulence and for other health exercises adapted to be carried out while in a lying position', protected by a US patent from 22 June 1915 (see Figure 5.2).[50] Abplanalp was careful to note that his particular system was equally suitable for men and women, and for all ages. His text, *Slimness and Health*, published around 1931 (the preface and fore-word were dated 1930), was both a 'reducing' manual to promote the virtues of weight loss and 'the hygienic, aesthetic and practical value of scientifically devised and graduated exercises'.[51] The apparatus was at the centre of the Abplanalp system expressed in *Slimness and Health*, although he also included many exercises which could be performed without such contraptions. Unlike other entrepreneurs, Abplanalp did not appeal to the patents as a way of bolstering his claims of expertise, relying instead on his personal experiences and those of his sons, and testimony from expert and lay followers. In his immediate postwar writings, Abplanalp was careful to delineate his system of

[45] Ibid.   [46] Nicholls, 'Youthful Old Age', 252.   [47] Abplanalp, *In Perfect Shape*.
[48] 'Arthur Abplanalp'.   [49] Abplanalp, 'The Hygienic Value', 42.
[50] Abplanalp, 'Exercising Apparatus'.
[51] Abplanalp, *Slimness and Health*. In a sign of the familiarity of the terminology, even by the early 1930s, Abplanalp described many of his exercises as 'ordinary physical jerks', noting that they might yield 'a youthful shape of figure' when followed diligently. Abplanalp, *Slimness and Health*, 25.

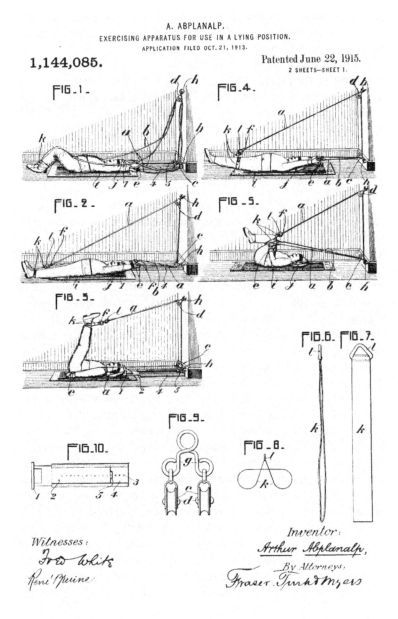

A. ABPLANALP.
EXERCISING APPARATUS FOR USE IN A LYING POSITION.
APPLICATION FILED OCT. 21, 1913.

1,144,085.

Patented June 22, 1915.
2 SHEETS—SHEET 1.

Figure 5.2 Abplanalp's devices were marketed as a way of extending his exercise regimen rather than an essential component.
Source: Arthur Abplanalp, 'Exercising Apparatus for use in a Lying Position', US Patent 1,144,085, 22 June 1915, 1

exercise from 'just another "system of physical jerks"', characterising his approach as both 'scientifically correct' and 'equally suitable for the healthy or the unfit, the young, the middle-aged and the elderly'.[52]

For *Slimness and Health* – a text which was for 'both sexes and all ages' – Abplanalp enlisted L. C. Dundas Irvine to write a foreword, endorsing the system of exercises. We last encountered Dundas Irvine in his capacity as critic of the centrality of atherosclerosis as the principal cause of ageing. In his foreword he identified the broad appeal of the exercises, which might give

benefit to the young who covet the endurance that wins the athletic cup, to the middle-aged who scan with dismay their increasing girth, and to the aged struggling against a fatigue which overcomes them ever earlier in the day.[53]

Abplanalp himself contended that '[n]othing renders the human body more ungraceful, is physiologically more useless and practically more troublesome than a burden of superfluous flesh.'[54] Whilst this might appear at first glance to be a manifestation of the 'cult of reducing', different stages of the life course were a central concern for Abplanalp, as 'when middle age approaches', levels of physical activity had a strong tendency to decline.[55] Physical culture advocates, medical practitioners and exercise gurus were all quick to note the self-evident benefit of continued exercise in later life. However, it is important to recognise that this existed in parallel with the growing popularity of abstention from the strains of modernity, including vigorous exercises. In the short story, *Turn Back the Clock!*, published in 1922 in *Pall Mall Magazine*, Mrs C. N. Williamson drew on a prevailing and delicate interpretation of young womanhood, through which Marian, who had 'taken a delicious rest cure, and looked years younger', was held up as an exemplar of femininity against her now 'elder' sister, Elizabeth, who 'felt a little – just a little – sad'. For Elizabeth, Williamson mused, '[e]verything seemed thoroughly over for her, now that her war-work was done.'[56]

More so, perhaps, than any other method of rejuvenation, the important role posited for highly specific exercise regimes demonstrates the extent to which the building of a healthy, youthful body was a desirable end in the early twentieth century. Even competing systems of vitality – such as the 'Vitalogy' promoted through the middle part of the nineteenth century in the United States by E. H. Ruddock (1822–1875), and perpetuated after his death by an enthusiastic following – acknowledged that bodies were 'made for vigor [*sic*], for the forthputting of all their faculties'.[57] Vitalogy, which emerged in

---

[52] Abplanalp, *In Perfect Shape*, xiii.   [53] Dundas Irvine, 'Foreword', 17.
[54] Abplanalp, *Slimness and Health*, 23.   [55] Ibid.
[56] Williamson, 'Turn Back the Clock!', 238.
[57] Ruddock was scathing in his criticism of '[p]ersons of extraordinary physical strength' who were both 'deficient in general health status [and] . . . short lived.' Ruddock, *Vitalogy*, 873–74.

parallel with new forms of alternative medicine in the latter stages of the nineteenth century, involved the adherence to natural laws of bodily synergy, but was still characterised by its promoters as a 'new science', which gave simple lifestyle instructions about 'how to live indefinitely'.[58] Amongst the sixteen tenets of Vitalogy – emanating from its self-styled 'Life Extension Institute' – was to 'seek out-of-door occupations and recreations ... stand, sit and walk erect, and to work, play, rest and sleep in moderation'.[59]

Rather than being displaced by the advent of hormone therapies, key figures within the physical culture movement continued to emphasise the efficacy of their everyday methods, which sought to promote an extension of the productive portion of life. The heightened profile and popularity of physical culture to extract maximal bodily efficiency was, in its infancy, a response to late nineteenth-century anxieties about decline. However, just as the interwar notoriety of rejuvenation sustained domestic electrotherapy for longer than has been supposed, so too were the gymnastics and calisthenics of celebrity fitness gurus imbued with new relevance in an era which placed increasing value on individual strength and productivity, as well as responsibility for health and vitality. Exercises which could be performed in the privacy of the home, and which demanded no special apparatus, held a broad appeal. For those who sought more highly ritualised, public expressions of athletic youthfulness, dedicated organisations established parallel forms of mass exercise.

"Movement Is Life": Mass Exercise for Young and Old

On 6 February 1937, the English Gymnastic Society staged a demonstration of their activities, in collaboration with a sister organisation from Denmark, at the Royal Albert Hall. Speaking at the event, Lord Dawson of Penn (1864–1945), President of the Royal College of Physicians and Physician-in-Ordinary to George V, addressed the assembled crowd, and noted the 'excellent work of the English Gymnastic Society', where women 'from youth to middle age and of all callings keep fit and young by a recreational training suited to their sex'.[60] Dawson opined that through these exercises women might achieve 'heath, vigour, confidence and content [natural greatness]', with the system on display – developed by Finnish instructor Kristina Elisabeth (Elli) Björkstén and adapted by Gladys Wright – praised for the effect of the 'movements and their beauty'.[61]

---

[58] Ibid., 875.   [59] Ibid., 873.
[60] 'English Gymnastic Society, Albert Hall, February 6th 1937', in 'Physical Training', Wellcome Library, PP/BED/B.3.
[61] Ibid.

Although Dawson's words of encouragement at the demonstration were doubtless well received by the participants, the omissions which he made from an earlier draft are perhaps just as striking. For example, one section which was struck through forcibly in his notes read:

Planning is needed more than generations ago. Then families were large, and the death rate was high and the strong ones did beset in their struggles and so the nation went forward. Now families are small. Unless therefore you secure high quality in these children, you are done. And to secure high quality, needs planning. And remember, in passing, that in their growth children need each other and single-child families mean less good quality and therefore are bad planning.[62]

In his capacity as Major-General in the Royal Army Medical Corps during World War One Dawson had, along with many of his contemporaries, recognised what he perceived to be the poor physical condition of soldiers, reflecting a badly maintained population more generally.[63] Reflecting on this at the annual meeting of the Academy of Physical Medicine in Boston in October 1936, Dawson's belief that physical training could overcome such weakness was evident:

There is a strong effort in this country [the United States] to save men the weakening of physique likely to result from unemployment. Recreative [sic] physical training makes that effort. Twenty-eight such men whose ages ranged between twenty and thirty had four months such training at the Lucas Tooth Gymnasium. A notable improvement in physique, purpose and hope resulted ... Build, movement, balance, grace, rhythm, quick response of body to mind, joyous energy; the result is heartening to look upon.[64]

Dawson reflected wider concerns that unemployment – a topic of profound socio-economic consequences in the Depression-era United States – was having a deleterious effect on the physical condition of working-age men.

For her part, Elli Björkstén (1870–1947), whose exercise regime formed the basis of the 1937 demonstration at the Royal Albert Hall, was a long-standing gymnastics teacher at Helsinki University Gymnasium who had pioneered non-military mass exercise, specifically those 'suitable' for women, from the first decade of the twentieth century. Her two-volume treatise on the subject, *Principles of Gymnastics for Women and Girls*, first appeared in English in 1932, and its continued popularity through the decade coincided with a

---

[62] Ibid.
[63] In a letter to *The Times* in November 1936, for example, Dawson noted with less-than-subtle eugenic undertones that 'the campaign for the bettering of national physique is arousing both interest and support.' Lord Dawson of Penn, 'The National Physique. Leaders of Youth. Good and Bad Breeding', *The Times*, 4 November 1936, in 'Physical Training', Wellcome Library, PP/BED/B.3.
[64] Dawson, 'Physical Education in England'.

dramatic expansion in organised group physical activity for women in Britain.[65] Much attention has been afforded to the Women's League of Health and Beauty (WLHB), established by Mary Bagot Stack in 1930, but that organisation was just one of many which sought to promote the individual, group and national benefits of mass exercise, many of which drew on existing forms of physical culture.

The WLHB may have become the dominant mass exercise force in 1930s Britain, but its origins were in more long-standing, conventional physical therapy. Mary Bagot Stack (1883–1935) had trained at the Institute of Physical Training in London, before establishing her own institution in Manchester, based on largely similar lines. Having visited India, where her daughter, Prunella, was born in 1914, Bagot Stack returned to Britain, taking over the prestigious training school in London formerly run by Mrs Joseph Conn.[66] Critically, the early descriptions of the WLHB referred to 'an international sixpenny health movement for business girls and busy women', calculated to be within financial reach of all, yet clearly demonstrating a conscious effort to target a more affluent, middle-class demographic.[67] At the demonstrations, both Mary and Prunella were held to be exemplars of the system which they practised. Forty-eight-year-old Mary, for example, was described as '[v]ery youthful looking, with marvellous vitality and enthusiasm, she looks years and years younger, and Prunella, who demonstrated some of the exercises, and has been brought up on them almost, is an exceedingly pretty and healthy young girl.'[68]

Membership of the WLHB increased dramatically shortly after its founding. As early as June 1930, in the run-up to the first public demonstration in Hyde Park, the *Leeds Mercury* reported that 'their number is increasing at an astonishing rate.' This was partly attributable to the contrast with '[o]rdinary setting-up exercises' which were 'so dull', but also because of the well-established 'health-and-beauty cult' which was already flourishing 'among the young people of Germany' and in several similar societies already active in Britain.[69] The public display by the WLHB coincided with the removal of an order barring women from bathing in the Serpentine, resulting in 'enormous competition amongst the girls of London' to be the first to swim across the

[65] Björkstén, *Principles of Gymnastics*.
[66] 'Health and Beauty – How to Cultivate and Develop it', *Belfast News-letter*, 6 October 1930, 5. Conn had herself developed a relatively simple, apparatus-free system of exercises, drawing heavily on the ideals of Sir Frederick McCoy, the Irish-born palaeontologist who spent much of his career at the University of Melbourne. See Fendley, 'McCoy, Sir Frederick (1817–1899)'.
[67] 'The Women's League of Health and Beauty. First Meetings in Ireland', *Northern Whig*, 8 October 1930, 6; 'Health for Sixpence', *Northern Whig*, 9 October 1930, 11.
[68] 'Health for Sixpence. Women's League Demonstration in Belfast', *Northern Whig*, 9 October 1930, 11.
[69] 'Health and Beauty', *Leeds Mercury*, 13 June 1930, 4.

water, their numbers notably swelled by WLHB members.[70] Bagot Stack herself was a vociferous and tireless promoter of the organisation, travelling to deliver speeches, invariably accompanied at demonstrations by Prunella.[71] These included return visits to branches such as those set up in Belfast where, just four months after its founding, 'the difficulty was to keep the membership within bounds.'[72]

The exercises promoted by the WLHB reflected both the trend towards calisthenics with limited or no equipment and a self-conscious femininity calculated to emphasise a graceful, effortless athleticism, organised to emulate the military drills so highly prized for men. Nor were these static in nature. Through the 1930s, for example, the exercises underwent significant changes. A twenty-six-second film fragment offers a glimpse into the first public demonstration of the WLHB in Hyde Park. With a brief inter-title proclaiming 'What the Park-keeper winked at! League of Health and Beauty provides a ravishing diversion in Hyde Park', the members of WLHB, watched by spectators filled the surrounding grass banks, performed stretching routines as well as quasi-balletic re-enactments of combat, wielding spears, bows and shields, accompanied by a band of musicians.[73] Subsequent demonstrations, such as those captured in the 1933 short 'Health and Beauty on Parade', which featured '1500 members of Women's League of Health and Beauty in [a] fine "do-this-and-keep-fit" display', also involved marches through the streets, in this case with delegations of WLHB members from branches as far afield as Liverpool, Belfast and Glasgow.[74]

In her accompanying book, *Building the Body Beautiful*, Mary Bagot Stack outlined 'a ten weeks' training course for women and girls ... designed to give the maximum benefit in the minimum of time.'[75] The exercises were, according to a report on the book in *The British Journal of Tuberculosis*, 'designed to assist in the establishment of Health, Grace, and Expression'.[76] The popularity of the WLHB and other forms of physical culture was set against the backdrop of significant discussion about 'modern youth'. As revealed, for example, in a formal debate hosted by the Junior Imperial League on 12 April 1937, it was far from clear whether 'modern youth was gradually becoming indolent and lazy' or if 'every spare moment was ... utilised for evening classes and exercise, showing an honest effort to improve health and mind'.[77] This was a

---

[70] 'Stage Stars in the Park. Who Will Be the First Serpentine Girl?', *Daily Herald*, 14 June 1930, 9.
[71] 'The Social Round – Another New Dance in Prospect', *Belfast News-Letter*, 3 October 1930, 7.
[72] 'The League of Health and Beauty', *Belfast News-letter*, 5 January 1931, 5.
[73] 'League of Health and Beauty Perform'.   [74] 'Health and Beauty on Parade!'
[75] 'Notices of Books', 192.   [76] Ibid.
[77] 'Is Modern Youth Decadent?', article clipping in 'Day Survey Respondent 512, March 1937 – December 1937', April 1937, 8, MOA.

self-conscious mirroring of similar such developments in Germany, recognised from the early 1930s by local press articles. The *Leeds Mercury* noted that, with reference to the early popularity of the WLHB, '[t]he health-and-beauty cult promises to become as powerful in this country as it is among the young people of Germany.'[78]

It is worth considering the extent to which the high-profile activities of the WLHB were genuinely representative of women's experiences of exercise in interwar Britain. Although reports of their demonstrations – capturing and defining female athleticism – were commonplace within the periodical press, daily reality was often very different. For example, Rose Jenkins, a short-hand typist and thirty-three-year-old divorced single mother, noted in her diary during March 1937 that on one particular morning her '[h]ealth [was] not good, due to too much wine the night previous'. When pestered by her seven-year-old son at 7:30 AM to do her morning exercises, she noted, 'I excused myself, by pleading headache.'[79] Over Sunday lunch on 12 September 1937, Theodora Bosanquet, from Hampstead in North West London, conversed with a friend, 'Prof. C.', who noted that 'exercise doesn't have any effect unless one both sweats and pants' and that it was '[h]arder to work up to sweating point in this colder weather.'[80]

The formalisation of morning exercises was, for some, however, highly routinised. On the morning of 12 October 1937, Edgar Hedley woke at 6:30 in the morning, slumbering in his basement room near King's Cross until 7 AM when his first activity on rising was to perform 'four Muller exercises'. This was followed by a 'rubbing exercise' after undressing and 'three more Muller jerks' after bathing.[81] On the same day, upstream on the River Thames in Chertsey, Leslie West left his bedroom 'with the intention of doing one or two physical jerks', only to be thwarted because the adjoining room was full of boxes as they had 'moved in yesterday.'[82] Hedley himself appears to have been a devotee of the Muller system, recording numerous other instances of performing such exercises in both mornings and evenings. Even on Christmas Day in 1937, after being woken at 6:30 in the morning by his three children, eager to share their stocking toys, Hedley did 'a few jerks' before joining his two older offspring to 'heave [his] wife out of bed'.[83]

[78] 'Health and Beauty', *Leeds Mercury*, 13 June 1930, 4.
[79] 'Day Survey Respondent 094', March 1937, 1, MOA.
[80] 'Day Survey Respondent 015, July 1937 – December 1937', 12 September 1937, MOA.
[81] 'Day Survey Respondent 318, August 1937 – April 1938', 12 October 1937, MOA. Hedley's routine – placing his bath in between different exercises – demonstrates that he followed Muller's instructions precisely.
[82] 'Day Survey Respondent 559, October 1937', 12 October 1937, MOA.
[83] 'Day Survey Respondent 318, August 1937 – April 1938', 25 December 1937, 1, MOA.

Indeed, by the late 1930s, it is apparent that J. P. Muller's name had become synonymous with daily exercises. On 1 August 1938, a national Bank Holiday, the junior bank clerk Dennis W. R. Frone of Loughton, Essex, was on a camping trip with his brother, 'a "Muller's Exercise" enthusiast' who 'hardly ever misses a morning without going through "My System".'[84] According to Frone, his brother followed the exercises with such devotion that he started 'snorting like a channel swimmer nearing the shore'; the diarist noted wryly that 'such grampus-like noises are not mentioned in the text-book.'[85]

It is difficult, if not impossible, to determine the exact nature of those physical jerks performed by diarists in their own homes, and the extent to which they aligned with or departed from those laid down by Muller. However, they were typically included in morning routines; Major F. Newhouse, a fifty-four-year-old chartered civil engineer who lived in Twickenham, included 'bath, shave, physical jerks' as his standard pre-breakfast regime (Newhouse also recorded that his breakfast included Yeast-Vite tablets, the supposed rejuvenating properties of which we have already encountered in the context of dietary supplements).[86]

An enquiry into the responses to various advertising topics from December 1938 reveals that the topic of 'national fitness' inspired. These included, from men, references to 'pretty girls; organised youth . . . [and] Health and Beauty', and for women '[k]eep-fit displays . . . Health and Beauty League, [and] [e]xercise without exercises'.[87] National fitness was both a set of grassroots practices designed to promote health and fitness, and a government initiative to cultivate a battle-ready population in the face of increasing German aggression.[88] Whether in the home, at mass demonstrations or as a central pillar of the burgeoning self-help genre, physical culture was a deeply enmeshed feature of British life by the outbreak of World War Two. Indeed, the propaganda film *The Lion Has Wings* – arguably the first such film made – released in late 1939 and produced by Alexander Korda, included mass youth physical culture as one of the exemplars of British civility, alongside bucolic shots of the countryside, cricket and donkey riding.[89]

Sports such as football and tennis continued to be significant features of exercise, yet in contrast to daily personal physical routines, they were rarely

---

84 'Day Survey Respondent 293, August 1937 – September 1938', 1 August 1938, 2, MOA.
85 'Day Survey Respondent 293, August 1937 – September 1938', 1 August 1938, 2, MOA.
86 'Day Survey Respondent 426, September 1937 – August 1938', 17 April 1938, MOA.
87 'Reactions to Advertising', December 1938, A-10, 42, MOA.
88 Zweiniger-Bargielowska, 'Building a British Superman'; Long and Marland, 'From Danger and Motherhood to Health and Beauty'.
89 Lou Alexander, 'BFI Screenonline'. The film was the subject of a mass observation file report in December 1939, when a cross-section of observers were asked to reflect on the meanings and significance of the hour-long film. 'The Lion Has Wings', December 1939, 2, MOA.

invoked by contemporary commentators as a means of achieving renewed youthfulness. Such activities were undertaken with social as much as health-related intentions, yet also for the 'sake of necessary exercise', as was the case with a game of tennis enjoyed in August 1937 by William Weleman, a student resident in Maida Vale who enjoyed 'perfectly satisfactory' overall health.[90] However, tellingly, at least some men, such as Boris Ford, were at pains to note that, in the case of a game of tennis, 'even this, spread over an hour, can be quite a manly enough exercise.'[91]

In her diary entries from autumn 1937, Naomi Mitchison, who described her health as 'singularly good for a woman of 39 who has borne six children', recalled the centrality of exercise in the restorative regimes practised at Norbury House Hotel, a 'very modern' spa hotel in the Worcestershire town of Droitwich Spa, and which hosted the St Andrew's Brine Baths.[92] On the morning of 12 November, she visited the on-site doctor's consulting room where she demonstrated her 'curative exercises' with the aid of a 'cheerful, upright, blonde expertress, who puts them right'.[93] This was followed by a morning at the brine baths, 'swimming and doing exercises', surrounded by other bathers and 'occasionally people showing one another how to do exercises'.[94]

Eugenic ideals, emphasising the necessity of a healthy youth, were as important a motivating factor as any in the expansion of mass exercise during the interwar period. It may seem paradoxical, however, that even those at the vanguard of the eugenic movement in Britain, such as C. J. Bond, acknowledged that 'an open-air life, regular exercise, and military training' might alleviate some of the 'defects' which had been identified in the 1917–18 report of Sir James Galloway's Commission, suggesting a quasi-Lamarckian model underpinning his eugenics.[95] In the 1928 Galton Lecture, Bond, a senior surgeon at Leicester Royal Infirmary, argued that the 'future of the race' depended on 'the possession of qualities of mind and body which will enable a people to respond to the good and to resist the bad influences in the environment'.[96] The ability of individuals to observe proper regimes of

---

[90] 'Day Survey Respondent 557, August 1937 – December 1938', 12 August 1937, 7, MOA. On some occasions, rather than restoring youthfulness, outdoor pursuits and sports were described in skin care adverts as the source of prematurely aged skin, largely due to sun damage (see Chapter 6).

[91] 'Day Survey Respondent 287, July 1937 – September 1937', 13 September 1937, 3, MOA.

[92] 'Droitwich Development Committee. Droitwich Spa Brine Baths and Medical Trust', c.1935, Worcestershire Archive and Archaeology Service, Worcester (WAAS), 3891/2/2; 'Droitwich Development Committee. Droitwich Spa Brine Baths and Medical Trust', 1936, WAAS, 3891/2/1; 'Brine Baths Closed for Good'.

[93] 'Day Survey Respondent 123, September 1937 – September 1938', 12 November 1937, 8, MOA.

[94] Ibid.   [95] Bond, 'Causes of Racial Decay', 10.   [96] Bond, 'Causes of Racial Decay', 18.

physical culture, therefore, lay at the heart of eugenic systems of racial renewal. This was, in the first instance, imagined to be a feature of youth and young adults, but it also spoke to a deeper underlying concern with the fitness of the population at large, including both young and old.

The rejuvenating exercises practised and promoted in the 1930s were of two broad kinds: those designed for specific age groups and others which were held as being universally applicable at any age. Frequently, though not exclusively, everyday tasks and physical activity were considered part of the latter. As H. C. Hopkinson, columnist for the physical culture magazine *New Health*, commented in 1936, '[l]arge numbers of septuagenarians still acquit themselves well in the hunting field, while among the poorer classes it is nothing unusual for men of over eighty to do many a hard day's digging in the garden.'[97]

At the same time, proponents of exercise regimes were keen to highlight the malleability of their programmes to the needs of all. In 1928, Lord Meston, former Secretary of the Finance Department of the Government of India, attended the opening of the twenty-fourth session of the British Institute of Physical Training (BIPT). The Institute, based at the Swedish Hall in London, promoted a system of physical jerks, suitable for all ages. In his address, Meston recounted his own experience of Vichy treatment and an encounter with 'a man who had had the monkey gland operation', noted their inferiority when compared to 'Major Cruden's rejuvenating exercises, because they are far better and renew our youth far more.'[98] George Cruden, an Aberdeen-based lawyer, had established a Physical Training College in the late nineteenth century, and the system of exercises which he promoted had gained a significant following, persisting into the interwar period.[99] Critically, however, the report on the activities of the BIPT noted that the ages of the pupils ranged from ten to seventy-eight, and amongst those participating in the exercises was a 'grandmother, . . . her daughter, and her grand-daughter, and the grandmother touched her toes and swung her Indian clubs and marched on her toes as gracefully as any young girl.'[100]

According to testimonials printed in promotional pamphlets for the BIPT, the exercises on offer, through classes, were suitable 'if you are Seventeen or Seventy years old'. Specific 'Classes for the Middle Aged' highlighted the attempts which Cruden made to appeal to a wide range of potential subscribers.[101] Other participants in the classes noted that, in common

---

[97] Hopkinson, 'Exercise for the Elderly', 26, in 'Old Age etc. (Third Series)', 1919–1955, PP/ FPW/B.7/3/1, Wellcome Library.

[98] 'Physical Jerks. Better than Monkey Glands', *The Scotsman*, 6 October 1928, 13.

[99] Thompson, 'The Acceptance of a National Policy for Physical Education', iv.

[100] 'Physical Jerks', *The Scotsman*, 6 October 1928, 13.   [101] Cruden, *The British Institute*, 14.

with attempts to move away from the 'formal, static and sombre' exercises favoured by the Swedish physical educator Pehr Ling (1776–1839), which had proven highly influential in German systems of physical culture from the 1840s, the BIPT provided also a 'cheery atmosphere . . . rather than a doleful, painful duty'.[102]

Many of the most prominent physical culture therapists, perhaps unsurprisingly, were quick to assert that their clients and those who had benefitted from following regimes of physical culture reached across the generations. Typical amongst these was T. W. Standwell, self-styled as a 'Consulting Specialist in Physical Culture and Dietetics' and, in 1950, 'Britain's foremost health consultant' who had 'specialised for over 30 years in the drugless treatment of nervous disorders in men, women, and children'.[103] In a promotional book likely published in the immediate aftermath of World War Two, *Do You Desire Health?*, Standwell asserted that '[t]here is practically no age limit' on his treatments. Indeed, for him it was 'a fallacy to consider that exercises should be given up when one reaches the age between 40 and 50.'[104] Critically, and in common with many other practitioners, Standwell highlighted the importance of tailoring exercises to life stage; 'movements must be adapted not only to age, but to physical condition.'[105]

Just as individual recipients of glandular therapy, successful dieters and domestic users of electrotherapy devices were celebrated for their devotion and resulting rejuvenated states, so too were older adherents of physical culture regimes held up as examples to follow. Emulating the transformational narratives of Eugen Sandow and Bernarr Macfadden, E. H. Ruddock's *Vitalogy* from 1929 recounted the case of 'Captain Diamond of San Francisco' who, at the age of 107, 'taught a class in physical culture and claimed to be able to walk 20 miles in a day without undue fatigue', despite having been 'weak and near the end' at the age of 70.[106]

Frederick L. Hoffman, who we encountered previously as an advocate of moderate eating habits, especially in those over the age of fifty, reserved special praise for appropriate physical activity in promoting longevity. For Hoffman, '[n]othing is more important than to keep the bodily machine in the best possible physical condition through wholesome recreational and physical

---

[102] Ibid., 19.   [103] 'Personal', *Birmingham Daily Gazette*, 21 January 1950, 2.

[104] Standwell, *Do You Desire Health?*, in 'Sexual Behaviour, 1939–1950', 12-16-C, 31, MOA.

[105] Ibid. Standwell's credentials in treating nervous diseases were established through his involvement in treating cases of shell shock arising from World War One. See Reid, *Broken Men*, 107–08. Standwell appears to be another example of a leading physical culture proponent who shaped practices through involvement in publishing. As others have noted, between 1930 and 1941 he published *The Superman*, a periodical which was devoted to finding and promoting 'men physically fit, Spartan in habit, who will not destroy the body with an excess of food, tobacco and alcohol'. Koureas, *Memory, Masculinity and National Identity*, 133.

[106] Ruddock, *Vitalogy*, 876–77.

exercise rather than through athletics or sports and pastimes which involve the risk of overstrain.'[107] This reflected broader anxieties, particularly amongst those who endorsed systems of physical jerks and individual and mass stretches, that those older men and women who participated in unregulated, unpredictable forms of exercise might be placing themselves at greater risk of physical damage.

The rejuvenation promised by advocates of physical jerks was both internal and external. Adherents could render their physiology more youthful, banish disease and infirmity, and also restore their external appearance and aesthetic to that of a younger person. Publications, including manuals and magazines, celebrated the physique of rejuvenated followers of these regimes, hailing individuals as emblems of dedication and purity. However, whilst the restoration of youthful good health was fundamental, presenting a rejuvenated body was by no means a subordinate aim. Nevertheless, there was a particular form of physical therapy – facial massage – which had as its primary goal the restoration of youthful good looks. Practised by almost all leading beauty culturists in the early twentieth century, we turn now to consider the significance of this hybrid form of 'treatment' which straddled the approaches of whole-body exercise and skin care.

The "Decrepitude of Furrows": Beauty Culture, Exercise and Massage

Writing on 'Ageing of the Skin' in a credible mainstream textbook on *Problems of Ageing*, published in 1939, Fred D. Weidman claimed that,

[i]f there is any part of the human body which literally thrusts the evidence of its advancing years upon whomsoever may look, it is the skin. A child knows the significance of wrinkles, gray hair and baldness. ... [E]mployers and prospective husbands and wives have learned to call upon the skin as the indicator in respect to youth.[108]

The celebration of physique in many manuals and periodicals emerging from the physical culture movement was not restricted to the bodies of athletic, lithe and youthful men and women. The face was considered a key site of possible rejuvenatory potential, with clear signs which might – notwithstanding a Romanesque figure hidden behind garments – reveal the 'true' age in an act of physiological betrayal. As well as the application of different products to the skin, considered in the following chapter, the use of facial exercises became an important mainstay of the arsenal of would-be rejuvenators. Manufacturers of these products almost universally recognised the importance of essential

---

[107] Hoffman, *Some Problems of Longevity*, vi.   [108] Weidman, 'Ageing of the Skin', 339.

preparatory steps in everyday hygienic practice; as Boots commented in their training manual for in-store demonstrators, '[t]he condition of the skin depends so much upon the whole process of living, a correct diet, a normal amount of suitable exercise, adequate rest, the care of internal conditions, and personal hygiene.'[109] Failure to follow these would render even the most advanced and expensive cosmetic or skin care products ineffective. Meanwhile, beauty advice columns in newspapers and women's magazines throughout Britain emphasised the inseparable effects of skin care products and their physical mode of application. In an article on 'stocking the beauty cupboard' in the *Lincolnshire Echo* in early 1935, for example, the anonymous author noted the benefits of astringent tonics for youthful radiant skin, but only 'if it is applied in conjunction with the correct facial massage and exercises'.[110]

As Jessica P. Clark has noted, the parallel emergence of beauty culture and physical culture in the late nineteenth century gave rise to facial massage as a key weapon in the fight against the appearance of signs of ageing.[111] Such physical manipulation was radically reconfigured in the interwar period in light of a social preoccupation with rejuvenation and youthfulness, even in the teeth of the Great Depression. On 1 January 1930, the prestigious women's magazine *The Bystander* carried a quarter-page advert for the Phyllis Earle's hairdressing services. 'Assisted by every scientific improvement', the establishment at 32 Dover Street in West London offered not just hairdressing but 'Inecto recoloration [*sic*] of grey hair, facial massage, manicure, chiropody and electrolysis'.[112] As well as the signs of ageing, the treatment promised to remove '[d]isfiguring blemishes or similar defects', highlighting the conflation of beauty with youthfulness.[113]

The campaign from Phyllis Earle – whose Institut de Beauté was a key feature the London beauty marketplace – continued throughout 1930 across a range of other high-profile periodicals, including *The Sketch*, *Punch* and *The Tatler*.[114] As well as high-profile purveyors of facial massage, local beauty culturists, such as Madame Kennard from Rugby and Miss A. H. Kendrick from Tamworth, also offered comparable services, often alongside violet ray treatments.[115] The regular contributor to the *Hull Daily Mail*, 'Babette', noted that, although '[g]irls in business have not too much time to spare

[109] 'Beauty Treatment Paper No. 1. Activities of Staff Training School and Demonstrators', 1938, WBA/BT/5/34/1/4, Boots Company Archive, 1.
[110] 'Stocking the Beauty Cupboard', *Lincolnshire Echo*, 7 January 1935, 3.
[111] Clark, 'Pomeroy v. Pomeroy'; Clark, '"Clever ministrations"'; Clark, *The Business of Beauty*.
[112] 'Hairdressing by Phyllis Earle', *The Bystander*, 1 January 1930, 61.
[113] 'Facial Massage', *The Sketch*, 19 March 1930, 59.
[114] 'Hairdressing by Phyllis Earle', *The Sketch*, 8 January 1930, 46; 'Hairdressing', *The Bystander*, 22 January 1930, 59.
[115] 'Women and Appearance', *Tamworth Herald*, 18 January 1930, 5; 'Miscellaneous', *Rugby Advertiser*, 17 January 1930, 6.

for facial massage[,] ... Hull is particularly well equipped with beauty parlours and salons.'[116] As well as facial massage, the proprietors of such establishments also offered 'throat massage' alongside treatments for the face and scalp, promising restoration of a youthful neck through physical therapy; many proudly declared that they used products from leading beauty magnates such as Helena Rubinstein.[117] The proliferation of small-scale, independent beauty culture specialists was conducted through and enabled by the extensive classified advertisement columns which expanded dramatically in the interwar period.[118]

Although facial massage itself was not a new feature of rejuvenation-linked practices, the specific techniques of massage became increasingly specific; this was equally the case for beauty culture practitioners and those who sought to apply these methods domestically. For example, in addition to the 'stroking, palming, rotating, digging into the muscles' which had been advocated previously, a new method from 'a famous beauty specialist' in Paris consisted of 'quick, light-fingered pinching, not rolling.'[119] The details of this particular method – communicated to readers of the *Yorkshire Evening Post* – were far more specific, and typical of instructions to women as to how they should undertake such routines:

The pinching and nipping should be quick, brisk and forceful. Begin under the chin, working both hands at once. Travel along the line of the jaw bone out to the ears. Come back to the chin again, and follow a line slightly higher. Then again on the chin, galloping up to the temples. It's fun.[120]

Discussion over the correct or optimum method of facial massage within the periodical press reveals substantial divergence. The rapid pinching, supposedly a cutting-edge method favoured in Paris – the European centre of beauty culture innovation in this period, revered within the British press – vied with 'the sharp vertical pat or slap guaranteed to bring up a glow of circulation, and replace worn tissues'.[121]

In some quarters, facial massage was highlighted as not just a typical but an essential part of women's armoury against the creeping signs of old age. In an uncompromising assessment, the regular beauty columnist of the *Northern Daily Mail*, reprinted in the *Northern Whig*, recorded that as a woman neared

---

[116] Babette, 'The Up-to-date Beauty Parlour' *The Daily Mail*, 21 March 1931, 6.
[117] 'Medical & Nursing', *West London Observer*, 14 February 1930, 14; 'Hairdressing', *Western Morning News*, 4 March 1930, 1; 'Binns' Service Week', *Hartlepool Northern Daily Mail*, 10 March 1930, 1; 'General Notices', *The Scotsman*, 15 March 1930, 1; 'Facial Massage and Beauty Culture', *Eastbourne Gazette*, 9 July 1930, 3.
[118] Cocks, *Classified*.   [119] 'Nipping for Beauty', *Yorkshire Evening Post*, 17 June 1930, 5.
[120] Ibid.
[121] 'How to Retain Health and Beauty', *Hampshire Telegraph and Post*, 15 August 1930, 24.

the age of fifty, she should 'decide once and for all whether she will grow old – or grow young!'[122] If the latter, it was critical to adopt 'the far less interesting lemon water, coffee, and dry biscuits' in place of pastries, exercise 'must be started at once' and facial massage was 'essential to remove the tiny wrinkles that have crept under the eyes, and to stimulate the tired muscles of the throat and face.'[123] Such perspectives exhibit an inherent tension: on the one hand, women were encouraged to mollify the signs of age, whilst on the other, they were reminded that there were limits to what might be achievable or desirable, as 'a picturesque disorder, charming in a young girl, becomes merely "messy" in a matron.'[124]

The object of these exercises was threefold: to remove fine lines, prevent the sagging of skin and 'correct any tendency to that nightmare of middle-age, a double chin'.[125] The facial massage was considered an important means of stimulating the 'formation of healthy new tissue' in the layer of fat under the skin.[126] For all that many advertisements trumpeted the affordability and efficacy of facial massage for a wide range of potential clients, the emphasis on the necessary precision of the treatment enabled some beauty commentators to recommend alternatives. Given that massage was expensive and had the potential to be 'definitely harmful', argued a beauty column across multiple major local newspapers in October 1937, readers who wished to preserve their complexions should instead employ 'a new beauty roller which rolls away wrinkles and lines, making the skin clear and healthy, radiating vitality ... banishing flabbiness, and restoring the face to its youthful contour'.[127]

The use of facial massage as a means of overcoming the signs of older age was by no means confined to women. As reported in their regular column 'Beauty Aids to Success' in March 1930, a representative from the *Daily Herald* made 'illuminating discoveries' that '[m]en are no longer content to grow old and wrinkled and grey ... [and] that it was now quite usual for men clients to have facial massage.'[128] The perception of massage as an appropriate and desirable form of physical therapy for men was enhanced during this period as a result of its successful application in cases of rehabilitation of war-wounded soldiers where it was used to 'restore wasted muscles and bring back to life useless limbs'.[129]

[122] 'At 50! Are you Growing Old or Young?', *Northern Daily Mail*, 14 October 1930, 2. This was reprinted as 'Her Infinite Variety. When She Is Fifty', *Northern Whig*, 29 October 1930, 11.
[123] 'At 50! Are you Growing Old or Young?', *Northern Daily Mail*, 14 October 1930, 2.
[124] 'At 50! Are you Growing Old or Young?', *Northern Daily Mail*, 14 October 1930, 2.
[125] 'Beauty Secrets from the East', *The Scotsman*, 13 March 1931, 5.
[126] 'Our Ladies' Page. Banishing Wrinkles', *Bournemouth Graphic*, 20 March 1931, 11.
[127] 'A Beauty Roller', *Sheffield Daily Independent*, 27 October 1931, 9; 'Help Yourself to Beauty', *Birmingham Gazette*, 30 October 1931, 4.
[128] 'Beauty Aids to Success. Wrinkles That Lose Man His Job', *Daily Herald*, 17 March 1930, 15.
[129] 'What Is Massage?', *Airdrie and Coatbridge Advertiser*, 22 March 1930, 7.

Nor were the links between employment and age restricted to men. In a lecture to the London College of Physiology in March 1930, Miss Stennings, the 'well-known "beauty expert"', argued that

City life does tend in the long-run to create paleness after a girl as reached, say, the age of twenty. The City air, the warm and sometimes muggy offices in which they work may attack a girl's complexion if she does not spend her hours of leisure in the open and in healthful exercise.[130]

The remainder of the lecture was devoted to the most appropriate make-up for business and leisure, yet for these hints and tips to be effective, 'moderate exercise in the fresh air' and 'gentle facial massage' were absolute necessities.[131]

When Boots launched their Number Seven range of skin care products in 1935, later joined by cosmetics, they produced a series of accompanying brochures and pamphlets about the new series, and about skin care in general. As well as maintaining a regular and consistent skin care regime, many of these highlighted 'a normal amount of suitable exercise' and facial massage as other means of achieving 'the preservation of natural Beauty' (see Figure 5.3).[132] Exercising, without overtaxing, muscles of the face was an important pillar of interwar beauty culture, applying ideas from whole-body exercise to retain the elasticity of the skin into older age.

Whilst massage was undoubtedly the preserve of the beauty specialist in this period, it was not exclusively located within that domain of expertise. On 12 July 1937, for example, P. Bibbings, who supplied specialist stationery to Cardiff Royal Infirmary, noted in his discussion of the 'very strong class distinction in the Hospital' that the stratification of status included 'Medical and Massage students'.[133] On the very same morning Mary Clayton, who was undergoing a course of 'electrical treatment (Faradism)' three times each week, was waiting in the 'massage department' at her local hospital near Battersea alongside another patient with arthritis who had 'given up hoping for miracles'.[134] Physical and electrical therapy were closely related and, in some cases, were united in single devices, notably electric vibrators which mobilised the force of electricity in the service of massage. In 1937, the manufacturers of the new model of the Pifco electric vibrator used promotional materials aimed at retailers to exhort the virtues of their product in promoting 'assimilation, . . . the circulation of the blood in the skin and the pores lying beneath'.[135]

---

[130] 'The Art of Make-up' Airdrie and Coatbridge Advertiser, 22 March 1930, 7.
[131] 'The Foundation of Beauty', Airdrie and Coatbridge Advertiser, 22 March 1930, 7.
[132] 'Beauty', 1935, 1, WBA/BT/11/40/4/1/1, Boots Archive.
[133] 'Day Survey Respondent 214, July 1937 – September 1938', 12 July 1937, 1–2, MOA.
[134] 'Day Survey Respondent 031, July 1937 – September 1938', 12 July 1937, 5, MOA.
[135] 'Pifco (new model) Electric Vibrator', Merchandise Bulletin, 27 September 1937, 5400.

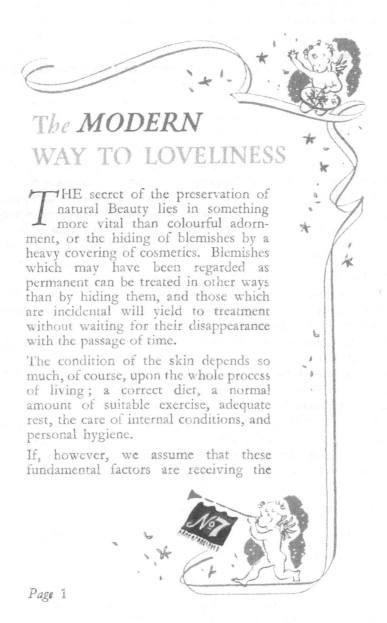

The MODERN
WAY TO LOVELINESS

THE secret of the preservation of natural Beauty lies in something more vital than colourful adornment, or the hiding of blemishes by a heavy covering of cosmetics. Blemishes which may have been regarded as permanent can be treated in other ways than by hiding them, and those which are incidental will yield to treatment without waiting for their disappearance with the passage of time.

The condition of the skin depends so much, of course, upon the whole process of living; a correct diet, a normal amount of suitable exercise, adequate rest, the care of internal conditions, and personal hygiene.

If, however, we assume that these fundamental factors are receiving the

Page 1

Figure 5.3 Brochures outlining beauty regimes often contextualised these within a broader sweep of lifestyle habits which were also said to influence the complexion.
Source: 'Beauty', 1935, 1, WBA/BT/11/40/4/1/1, Boots Company Archive

In addition to its manifestation within mainstream medical practice, massage carried out by beauty culturists was in some senses an unremarkable daily activity. Recording her activities on 12 August 1937 as comprising a 'fairly typical day', Laura Chamberlin, who adjudicated requests for public assistance for London County Council, paused on her return home at Charing Cross Station and 'rang up [a] "beauty culture specialist" to make an appointment for a face massage on Saturday morning'.[136] Such activity reflected earlier advertising which claimed that 'a good Facial Massage is not a luxury so much as a real necessity' given that soap and water alone cannot 'tone, soften, and rejuvenate the skin and complexion'.[137] Others noted the proliferation of 'the usual manicure and facial massage', almost always advertised alongside the hugely fashionable 'permanent wave', highlighting the ubiquity of such treatments.[138]

The everyday environment of the beauty parlour, far from constituting a joyful space, was largely a serious one. As 'Prunella', the fashion correspondent of *The News*, noted in May 1930, 'I used to think a dentist's surgery was the most melancholy rendezvous ever invented. That was before I became a beauty parlour client.'[139] In a column which appeared alongside 'special exercise hints for ladies' by John Gravener, Prunella recounted that whilst being 'massaged beneath the chin ... the attendant nymphs in the modern Temple of Venus' were singularly dismissive of humour or light-heartedness on their premises, and especially during treatments.[140] The proliferation of possible treatments, for both women and men, was the subject of some controversy, with a widely circulated sketch in local newspapers from December 1939 wryly noting that one barber persuaded a male customer to have not just a shave but also 'a haircut, shampoo, facial massage, singe, seafoam, electric buzz, tar spray, and tonic rub', by which time 'he needed another shave!'[141]

The expanse and prevalence of such rejuvenating physical beauty therapies was also reflected in advice columns for women in both newspapers and magazines; 'every woman under 50 is trying to look like a girl of 17', chided the *Belfast Telegraph* in an article from March 1936.[142] Similarly,

---

[136] 'Day Survey Respondent 026, June 1937 – November 1937', 12 August 1937, 2 and 5, MOA.
[137] 'The Beauty Parlour', *Hartlepool Northern Daily Mail*, 2 April 1930, 6.
[138] 'Table Talk. The Cult for Dyed Eyelashes', *The News*, 5 June 1931, 12; 'Fashions. Hairdressing', *Yorkshire Post*, 11 August 1931, 1; 'Bubbling Over with Love', *Motherwell Times*, 11 September 1931, 1.
[139] Prunella, 'Seeking Beauty', 19.
[140] Prunella, 'Seeking Beauty', 19; Gravener, 'How to Keep Your Health', 19.
[141] 'Needed Another', *Lincolnshire Free Press*, 25 December 1939, 10.
[142] Far from being a critique of such practices, the article very swiftly moved to offer advice to women about how they might make use of what they termed 'facial "jerks" ... to ward off, for a few years at least, this encroaching horror of old age'. Such exercises included both stretches to ensure that the backbone remained supple as well as simple movements to avoid sagging of the tissue around the cheeks and throat. 'Warding Off Age. Hints on Keeping Young', *Belfast Telegraph*, 28 March 1936, 5.

manufacturers of even the most humble of products, such as toilet soaps, sought to persuade consumers that these inexpensive bathroom essentials could confer the benefits of more costly beauty treatments. A major advertising campaign for Eve toilet soap during early 1937 claimed that every wash could be made 'a complete facial massage [to] refresh your skin, tone up the tissues, renew your youthful loveliness'.[143]

As well as using particular products, or visiting a specialist, to achieve a rejuvenated state, beauty columns also advised women how best to replicate these effects for themselves. In this respect the social practices of mass beauty therapy – in the salon – had a domestic analogue in much the same fashion as the mass physical culture organisations had theirs in the form of morning exercises. In her provocatively titled article, 'One Chin Is Enough!', the beauty writer Jane Jacquin described massages which she claimed could produce 'a stimulating and rejuvenating effect' on 'fleshy chins', as well as advocating the use of '[a]n elastic chin strap . . . [to] hold the muscles of the face and chin in firm contour'.[144] The supposed motivation for women, so the advertising materials and 'self-help' literature claimed, was, as Jane Turner put it writing about facial massage in the *Sussex Express* in 1935, 'a special desire to feel one's best'.[145] This was, as we shall see in the following chapter, entirely typical of exhortations at the time, with a strong emphasis on rejuvenation and beauty culture as a fundamental aspect of womanly duty.

Whilst the numerous contrivances and contraptions designed to alleviate sagging skin around the neck might perhaps best be regarded as historical relics, both facial massage and the many closely related modes of applying skin care products endured as a legacy of the period. For example, an internal Boots promotional pamphlet from the mid-1960s reminded store assistants that

[a]lmost as important as using the correct preparation for each type of skin is applying the preparation in the right way. Basically, the movement should always be an upward one. This helps life the skin, keeping it firmer and younger looking – and looks much more attractive in the process![146]

Many of these practices of physical therapy relied on the harmonious interaction between skin product and mode of application. However, some of the most high-profile figures in beauty culture during the interwar period also

[143] 'While Her Complexion Is Still Soft and Lovely. . .', *Daily Herald*, 23 March 1937, 9. For another example from this campaign, see 'Now – While She Is Still Lovely', *Belfast Telegraph*, 28 April 1937, 14.

[144] Jane Jacquin, 'One Chin Is Enough!', *The News*, 2 August 1935, 14. The article was published across numerous local newspapers. Jane Jacquin, 'One Chin Is Enough!', *Linlithgowshire Gazette*, 2 August 1935, 6.

[145] Jane Turner, 'Christmas Topics and Tips. Face Massage', *Sussex Express*, 20 December 1935, 23.

[146] 'A Guide to Selling Beauty: Number Seven', c.1965, 17, WBA/BT/11/34/2/1, Boots Archive.

sought to establish their expertise in the domain of exercise in its own right, none more so than Elizabeth Arden.[147] In 1924, keen to capitalise on in-salon exercises which had proved to be popular, Arden issued an eighteen-page pamphlet, *The Elizabeth Arden Exercises for Health and Beauty*, which outlined the key principles of six core exercises which would 'keep every tissue functioning gaily and eagerly …[,] set the blood to dancing like an elixir of spring in your veins … [and] keep the keen lines of youth in your figure – and the joy of youth in your heart'.[148] The six exercises in question cut across a broad swathe of scientific perspectives on the causes underpinning premature ageing and ill health. For example, drawing on popular theories of intestinal stasis derived from Elié Metchnikoff, Arden claimed that 'effete matter filling the intestines sends ugly toxins through the system to dull the mind and cause depression; to poison the blood … and lay the body open to infection and ills.'[149] Although basic sketches of the exercises appeared in the brochure, the overwhelming focus of the content was the rationale and purpose underpinning them. Indeed, it is difficult to imagine how a reader previously unfamiliar with this set of exercises would have been able to perform them without seeking further information; the intention was therefore perhaps to encourage a visit to Arden's salon rather than to enable the practice of the exercises in the privacy of one's home, an approach which contrasted sharply with that of J. P. Müller.

Legacy and Conclusion

In 1960, Roland Evin Hovarth, author and health-food writer, noted that 'exercise is slowly becoming a necessary daily practice in order to achieve rejuvenation of your physical and mental systems.'[150] He was, of course, conveniently ignoring a lengthy history of exercises whose promoters had claimed for them to have rejuvenating effects on body and mind. Hovarth had his own agenda: to enhance his priority claim over a system of exercise which was suitable for 'men and women of any age', and which should last for at least one hour each day after the age of twenty, as 'anything less will result in physical deterioration', notwithstanding the highly significant and diverse contributions of his forerunners.[151]

---

[147] A fuller consideration of Arden's career and skin care products is reserved for the following chapter. Suffice to say here that by the late 1920s Arden – Florence Nightingale Graham (1878–1966) – had established her company, underpinned to a large extent by her own image as the archetypal American beauty, as a leading international house of beauty culture. For a lucid and entertaining account of Arden's life and professional activities, and in particular her rivalry with Helena Rubinstein, see Woodhead, *War Paint*.

[148] *The Elizabeth Arden Exercises*, 2.   [149] Ibid., 6.

[150] Hovarth, 'The Key to Rejuvenation', 36.   [151] Hovarth, 'The Key to Rejuvenation', 39.

Public manifestations of exercise in the interwar period, whether mass physical culture, sport or more singular facial massage, have attracted considerably more scholarly attention than domestic practices.[152] In her writing on the place of yoga within the activities of The Women's League of Health and Beauty, Patricia Vertinsky has argued that these specific practices became increasingly aligned with 'the national imperatives of fitness regimentation' and detached from the aspects of yoga which promoted bodily freedom and autonomy.[153] On this reading, the initial focus of the WLHB on female emancipation gradually gave way to a pragmatic alignment of bodies with racial fitness and national security. However, as I have explored here, when we examine the attitudes of this organisation with an appreciation for the body as a four- as well as three-dimensional entity – intimately connected with temporality – a rather different picture emerges. Instead, we see that from its very inception the WLHB promoted a form of physical culture which emphasised the importance of youthfulness as a key feature of successful femininity. Their message was sufficiently effective that, despite the assertion emerging from mass observation during World War Two that 'the youth movement as it existed before the war has been completely smashed', including opportunities for getting 'any fresh air and exercise', the WLHB continued actively thereafter.[154]

Similarly, whilst Ina Zweiniger-Bargielowska has shown convincingly that the relationship between 'manliness, physical fitness and patriotism in interwar Britain' was cemented by physical culture, the acknowledged importance of youth movements and ideals in her narrative is cast generally in sociopolitical rather than demographic or biological terms.[155] The impact of mass displays of male and female athletic prowess also served to throw into sharp relief the imperative for the older generations and the prematurely aged to aspire to a state of physical rejuvenation. As a consequence, the activities of the WLHB arguably also fanned the flames of commercial enterprises which promised quick, painless and private rejuvenation of the body.[156] The advice of physical culture magnates such as Sanford Bennett, Bernarr Macfadden and Eugen

---

[152] One of the most prominent exercise systems of the nineteenth century, developed by Per Henrik Ling, was invariably presented by authors as a means of coordinating physical education in schools and other institutions. The American physician Mathias Roth, who was based at the Hahnemann Hospital in Philadelphia, argued that the Ling system should be 'introduced with the greatest advantage into every school and seminary ... [as] part of sound and good education'. Roth, *Movements or Exercises*, i.

[153] Vertinsky, '"Building the Body Beautiful"', 535.

[154] 'Clubs: 1940–41 (and Church)', 51-2-I, in 'YOUTH 1937–1943', MOA, 2.

[155] Zweiniger-Bargielowska, 'Building a British Superman', 596.

[156] As we saw in earlier chapters, many products which claimed to exert rejuvenatory effects on the body demanded an occasional physical discomfort, or at least invasion of the body, often under the gaze of an attendant.

Sandow was variously recognised as being of a practical, sensible nature and dismissed for 'the erotic appeal' inherent in their narratives of masculinity and 'vitality'.[157] Against all of these, however, was the emergence of an extensive, private, domestic culture of rejuvenating exercises and physical beauty therapies, practised in the home and often drawing on longer-established methods such as those of J. P. Müller.

Critically, exercise provided both the means and motivation for achieving a renewed or continuing state of youthfulness both within and on the surface of the body. As Charlotte Macdonald has put it, '[i]n the language of health and beauty was a language of inner vitality and outer radiance, a modern formulation of the individual as a "self" equipped to embrace the exciting but uncertain possibilities of the "modern world".'[158] The pursuit of structured exercise regimes, whether privately or en masse, served to enhance the desirability of youth, whilst simultaneously offering both men and women a route for realising these ambitions and an indicator of success. Additionally, we can see clearly in the activities described in this chapter the origins of contemporary movements such as active ageing. The imperative to remain mobile and engage in activities designed to keep the body in motion at regular intervals were fundamental to regimes of rejuvenatory exercise in the interwar period. The highly specific routines which became especially popular with self-proclaimed exercise specialists served to reinforce the importance of practising such regimes under supervision, exerting a correspondingly greater control over bodies, even through the medium of text. Concerns about unhealthy, unproductive and prematurely aged bodies stemmed from nineteenth-century anxieties over human degeneration and World War One, and were exacerbated by Depression-era economic hardship and the revitalised physical prowess of Germanic youth. As a consequence, exercise became a focal point for addressing socio-economic struggles, with the aim being nothing less than the restoration of a superior state of physical and mental productivity in both young and old.

As Susan Grant has argued for the same period, physical culture was itself a central feature of the Soviet project from the outset.[159] Meanwhile, individuals such as Bernarr Macfadden and Eugen Sandow cultivated an international following, and their claims to expertise expanded far beyond exercise regimes; Macfadden even self-published the *Physical Culture Cook-book* in 1932.[160] By focussing on British appropriation of and responses to rejuvenating physical culture in the 1930s, we see an apparent contradiction: the practice was both held up as a national enterprise and recognised as a feature inseparable

---

[157] Fishbein, *The Medical Follies*, 173.   [158] Macdonald, 'Body and Self'.

[159] Grant, *Physical Culture and Sport*; Grant, 'Bolsheviks, Revolution and Physical Culture'.

[160] Macfadden, *Physical Culture Cook Book*.

from other national contexts, especially Germany under National Socialism. At the same time, in line with Broderick D. V. Chow's observations, physical culture was itself 'an *anxious* performance of masculinity'.[161] By recognising that these practices were intimately aligned with the aged and ageing body, we see that such anxiety was not limited to masculinity, but stemmed from a keenly felt sense of decline in both men and women.

Facial exercises too became an essential part of maintaining a youthful look, reflecting a rise in the scientisation of beauty regimes. In Chapter 6, we will see how care for the body extended to presenting a more youthful face to the world. As well as creating a rejuvenated physiological state, with a 'younger' body, the interwar period also witnessed the development of a mass market for products which claimed to cover, remove or replace the effects of ageing on the skin, or induce the skin to resist the onset of older age. In this enterprise, manufacturers drew extensively on many of the fashionable biological substances of the age, including hormones and vitamins, in order to persuade consumers of the efficacy of their products.

---

[161] Chow, 'A Professional Body', original emphasis.

> If a woman can make herself more pleasing, more beautiful with make-up of
> any kind, it is her duty to use make-up for that purpose.[1]

Dr William Brady, who penned the above words, was the public face of
medicine for many residents of Milwaukee during the 1930s. In his regular
column for the *Milwaukee Sentinel*, he answered readers' questions about
health and used his experience in this capacity to issue a twenty-six-volume
collection of popular pamphlets on a wide range of topics, from care of the feet
and diabetes to dieting and, in the instance quoted above, *The 7 Keys to Vite*.[2]
Brady went far beyond conventional medical advice in his definition of 'vite',
which meant, he claimed,

preservation of the characteristics of youth, better-than-average nutritional condition
as manifested in lower death-rates, better growth and development, extension of the
prime of life in both direction, material improvement of the life expectation of adults,
higher average level of positive health thruout [*sic*] the life cycle, greater pep, more
vitality, the highest degree of natural immunity, an adequate fund of reserve power to
tide over emergencies and strains, the resiliency of the untamed animal or the
primitive savage.[3]

Brady could be describing the claimed effects of any number of the diverse
rejuvenation methods we encountered in previous chapters, whether physical
jerks, vitamin-rich foods or hormone surgery. Most striking, however, is that
despite his claim that wrinkles and many other signs of ageing could be
mitigated by simple lifestyle changes, he also favoured the use of modes of
cosmetic concealment and promoted it in his writings. By the time that he
was writing in the mid-1930s, an increasing proportion of women in the
Anglo-American world (and it was almost exclusively women) were practising daily cosmetic routines in a marketplace filled with skin care products
which claimed rejuvenatory effects. Indeed, beauty culture in its broadest
sense was, according to Ina Zweiniger-Bargielowska, 'no longer a privilege

---

[1] Brady, *The 7 Keys to Vite*, 21–22.   [2] Brady, 'Your Health', 5.
[3] Brady, *The 7 Keys to Vite*, 7.

of the wealthy and leisured during the interwar years'.[4] Zweiniger-
Bargielowska has a star witness in the form of Helena Rubinstein, arguably
the most influential figure in interwar beauty, who, in her 1930 commentary,
The Art of Feminine Beauty, noted that a 'great democratization' had
occurred, highlighting the 'duty' and 'virtue' inherent in the practice of
beauty culture.[5] Similarly, in August 1930, a commentary on the 'present-
day cult of beauty preparations' in the trade publication *Retail Chemist* noted
that the 'increase in world consumption of cosmetic preparations during the
past decade or so assumes tremendous proportions – having been computed
in fact at six or sevenfold.'[6]

Set against this highly significant expansion of the use of cosmetic products, my focus here is on the generation and public life of specific products
and classes of products which claimed to produce rejuvenating effects, rather
than on the wider context of developments in beauty culture and female
aesthetic: the subject of an excellent recent study by Jessica P. Clark, which
focusses closely on London.[7] The refinement of a genuine mass market for
skin care in the interwar period was accompanied by increasing efforts on the
part of manufacturers to target different stages of the life course with age-
specific products and methods. As we shall see, the rejuvenation of the skin
through both surgical and cosmetic means remained a highly contested
space, whilst new scientific ideas about the skin and its relationship with
nutrition and hormones were key sources of ammunition for those wanting to
expand and exploit such a lucrative market. Following a roughly chronological structure, I argue that the vehicle of skin care products was largely
responsible for the continued popularity of and fascination with hormones,
long after many of the key medical advocates of these substances had rowed
back from their earlier, often bold claims. We begin with some consideration
of the important pre–World War One context and early cosmetic, aesthetic
surgery, before examining how the dynamic medico-cultural landscape of the
1920s influenced product development and advertising strategies through the
1930s and beyond World War Two. As Nancy Tomes has recently argued for
the context of the United States, the parallel emergence of modern medical
practices and professional advertising had a profound effect on consumers of
devices, home remedies, treatments and products.[8] The case of rejuvenating
skin creams highlights how this process was also profoundly influenced by
more general sociocultural factors, such as demographic change and the
emergence of professional beauty culture, and the popularisation of scientific
views of bodily control.

[4] Zweiniger-Bargielowska, *Managing the Body*, 244.   [5] Ibid.
[6] 'Modern Cosmetic Vogues', *Retail Chemist*, August 1930, 266–71, 266.
[7] Clark, *The Business of Beauty*.   [8] Tomes, *Remaking the American Patient*.

From Beauty Culture to Surgical Practices

> It had taken no miracles of plastic surgery to rejuvenate these two – just hard, faithful work, good sense and faith. Everything about them bespoke vigor, freshness and youth. They moved as though they were glad to be alive, and it made one glad to look at them.[9]

As Jessica P. Clark has argued in her work on *fin-de-siècle* Britain, the emerging figure of the beauty culturist as expert in the care of the skin and, at least to some degree, its biology was pivotal in establishing the female aesthetic as an object of contention in the early twentieth century. However, this new class of 'expert' did not appear suddenly or smoothly, attracting both positive and negative comment in the periodical press during the late nineteenth century.[10] At its heart, this process was concerned with establishing who had the authority to determine the most effective regimes for maintaining female beauty.

In the late Victorian period the nature of the female aesthetic was rooted in an appreciation for the classic 'English rose', a trend which both emerged from and fuelled a proliferation of skin whiteners. A number of these, such as Aspinall's Neigeline, promised not only a paler complexion (equated with beauty) but also to make 'the old young and the young younger' (see Figure 6.1). Images such as these did not universally conform to typical representations of idealised female beauty. In this case, although the before-and-after imagery clearly conveys the impression of younger-looking skin, the clothing and hair remain unaltered, directing the attention of the viewer to those things which do change: removal of wrinkles, and more clearly defined mouth and eyes. Older women, the advertisement suggested, could retain key aspects of their identity whilst simultaneously recapturing a youthful visage. Neigeline was in many ways a product typical of the years around 1900, claiming paradoxically to be priced 'within the reach of all' but also targeted specifically at skin 'irritation' from the sun during archetypal upper- and upper-middle-class pursuits, including 'Yachting, Racing or Tennis'.[11]

It is no exaggeration to suggest that the British cosmetic and beauty culture landscape prior to the turn of the twentieth century, perhaps even more so immediately prior to World War One, was thriving.[12] Salons such as Mrs Pomeroy's in Bond Street, Eleanor Adair's premises in New Bond Street and the Phyllis Earle Institut de Beauté, which offered therapies using Kemolite, a radio-active mask, 'prepared in the wonderfully equipped laboratories under

[9] Burbridge, *The Road to Beauty*, 131.
[10] Clark, '"Clever Ministrations"'; Clark, *The Business of Beauty*.
[11] 'Neigeline', [1895], 'Skin Care Ephemera. Box 1', EPH625:1, Wellcome Library.
[12] Browning, *Beauty Culture*.

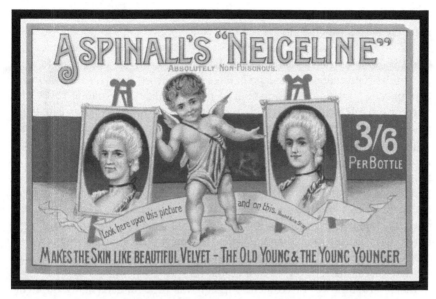

Figure 6.1 Advertisement for Aspinall's Neigeline highlighting its beneficial action on the complexion and rejuvenating effects.
Source: 'Aspinall's "Neigeline"' (March 1895), Beauty Parlour 3 (33) – Cosmetics, John Johnson Collection, available online at: http://gateway.proquest.com/openurl?url_ver=Z39.88-2004&res_dat=xri:jjohnson:&rft_dat=xri:jjohnson:rec:20080218142229kw, accessed 26 January 2018

the supervision of chemist-cosmeticians … [and administered in] surroundings of daintiness, restful charm and hygienic cleanliness', established London, and the area around Bond Street in particular, as the centre of British cosmetic fashion and style.[13] Here, before the arrival of Elizabeth Arden's semi-mythical experiences for women 'behind the Red Door' of her exclusive salons, innovations in product, marketing and customer experience laid the foundations for models replicated elsewhere across the country.[14] By the end of World War One, dedicated emporia had sprung up around Britain, promising to preserve and protect the youthful charm of women, often, though not always, with claims of scientific authenticity for their methods. Mrs Turk, who oversaw an emporium in Cheltenham dedicated to the 'Fountain of Rejuvenation and Perennial Youth', for example, claimed to 'circumvent the ravages of Father Time' and contribute to 'that high average of good looks and delicate complexion for which Cheltenham ladies are noted'.[15]

[13] Marsh, *Compacts and Cosmetics*, 65; Clark, *The Business of Beauty*.
[14] Clark, '"Beauty on Bond Street"'; Clark, 'Pomeroy v. Pomeroy'.
[15] 'Shopping in the Promenade', *Cheltenham Looker-On*, 13 December 1919, 23.

In addition to these 'soft' rejuvenation options of the everyday, domestic kind, the 1920s saw the emergence of a concerted attempt to popularise new forms of aesthetic surgery. Although such practices – which constituted an effort by cosmetic surgeons to assert their professional credentials – form a part of the rejuvenation landscape in the early interwar period, I discuss them here only in passing. The formation of the American Association of Plastic Surgeons in 1921 can be read both as an attempt by members to insulate their practices from charlatans and so-called quacks and as an opportunistic foray in response to growing demand for medically unnecessary procedures to enhance appearance.[16] On both sides of the Atlantic, cosmetic surgery for aesthetic purposes existed in parallel professional and fringe forms during the interwar period – according to Elizabeth Haiken, it was not until after World War Two that the then-established group of plastic surgeons were able to finally 'oust the quacks'.[17] However, many cosmetic surgeons operating at the periphery amassed significant wealth and, despite battling professional attempts to discredit their work, aroused great interest amongst potential consumers; their tools of surgery became arbiters of aesthetics.

Belief in the power of cosmetic surgery was of a fundamentally different kind to that which motivated consumers of skin creams. Men and women who went under the knife were trusting not only in the power of science but also the skill of the surgeon; rejuvenation in this way was as much a mechanical as a physiological process. By way of illustration, it is useful to consider briefly the work of one of the leading – and most controversial – practitioners in aesthetic facial surgery in the interwar period, Charles H. Willi, before returning to the domestic rejuvenation practices which are my main concern.

Willi was one of a number of London-based plastic surgeons who explored how new procedures might enable the recreation of a more youthful appearance. A Swiss citizen with, at best, spurious medical credentials, who spent over fifty years practising in London, Willi drew on techniques which had been developed by Harold Gillies and his collaborators during World War One, coupled with novel use of diathermy in order to avoid having to use the surgical instruments which he was singularly unqualified to handle. He established a successful practice extrapolating these approaches to cases of cosmetic improvement and built up an incredible fortune by working alongside qualified doctors and defending his work through the courts.[18] Even in the mid-1920s, arguably before the peak of skin care product proliferation, Willi and his compatriots were at the height of their public visibility and positioned

---

[16] Haiken, *Venus Envy*.   [17] Ibid., 145.

[18] Willi, *The Face*. This synthetic volume ran to at least three editions: Willi, *The Face*, 3rd edition. For a fascinating and entertaining biographical account of Willi's life, see Ludovici, *Cosmetic Scalpel*.

themselves against an emerging kind of expert – the beauty specialist – who had generally relied on 'face massage ... beauty creams, and skin foods' and whose treatments, according to Willi, had been of 'very doubtful benefit'.[19] In contrast, he saw a bright future for cosmetic surgery designed to restore beauty and youthfulness – properties which Willi saw as intimately connected.

Willi both resisted the attempts by beauty specialists to claim scientific authority over the physiological condition of the skin and extended the reach of his own expertise beyond surgery to the social function and significance of attractiveness. To pick out just one example, in his 1926 treatise, *Facial Rejuvenation; How to Idealise the Features and the Skin of the Face by the Latest Scientific Methods*, he considered the question: '[w]hy does a woman dread the loss of her good looks?', concluding that although '[r]eal love takes no heed of wrinkles or faded cheeks ... A beautiful woman is a woman armed' against the prospect of being spurned by a shallow lover who might be 'attracted by another, a girl whose white hands had never known a menial task'.[20] There is a clear English aesthetic visible in Willi's work, with references to pale skin and 'pure and eloquent blood'; indeed, he explicitly referenced 'young Englishwomen whose health and physique make them as beautiful as Greek statues'.[21]

Maintaining skin health and beauty was not just dependent on the appropriate deployment of surgical intervention. Even Willi, who prized the efficacy of such intervention above 'oils, cold creams, ointment [and] pastes', noted that 'beauty of skin is mainly a question of general health.'[22] Amongst the products which he did recommend was 'good soap', singling out his own Hystogen Institute in London (also known as the 'Hystogène Institute' and 'Institute of Facial Perfection') as purveyor of 'three preparations excellent for this purpose'.[23] Although we might have reasonably expected advertising for skin care products to play on striking gender differences in perceptions and experiences of the ageing process, this theme was also strongly evident in surgical practice. Willi, for example, noted that '[f]or women, of course, the fat-filling method as a means of prolonging or restoring youth and beauty is a particular boon, but even men, who may value less the skin that indicates youth and that clads beauty, sometimes feel that certain wrinkles belie their vigour, and in the interests of their business may be glad to remove them.'[24]

According to advertisements, at the Hystogen Institute, variously claimed to have been founded in 1907, 1910 or 1911, clients could expect 'to remove immediately, painlessly and permanently, the marks of age, worry or ill-health

---

[19] Willi, *Facial Rejuvenation*, v.   [20] Ibid., viii–ix.
[21] Ibid., 20. See also Carden-Coyne, *Reconstructing the Body*, 228. Carden-Coyne identifies in this characterisation by Willi as 'classicism met sexual allure and modernity in marketing'.
[22] Ibid., 35 and 47.   [23] Ibid., 52.   [24] Ibid., 92.

from the face by a simple scientific process'.[25] Willi advertised almost exclusively to women, generally through high-end fashion magazines, and noted the 'approved scientific principles and facts' underpinning his treatments.[26] The adverts frequently appeared alongside articles praising habits of domestic aesthetic improvement, such as 'care of the skin and complexion ... [through] commonsense and precaution'.[27]

In many respects, Willi was to cosmetic surgery what Otto Overbeck was to electrotherapy. Both used unconventional, controversial means of establishing authority and exploiting the marketplace, including the pretence of medical or scientific credentials, advertising through periodicals, extensive use of personal testimonials and attempts to secure patents against their inventions (in Willi's case, a device suitable both for 'correcting' a double chin and reducing the lower abdomen).[28] Although, as we saw in Chapter 4, Overbeck's invention attracted controversy, he did not ultimately go through the same public legal wrangles which, in the case of Willi, proved to be at least moderately damaging of his reputation.[29]

In the mid-1920s, when very few, if any, medical practitioners were willing to denounce wholesale the possibility of rejuvenating the human organism by hormonal means, specialists in facial rejuvenation were attempting to place increased emphasis on the restoration of youthful appearance over actual physiological rejuvenation.[30] Willi argued that the kind of rejuvenating effects observed through hormone treatment could not last, as '[w]e cannot make a man young again simply by adding to his blood the secretion of the thyroid or of any other gland ... it is better and more simple to treat the skin directly.'[31]

Whilst in Britain Willi's chief object was to restore the authority of medical practitioners over the domain of the skin, the American physician Morris Fishbein went further, claiming that 'it is quite impossible to feed the skin by rubbing in fats or creams of any kind.'[32] Fishbein, who spent over twenty-five years as editor of the *Journal of the American Medical Association* from 1924, gained a reputation for unmasking quacks and, as he saw it, protecting medical consumers and patients from what he characterised as the spurious claims of many medical advertisements.[33]

---

[25] 'Why Should a Woman Look Old?', *The Bystander*, 5 March 1919, 518. Willi arriving in London in 1910 and it is most likely that the institute was established in either 1910 or 1911. Willi, *Secret of Looking Young*.

[26] 'Rejuvenated', *The Bystander*, 12 December 1923, x.

[27] 'Fashions Fancies', *The Bystander*, 5 March 1919, 518–20, 518.

[28] Willi, 'Appareil pour la réduction'.   [29] Ludovici, *Cosmetic Scalpel*, 75.

[30] Willi, *Facial Rejuvenation*, 156.   [31] Ibid., 158.

[32] Fishbein, *The New Medical Follies*, 88.

[33] 'Dr Morris Fishbein Dead at 87; Former Editor of A.M.A. Journal', *The New York Times*, 28 September 1976, 40.

We move now to explore how *care* of the skin – the principal mediator of our interactions with other human beings and the world – came to dominate the rejuvenation landscape in the late interwar period.[34] Despite the efforts of figures as diverse as Willi and Fishbein, in their own ways, to preserve this as the domain of medicine, expertise over the skin, its ageing, physiology, care and rejuvenation became just as firmly located in manufacturers of skin creams and purveyors of beauty treatments as in surgeons and dermatologists. The incidence of everyday, domestic, preventive skin care measures far outweighed the effects of Willi's calculating scalpel. As well as long-established themes in cosmetics about the preservation and restoration of female beauty, a range of new products in the rejuvenation marketplace nevertheless drew on claims of scientific authority to cement this perception. As we shall see, whilst the marketplace may have been transformed, this rested as much on the re-appropriation and repurposing of existing products as the introduction of novel methods. The reimagining of so-called 'skin foods' – products designed to nourish and protect the skin – as substances which could preserve the face from the effects of ageing was paralleled by the mobilisation of both vitamins and hormones as agents of epidermal rejuvenatory potential, all cast as 'modern'.

The Modern Way to Loveliness: Scientising Beauty Culture

> If you can show me a woman who doesn't want to look young and beautiful – well, I'm afraid she isn't in her right mind. Women all want it – and we admit that they do! That's where men and women are different. Men hate to grow old – but they don't like to say so.[35]

The beauty culture advocated by Helena Rubinstein, quoted above in a 1922 newspaper interview, her great rival Elizabeth Arden, and other cosmetic giants of the early twentieth century transcended national boundaries. Although ostensibly a feature of the American (and in particular, the New York) beauty landscape, their innovations in products and marketing were developed in consort with ideas emerging from the European context, distilled through American high society and the marketing expertise of Madison Avenue, and reflected out through an international network of salons.[36] By the early 1930s, a wide range of products such as skin foods, firming lotions

---

[34] Benthien, *Skin*, 1; Connor, *The Book of Skin*.
[35] Gray, 'People Who Want to Look Young', 32.
[36] For biographical accounts of both Rubinstein and Arden, and their impact on global beauty culture, see: Fitoussi, *Helena Rubinstein*; Brandon, *Ugly Beauty*; Woodhead, *War Paint*; O'Higgins, *Madame*. Helena Rubinstein penned an autobiography later in her life. See: Rubinstein, *My Life for Beauty*.

and oils were already established in the skin care market alongside older popular preparations such as cold and cleansing creams.[37]

The emerging mass market for, and specific British relationship with, these products was a source of considerable anxiety for pharmacists and chemists. Much like Norman Haire's assertion that there was a distinct lack of meaningful engagement with practices of hormone rejuvenation, as we saw in Chapter 2, the trade community doubted the level of British interest in cosmetic products, or even the need for these. As one correspondent noted in the trade journal *Retail Chemist* in 1930:

[c]osmetics is a subject upon which British authorities have written little, if at all. Not so their Continental confrères, however, who, on the contrary, provide not only technique of an exceptionally high quality, but also have no unnatural shyness in publishing their results.[38]

Retail Chemist was the most widely-circulated and influential periodical of its kind in Britain, and it provided a forum for discussion which reveals mixed attitudes towards the growing influence and use of skin care products amongst front-line retailers. For example, the pharmacist William F. Pleasance, joint proprietor of the London-based firm Blackaller and Pleasance, argued that '[t]he present vogue [for large-scale use of cosmetics] very largely originated in American ... [I]t must be admitted that as a nation English women are fortunate in the possession of complexions which are second to none, and it would be the more deplorable if the use of toilet articles were not kept within reasonable bounds.'[39] The 'Anglo-Saxon skin, lovely at its best, but super-sensitive, delicate and difficult', was widely regarded as requiring specially prepared treatments.[40]

Notwithstanding these concerns, the closely-related topics of complexion, toilet articles, cosmetics and skin care products were a source of considerable interest for the national network of retail pharmacists. At the outset of the 1930s, for example, a leading article in *Retail Chemist* noted that '[o]f all the various sections into which toilet products generally may be classified, none enjoys a more constant demand or is of greater importance than skin creams. As us well known, every woman regards a clear, healthy-looking complexion as her natural birth-right, and will go to endless trouble to preserve that which

---

[37] Companies manufacturing skin foods in the late 1920s included Tokalon, Boots (though their Les Fleurs range), Yardley, Coty, Vinolia, Pomeroy and Apiella, to name just a few. See: 'Tokalon Skin Food', *The Chemist and Druggist*, 10 August 1929, 21; 'Pomeroy Skin Food', *The Chemist and Druggist*, 6 July 1918, 20; 'Royal Vinolia Vanishing Cream', *The Chemist and Druggist*, 29 June 1918, 27.

[38] 'Comments of the Month', *Retail Chemist*, October 1930, 338–9, 339.

[39] William F. Pleasance, 'Are Modern Cosmetics Harmful?', *Retail Chemist*, August 1930, 286.

[40] 'The Making of a Good-Looking Woman', *Britannia and Eve*, 1 January 1935, 41.

she has, or to make amends for any condition'.[41] Nor was the development of new products solely the preserve of the beauty culturist. By the 1930s the mobilisation of scientific expertise around the endocrine system in the manufacture and, critically, marketing of skin care products was a commonplace, though not universal strategy amongst corporations in both Britain and the United States. As highlighted in a digest of 'Current Medical Topics' in May 1931, '[a]lready in industry, business and profession, the biologist is considering the application of science. . . . [T]he endocrine glands would appear to offer the most hopeful and promising of the reagents'.[42]

This link between hormones and skin care became an important aspect of beauty culture from the late 1920s onwards. If that propagation was due to continued fascination with surgical intervention and the skilful orchestration of the Steinach and Voronoff sets, the maintenance of hormones' preeminent position in the public arsenal of rejuvenation through the 1930s and beyond World War Two arguably owed far more to the repurposing of these substances in skin care products. In 1928 the American beauty magnate Helena Rubinstein passed judgement on Alexis Carrel's talk to the Third Race Betterment Conference, held at the Battle Creek Sanatarium, Michigan. In his paper, Carrel dismissed the possibility of everlasting life, arguing that mortality was the necessary price we paid 'for the possession of our brains'.[43] As reported in the *Brooklyn Daily Eagle* on 19 January 1928, Rubinstein, who was on the brink of selling her multimillion dollar cosmetics business to Lehman Brothers, noted the success of Voronoff and Steinach's treatments in men, but lamented the limited applicability to women. However, she claimed, in Paris the use of a new 'skin serum' was yielding remarkable rejuvenation results.[44]

After the Wall Street Crash of 1929, Rubinstein bought back a controlling stake in her business at a fraction of the cost and almost immediately entered into the hormone cream market. She was not the first to attempt a mass-market hormone cream but she had been concerned with scientific rejuvenation research for a decade, having claimed at least as early as 1922 that she had spent time 'working with Doctor Kapp, of Berlin and Vienna, one of the physicians engaged in these experiments [with monkey glands].'[45] Rubinstein argued then that 'even without resorting to monkey glands, ninety-nine women out of a hundred could look younger than they do.'[46] As has been well-documented, by 1932, Rubinstein had determined to launch her Hormone

---

[41] 'Perfumery: Complexion and Toilet Creams', *Retail Chemist*, May 1930, 122–5, 122.
[42] 'Current Medical Topics', *Retail Chemist*, May 1931, 196–7.
[43] Carrel, 'The Immortality of Animal Tissues', 313.
[44] Beckley, 'There Is No Eternal Youth', 5.
[45] The experiments in question involved the use of 'transplanted monkey glands, or by inoculation of a serum made from these glands.' Gray, 'People Who Want to Look Young', 32.
[46] Gray, 'People Who Want to Look Young', 32.

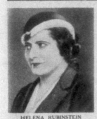

AN AMAZING DISCOVERY—
A TRIUMPH of BEAUTY SCIENCE!

Helena Rubinstein, beauty authority and pioneer of scientific beauty culture, has for thirty years, as chemist and dermatologist, collaborated in the researches of leading physicians in the most famous laboratories of Europe. She now

triumphantly presents her amazing discovery, the HORMONE TWIN CREAMS, which actually recreate Nature's own regenerative elements, the vital glandular secretions of youth.

HORMONE CREAMS RECREATE VITAL
GLANDULAR ELEMENTS of "FIRST YOUTH"

HELENA RUBINSTEIN

In "*first youth*" the cellular structure of the skin and underlying tissues is constantly recreated by the hormones, the vital glandular secretions. They keep the contours firm and rounded, the skin fine, clear, soft and radiant. It is the deficiency of these hormones which causes the dread signs of age to appear.

NEW METHOD of
SUPPLYING REJUVENATING HORMONES

An utterly different treatment! By simple application to the skin these Hormone Twin Creams supply the biological substances, the actual glandular secretions, which regenerate the skin. Used in conjunction with your daily Helena Rubinstein Home Treatment the Hormone Twin Youthifiers, two supplementary glandular feeders, a day and night cream, penetrate the skin and underlying tissues and eradicate all signs of age. . . . Simply, quickly and privately the deficiency of hormones can be supplied and the tragedy of aging faces, necks and hands avoided. The Hormone Twin Creams supply actual hormones throughout the cellular structure and, correcting lines, wrinkles, sallowness and flabbiness, they bring back the lost loveliness of authentic youth! The price of the two Hormone Creams is 2½ guineas.

A SPECIAL SALON OFFER

So that everyone may experience the sensational rejuvenating effects of the Hormone Twin Creams, they will be used in all Courses of Salon Treatments WITHOUT EXTRA CHARGE... Write or telephone (Regent 5232) Madame Ceska Rubinstein, the sister and associate of Madame Rubinstein, for consultations or appointments.

PARIS   CANNES
MILAN   BERLIN
VIENNA COPENHAGEN

helena rubinstein LTD.
24 GRAFTON STREET, LONDON, W.1

ESTABLISHED 1902—
ALL PREPARATIONS
MADE IN ENGLAND

Figure 6.2 The first British advertisement for Helena Rubinstein's Hormone Twin Youthifiers. ('An Amazing Discovery – A Triumph of Beauty Science', *The Bystander*, 4 May 1932, 245.)

Twin Creams (more popularly known as the Hormone Twin Youthifiers) in Britain, a year after they had burst into the American marketplace.[47] In her newspaper advertising (see Figure 6.2), Rubinstein styled herself as a 'beauty authority and pioneer of scientific beauty culture ... chemist and dermatologist [who had] collaborated in the researches of leading physicians in the most famous laboratories of Europe.'[48]

From the outset the promotional strategy developed by Rubinstein, long before her notable partnership with advertising legend David Ogilvy in the 1940s, was to align the action of the cream with the scientific language of endocrinology.[49] Thus, the (unnamed) hormone(s) in the cream acted on 'the cellular structure of the skin ... [by replacing] vital glandular secretions' lost with age which 'regenerate the skin.'[50] The simple message to potential customers was that '[h]ormones, the chief stimulators of skin and tissue

[47] Bennett, 'Rubinstein and the Rejuvenationists'.
[48] 'An Amazing Discovery – A Triumph of Beauty Science', *The Bystander*, 4 May 1932, 245.
[49] Fitoussi, *Helena Rubinstein*, chapter 27.
[50] 'An Amazing Discovery – A Triumph of Beauty Science', *The Bystander*, 4 May 1932, 245.

renewal, are plentiful in healthy youth, but lacking in older, or even merely fatigued persons. This loss is the main cause of facial degeneration.'[51]

The following year, in the same publication which carried this first advertisement – *The Bystander* – a half-page article by 'Maquillage' claimed that Rubinstein (described here as 'a chemist and dermatologist' as well as a beauty magnate) 'imprisons the elements of first youth in twin pots of a new rejuvenating cream.'[52] Mirroring some of the earlier medical hyperbole surrounding the endocrine system, as well as Rubinstein's own promotional material, the author argued that 'these vital glandular secretions are the very life essence.'[53] Underlying this was the assumption that the 'regulated supply of the vital glandular extracts will rejuvenate and restore health and vitality', a fact 'acknowledged and proved' by earlier medical research.[54] Subsequently trend-setting publications including *Tatler* lauded the Rubinstein creams, which occupied '[p]ride of place' in the daily toilet routine.[55] These supposedly independent assessments by publishers of great prestige bestowed further socio-cultural capital not only on Rubinstein, but also to wider hormone-based products and marketing claims.

As might be expected with such a high-profile figure in the cosmetic landscape, Rubinstein's intervention in the market of hormone creams legitimised such practices and provided the latest advertising model for claiming scientific authority over the skin, skin care products and even whole-organism physiology. In subsequent years a range of similar products, all claiming to rejuvenate the skin, were launched on the British market. These included the Juvigold Tonic Life Elixir, produced by the Middlesex Laboratory of Glandular Research Ltd., which was described in promotional materials as 'a balanced ductless-gland food', to be taken orally.[56] In contrast to the Hormone Twin Youthifiers, the manufacturers of Juvigold Tonic did not claim that the preparation included actual hormones, but rather 'gold, platinum, palladium, brain and spinal cord extracts', all of which were calculated to promote the natural

---

[51] 'Beauty that Outlasts the Years', *Tatler*, 12 June 1935, viii.
[52] 'Maquillage', from the French for 'makeup', was a common term in periodicals for discussion and promotion of cosmetic products, reflecting a wider social environment where France, and Paris in particular, was seen as the leading centre for innovation in cosmetics. See, for examples: 'Maquillage', *The Globe*, 21 June 1911, 14; 'Milk and Roses', *Belfast News-Letter*, 11 February 1931, 5; 'Maquillage', *Yorkshire Post and Leeds Intelligencer*, 28 October 1938, 6. Indeed, the author's column – 'The Gentle Art of Being Beautiful' – was a regular feature in *The Bystander*, which often featured discussion on youthfulness. See, for example, the claim that 'a woman is as young as her eyes'. Maquillage, 'The Gentle Art of Being Beautiful', *The Bystander*, 13 September 1933, 498.
[53] Maquillage, 'The Gentle Art of Being Beautiful' *The Bystander*, 25 May 1932, vi.
[54] Maquillage, 'The Gentle Art of Being Beautiful' *The Bystander*, 25 May 1932, vi.
[55] 'The Highway of Fashion', *The Tatler*, 3 July 1935, iv.
[56] 'The Chemist's Buying Review', *Retail Chemist*, August 1934, 251–2, 252.

activity of the ductless glands to restore and revitalise.[57] Rather than a direct replacement of hormones, therefore, Juvigold was a product conceived to work in harmony with the endocrinological apparatus of the female of the body.[58] Another, the Hormone Cream produced by Elizabeth Bock, was part of a range of products – including 'Strawberry Cream Mask', 'Anti-Wrinkle Cream' and 'Alimenteau Cream' – which provided 'speedy removal of wrinkles and tired lines' and contained 'important tissue-building properties which rejuvenate and regenerate the skin.'[59] The allure of the hormone market was tempting even to those companies who had not previously countenanced such ventures. For example, the 'candle-making' firm J. C. and J. Field (established in London at least as early as 1642) began producing toilet preparations in 1935, launching the 'Nell Gwyn Beauty Aids' range which featured a rejuvenating skin food.[60]

Variations on the claim that hormone creams could 'not only transform an ageing complexion but reveal hidden loveliness in every type of skin' were deployed extensively in advertisements, with some, such as Calypso Cosmetics who manufactured Vitagland Hormone Cream (also known as 'Vitagland Rejuvenation Cream') from 1935, even going so far as to assert that their preparation would make users '*feel* and look many years younger.'[61] Reports reveal that store managers at Boots chemist branches received 'hundreds of enquiries asking where the item referred to [Vitagland Rejuvenation Cream] can be obtained.'[62] Feature articles in the periodical press served to reinforce these messages through the mid-1930s. For example, an anonymous article in *Britannia and Eve* noted in 1935 simply that '[a]bsorbing hormones through the pores has a marvellous effect in preserving and restoring youthful beauty.'[63] Such commentaries abounded with reverence for scientific expertise behind these preparations, which went far beyond the claims made by advertising for more traditional skin foods, which were presented as agents capable of restoring lost moisture, but not intervening physiologically with the skin and its structures.[64] Other companies, such as the large cosmetics manufacturer Dubarry insisted that their products, in this case 'Nuglandin Cream: the

57 'Amazing New Tonic', *Daily Herald*, 29 August 1934, 16.
58 'Juvigold Ductless Gland Tonic', *Merchandise Bulletin* 452, 7 October 1935, 4419.
59 'Now is the Time for Complexion Care', *Tatler*, 19 September 1934, xvii; 'Now is the Time for Complexion Care', *Britannia and Eve*, 1 October 1934, 117.
60 'Patents', *Merchandise Bulletin*, 14 March 1935, 4068-9, 4069.
61 'Recapture Youthful Beauty by Rejuvenation of the Skin from Within', *Britannia and Eve*, 1 January 1935, 109, my emphasis; 'Vitagland Hormone Beauty Cream', *The Bystander*, 6 February 1935, i.
62 'Patents', *Merchandise Bulletin*, 21 March 1935, 4109-11, 4111.
63 'A Cream That Makes You Young', *Britannia and Eve*, 1 December 1935, 41.
64 'An Ideal Skin-Food', *Punch*, 25 June 1930, xxv, EFL/CP/PO/5/1/19, Unilever Archives, Port Sunlight.

marvellous skin rejuvenator', drew on the work of 'famous Skin Doctors in England, Germany and America'. Imagery for Nuglandin drew heavily on a Japanese aesthetic, highlighting an approach rooted in exoticism rather than the popular theme of British naturalism (see Figure 6.3).

Hormone creams were also marketed in contrast to mechanical rejuvenation interventions of the time, offered by the likes of Madame Manners, which promised 'permanent face rejuvenation . . . [and] beauty in one visit'. Instead, customers of Rubinstein, Calypso and Elizabeth Bock need not subject themselves to the treatment table.[65] The lack of necessity for the consumer to make a special trip to visit a beauty culturist or, worse, a medical practitioner or surgeon, was held up by manufacturers as a major advantage of their easily-absorbed, easily-applied creams. These products were part of a 'fool-proof home treatment' and accompanied with detailed instructions for use.[66] The opportunity to employ the results of endocrine science – 'valuable glandular components, which give back youth and vitality to the skin' – in a domestic setting was calculated to empower women, making the latest innovations available at a fraction of the cost of salon treatments, let alone surgery.[67] When the alternative youth-bestowing treatments came via the scalpel or face-peels which frequently were described as 'an entirely new torture', the appeal of luxurious, rejuvenating face creams becomes quite apparent.[68]

Not all were enthused by the availability of powerful hormones in a manner so readily accessible to domestic users. As a major editorial feature in *Retail Chemist* cautioned in 1935:

[w]e are as yet woefully ignorant of all the possible changes that may take place when such potent glandular preparations are used in an unbridled manner by the general public and . . . if the instructions state that the preparation should be used "a small quantity to be rubbed in daily" the user will in all probability take a large amount and massage it in three or four times daily so as to achieve a quicker result.[69]

Some manufacturers were content to produce products containing hormones, but shunned extensive advertising campaigns, perhaps fearing repercussions if their claims were found to be false, or just concerned about the association between their brand and this novel product. For example, Pains & Byrne, the

---

[65] 'Permanent Face Rejuvenation by the Manners Treatment', *The Tatler*, 15 June 1932, xv. The Manners Treatment was advertised extensively from the late 1920s through the 1930s. Manners rapidly dropped the description of her treatment as 'plastic facial rejuvenation' and became progressively more vague about what exactly was involved. See: 'Plastic Facial Rejuvenation by the Manners Treatment', *The Tatler*, 20 February 1929, e; 'Permanent Face Rejuvenation by the Manners Treatment', *The Sketch*, 3 December 1930, 18;
[66] 'A Cream that Makes you Young', *Britannia and Eve*, 1 December 1935, 41.
[67] 'Secrets of the Salon: A Beauty Questionnaire', *Britannia and Eve*, 1 August 1932, 54–5, 54.
[68] 'Beauties and Beautifiers', *The Sphere*, 24 December 1932, 522-3, 522.
[69] 'The Skin', *Retail Chemist*, August 1936, 250-2, 252.

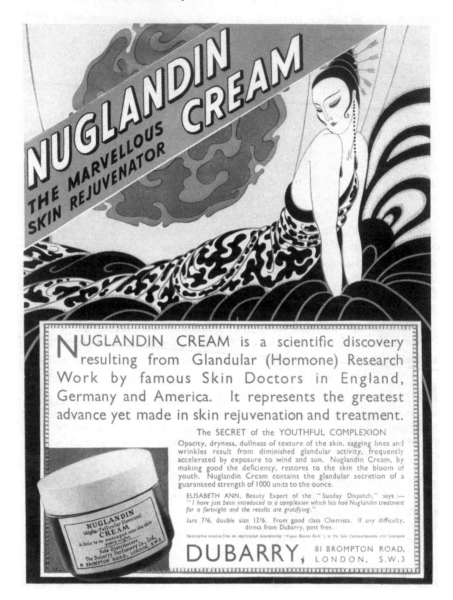

Figure 6.3 A 1936 advertisement for Dubarry's Nuglandin Cream, printed in the high-end British periodical *The Tatler*. ('Nuglandin Cream', *The Tatler*, 4 March 1936, 35.)

medical manufacturing firm, introduced 'Nuages', a new 'Skin Hormone Cream', in 1935, but the trade literature noted that 'it is not being advertised', despite being sold throughout the country in Boots stores.[70]

A number of the most significant names in beauty culture also shunned the use of hormones in their products and therapies. Elizabeth Arden, for example, relied instead on promoting her range of rejuvenating treatments as in synergy with nature, eschewing the scientised language and claims of Helena Rubinstein. Arden's promotional material of the mid-1930s abounded with promises that rejuvenation could be achieved, and youthfulness sustained, '[n]ot through complicated rituals that soon grow to be a burden; but by three daily steps that bring out latent loveliness: Cleansing, Toning and Soothing.'[71] The slogan 'Farewell to Age' underpinned a major Arden advertising campaign across Britain during 1935; on this occasion, consumers were urged to visit local chemists where 'Miss Arden's Representative' would 'keep you young and make you lovely . . . by a quick, home treatment adapted to your personal needs.'[72] In contrast to the argument advanced by Searing and Zeilig that *'Elizabeth Arden* was among the first in the 20th century to imply that the user could look younger through the use of cosmetics', Arden was in fact treading a very familiar path, adapting her messages to fit an expanding but well-established public fascination with youthfulness.[73]

Arden's advertising also drew on the mythical treatments, carried out in luxurious surroundings, available at her exclusive salon at 25 Old Bond Street in London. By promising a series of beauty treatments, not to mention exercise programmes, tailored to the individual physique, complexion and age of her clients, Arden highlighted the importance of personalised, not universal, rejuvenation. The promotional material from the mid-1930s promised to turn 'the years back, removing their traces from your face and your body; leaving you the wisdom you have gleaned during that time, so that your new beauty and youth mean more to you than they ever could have.'[74] Through advertising in exclusive periodicals such as *The Tatler* and *The Sketch*, 'women who place themselves in Elizabeth Arden's hands' could be made not only more youthful

---

[70] '"Nuages" Skin Hormone Cream', *Merchandise Bulletin*, 30 December 1935, 4526.

[71] 'Farewell To Age - by Elizabeth Arden', *Harper's Bazaar*, 1933, Ad*Access Collection, Duke University Library, BH1419.

[72] 'Farewell to Age!', *Lancashire Evening Post*, 23 April 1935, 8. Similar adverts appeared in the local press elsewhere. See: 'Farewell to Age!', *Lincolnshire Echo*, 1 February 1935, 4; 'Farewell to Age!', *West Sussex County Times*, 22 February 1935, 8; 'Farewell to Age!', *Chichester Observer*, 26 June 1935, 6; 'Farewell to Age!', *Sunderland Daily Echo*, 13 April 1935, 8; 'Farewell to Age!', *Worthing Herald*, 15 June 1935, 14.

[73] Searing and Zeilig, *'Fine Lines'*, 11, original emphasis.

[74] 'Sweeping the Years Away. . .', *The Tatler*, 18 April 1934, 125.

but also remain 'beautiful to the last day of your life', with more details available in the accompanying pamphlet, *Sweeping the Years Away*.[75]

In common with Arden, French company Innoxa, who began to expand into the British market in the late 1920s, claimed that their products would 'give the skin an astonishingly healthy and young appearance' as they were derived from 'the prescriptions of an eminent French Skin Specialist'.[76] Innoxa, which became a defacto British company when manufacturing was switched there permanently following the outbreak of World War Two, drew on supposed scientific pedigree, but without recourse to hormones.[77] Promotional material as far afield as Singapore and Australia listed the company's Bond Street premises as the principal address.[78] In common with many brands, the scientific basis of Innoxa products was a critical aspect of their marketing strategy. The creams, developed originally by 'Dr Francis Debat, noted French Dermatologist,' had a 'scientific basis' and were originally intended 'to cure various skin conditions' rather than act as purely cosmetic products.[79]

Products which claimed to rejuvenate the skin were therefore highly diverse, from those wedded directly to the supposedly latest scientific findings in endocrinology and dermatology – such as those promoted by Helena Rubinstein – to others which through omission of such language highlighted their natural, synergistic action on the body. It was in this context that the British retail pharmacy and chemist company, Boots, set about devising a range of skin care products for a new 'Beauty Series'.[80] Rather than simply concealing blemishes on the skin, these complementary preparations were designed to offer 'the finest beauty treatment that money can buy in one's own home.'[81] The range of products, known as the Number Seven series, included hand lotion, cleansing cream, foundation cream, face powder and fragrance spray, all of which were marketed as a complete system of skin care and which were to be used in the home following specific instructions.[82] The series was extended to include cosmetic products in 1936. Most significantly for our purposes, amongst the list of preparations was a 'skin food' which, it was claimed, 'fills out hollows and preserves the flesh of the face and neck in a

[75] 'So Often. . .Life Begins at Forty', *The Tatler*, 27 June 1934, 605.

[76] 'Innoxa Beauty Preparations', *Exeter and Plymouth Gazette*, 7 June 1927, 4.

[77] 'Innoxa Complexion Powder', *Border Watch*, 10 June 1937, 3; 'Innoxa Beauty Demonstrations' *Warwick Daily News*, 12 October 1937, 3; 'Innoxa Preparation. Visiting Beauty Specialist', *Johnstone Advocate*, 20 June 1939, 6; 'Aid to Beauty. "Innoxa" Products', *Cairns Post*, 1 September 1938, 3.

[78] 'Innoxa Week. Learn to Grow Lovelier', *Strait Times*, 3 April 1938, 21;

[79] 'Innoxa Preparations', *Townsville Daily Bulletin*, 6 October 1936, 3.

[80] 'Formula Committee Minutes', 18 July 1924, 5349, 743, Boots Archive.

[81] *The Number Seven Ways to Loveliness*, 1949, 4, A30/3, Boots Archive.

[82] 'Formula Committee Minutes', 2 January 1935, 5489, 744, Boots Archive.

condition of healthy youth'.[83] More than this, the cream contained 'the oils necessary for deep tissue building', demonstrating a clear connection between the preparation and the underlying physiology of the skin.[84] In an era where differences in skin types were fast becoming features of advertising material for both cosmetic and skin care products, the promotional literature of the Number Seven Skin Food noted that it was suitable for both dry and oily skins. Significantly, promotional material claimed that 'excessive oiliness' was 'a symptom of incorrect gland adjustment', highlighting the prominence of glandular explanations for medical conditions within the public sphere during this period.[85]

The development of rejuvenation narratives was not just about introducing new substances into skin care regimes. Manufacturers also reimagined long-standing products and reframed them as active contributors to a youthful visage. This was partly realised through the imagery of advertisements, which emphasised the significance and centrality of youthfulness and also high-lighted the ceaseless battle against the years. In many of these, female beauty and charm acted as proxies for youthfulness, the implication being that loss of these was synonymous with older age (see Figure 6.4). Skin foods were far from new products in the 1930s – they were rather an established part of everyday beauty regimes as a richer, more nourishing alternative to cold cream, alongside the staples of the powder room such as toner and lipstick. There was no typical formulation for skin foods. Whilst the production of cold or vanishing creams had reasonably stable methods and ingredients, a wide range of petroleum products, oils, waxes and extracts were included in products labelled as skin foods.[86] Skin foods, claimed by manufacturers as nourishing and easily absorbed, frequently referenced two physiological fea-tures of the skin: the underlying fatty tissue and the body's glandular structure. Advertising material for the long-lived and popular Pomeroy Skin Food, for example, noted that it provided 'systematic feeding of these glands ... [resulting] in the disappearance of wrinkles and lines, the filling out of hollows, and a more graceful contour.'[87]

At Boots, the management of products fell to the Formula Committee, which convened on a weekly basis and made recommendations to the Execu-tive for new lines, explored alterations to existing ranges, and acted on suggestions and complaints from staff and customers.[88] Unlike specialist cosmetics and skin care manufacturers, the members of the Committee took

---

[83] *Beauty Booklet*, 1935, 20, A30/48, Boots Archive.   [84] Ibid.   [85] Ibid.
[86] According to Melendy, skin food worked precisely because it nourished 'the fattening qualities' in the skin and acted to 'build up the underlying tissue.' Melendy, *Perfect Womanhood for Maidens-Wives-Mothers*, 323.
[87] 'Pomeroy Skin Food', Beauty 3, EPH 136:11, n.d., Wellcome Library.
[88] Hornsey, '"The modern way to loveliness"'.

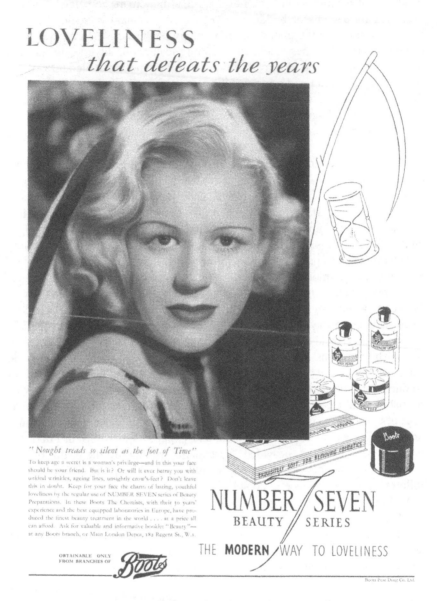

LOVELINESS
that defeats the years

" Nought treads so silent as the foot of Time"

To keep age a secret is a woman's privilege—and in this your face should be your friend. But is it? Or will it ever betray you with unkind wrinkles, ageing lines, unsightly crow's-feet? Don't leave this in doubt. Keep for your face the charm of lasting, youthful loveliness by the regular use of NUMBER SEVEN series of Beauty Preparations. In these Boots The Chemists, with their 50 years' experience and the best equipped laboratories in Europe, have produced the finest beauty treatment in the world . . . . at a price all can afford. Ask for valuable and informative booklet "Beauty"— at any Boots branch, or Main London Depot, 182 Regent St., W.1.

NUMBER SEVEN
BEAUTY SERIES

THE **MODERN** WAY TO LOVELINESS

OBTAINABLE ONLY FROM BRANCHES OF *Boots*

Figure 6.4 A typical advertisement in the British for Number Seven products. The less-than-subtle references to the inevitable passage of time are represented by the hourglass and, in a rather sinister turn, Death's scythe, as well as mentions of the scientific purity of the products, based on '50 years' experience'. Campaigns of this kind were common to many skin care manufacturers. Source: 'Loveliness that Defeats the Years', WBA/BT/11/45/1/1/10, c.1938, Boots Company Archive

decisions about a far wider range of products, including disinfectants and other proprietary domestic preparations. Consumers were not passive recipients of products, even those whose production and marketing was tightly controlled by a large manufacturer such as Boots. Specific suggestions for modifications to the Number Seven came from customers on a regular basis; for example, between October 1935 and January 1936, the Formula Committee noted that Mrs B. Nichols requested that the creams be issued 'in lighter containers for travelling', an employee at Boots Branch 987 suggested 'that we should issue a Sulphur Skin Lotion', and the regularly convened Staff Training School pressed for the Formula Committee to introduce 'miniature tubes of the creams for demonstration purposes'.[89] By April 1936, miniature tubes were indeed available for in-store demonstrators.[90]

Amongst the new range of products, Number Seven Skin Food was particularly problematic for the Formula Committee, with numerous complaints of a resulting 'rash or irritation' first coming to light in May 1935, almost immediately after the range was launched.[91] The reported effects ranged from 'burning and acute irritation' to 'a good deal of irritation and inflammation', with one customer reporting that 'it took the skin off her face and she had to have medical treatment.'[92] This caused some initial concern and a protracted rethink about the product ingredients.[93] In an effort to eliminate potential cases of skin irritation during the course of their investigations, the Formula Committee introduced a modified base cream for the whole of the Number Seven range and tested further experimental versions of the skin food on 'people known to be susceptible to the original product' from amongst the Boots staff.[94] After a successful – and rather informal – trial of this revised formulation on '[t]wo girls at [Boots offices in] Beeston' who had previous experienced an adverse reaction, the new Number Seven products were introduced in January 1936.[95]

Over the following months, the Formula Committee spent considerable time discussing the matter. For example, despite the issuing of a revised formulation the previous month, in February 1936 the Committee noted that further complaints about the 'the Skin Food were causing some concern'. After discussing the question 'from all angles', and contemplating recalling the entire flagship range of products, they determined instead to pull just the Skin

[89] 'Formula Committee Minutes', 15 October 1935, 5755; 1 January 1936, 5830; 10 February 1936, 5889, 744, Boots Archive.
[90] 'Formula Committee Minutes', 29 April 1936, 5998, 744, Boots Archive.
[91] 'No7 Complaints', 1935, 1, WBA/BT/9/22/20/34, Boots Archive.
[92] 'No7 Complaints', 1935, 2-3, WBA/BT/9/22/20/34, Boots Archive.
[93] 'Formula Committee Minutes', 22 October 1935, 744, 744, Boots Archive.
[94] 'Formula Committee Minutes', 27 November 1935, 5793, 744, Boots Archive.
[95] 'Formula Committee Minutes', 1 January 1936, 5930; 15 January 1936, p. 5849, 744, Boots Archive.

Food and offer 'some suitable explanation ... to the Branches'.[96] Despite further modifications of the perfume, by May the Formula Committee were receiving 'an alarming number of complaints on Skin Food'; the following month, 'the complaints had not in any way diminished.'[97]

Despite the fact that numerous modifications were unsuccessful in preventing reactions on the skin, a short report from the Formula Committee noted that 'the Skin Food has been the most successful member of the Number 7 Series from the sales point of view.'[98] This observation, made in December 1936, came against the backdrop of a major investigation into the effects of the product. The previous month the Formula Committee had canvassed 'reports from over 800 toilet assistants' on the effects of the skin food, of whom '16% ... made complaints of varying degrees of seriousness about the effect of the product on their skins, and well over half of these complaints appeared to deserve being taken seriously.'[99] The investigation also revealed a critical change in consumers' relationships with their own skins. As the report on the adverse effects of the Number Seven products noted,

A strong demand appears to be arising among the Retail staff, especially those engaged in beauty treatment, for the issue of two skin foods, one labelled for one type of skin, and one for another. The heads of the Beauty Parlours point out that they have great difficulty in convincing customers that a single skin food, which forms the basis of the Number Seven treatment, can adequately cater for all types of skin, especially when we admit by marketing a variety of preparations, that different types of skin need different foundations.[100]

In common with many other manufacturers of cosmetic and skin care products, World War Two had a very significant impact on Boots' ability to source sufficient quantities of the raw materials required for their products.[101] In the case of the Number Seven skin food, the early 1940s saw the cessation of supplies of triethanolamine, almond oil and petroleum jelly; in response, the Formula Committee recommended the substitution of liquid paraffin and lanoline, and this new preparation continued to be used in the immediate postwar years.[102] Indeed, in 1948, the Toilet Sub-Committee, whose responsibilities

[96] 'Formula Committee Minutes', 26 February 1936, 5917, 744, Boots Archive.
[97] 'Formula Committee Minutes', 20 May 1936, 6028; 10 June 1936, p. 6064, 744, Boots Archive.
[98] 'Formula Committee Minutes', 2 December 1936, 6264, 743, Boots Archive.
[99] 'Report: Number Seven Skin Food. M.R. 102. The Present Position', 27 March 1937, 1, WBA/BT/9/22/20/34, Boots Archive.
[100] 'Report: Number Seven Skin Food. M.R. 102. The Present Position', 27 March 1937, 3, WBA/BT/9/22/20/34, Boots Archive.
[101] For a wider discussion of this, see Mason, 'The Impact of World War II'; Jones, *Beauty Imagined*.
[102] 'Formula Sub-Committee Minutes', 8 July 1941, 421; 'Formula Sub-Committee Minutes', 18 January 1943, 859, No7 Extra Rich Skin Food Product File, 843/24, Boots Archive.

were not as far-reaching as the Formula Committee, were still receiving complaints that the Skin Food was not 'sufficiently greasy'; their efforts to revert wholesale to the prewar formula were hampered by the now prohibitively high cost of almond oil, and the product had therefore been irrevocably altered by the availability of its components.[103]

Notwithstanding the challenges experienced by Boots when introducing a new product into a rapidly expanding, and increasingly discerning and diverse marketplace, skin foods remained popular and long-lived products. Boots claimed that the Number Seven extra-rich skin food, which had been developed during the late 1930s but was not put on the market until the early 1950s, contained 'age-defying ingredients that soothe and soften the skin and ward off lines and wrinkles', demonstrating the persistence of lines and wrinkles as key indicators of ageing.[104] The product was originally devised by the Formula Committee 'not to overcome the difficulties of sensitivity [to other products], but as [a] logical sales asset, following present practice of Foundation Cream in two varieties'; its development was designed to combat some of the teething problems of the original Number Seven skin food, but introduction was halted by the outbreak of war.[105] Intriguingly, by the time this suggestion reached the Toilet Subcommittee in September 1938, the rationale for developing a new product had seemingly shifted from exploiting a gap in the market to catering for different skin types, revealed at least in part by the experience of (exclusively female) store-based toilet assistants. Now, instead of identifying a possible commercial opportunity, the Formula Committee justified issuing a new type of skin food in terms of customer necessity, suggesting 'an alternative Skin Food which would be more suitable for individuals with dry skins. It had been felt for some time ... that one Skin Food is unsuitable for all skins.'[106]

The skin care products of the Number Seven range were designed primarily to alter outward appearance. The marketing claims went beyond simply covering up the signs of ageing, however; these skin care products were marketed with the view that 'make-up on its own is not enough.'[107] Whilst the rejuvenation practices associated with hormones (whether invasive or non-invasive) offered seemingly universal solutions, applicable to all, the use of a daily skin care regime was far more personalised. For each skin type there was

[103] 'Toilet Sub-Committee', 28 July 1948, 394, No7 Extra Rich Skin Food Product File, 843/24, Boots Archive.

[104] 'New ... Better and Lovelier Number Seven', 1953, 2, A30/16, Boots Archive.

[105] 'Formula Sub-Committee Minutes', 25 May 1938, 6789, No7 Extra Rich Skin Food Product File, 843/24, Boots Archive.

[106] Formula Committee, 'No.7 Skin Food for Dry Skins', 19 September 1938, No7 Extra Rich Skin Food Product File, 843/24, Boots Archive.

[107] 'A Guide to Selling Beauty: Number Seven', c.1965, 31, A30/14, Boots Archive.

a combination of products especially calculated to reduce the outward appearance of ageing. By the early 1960s, the idea that different skins required different treatment had become a fundamental and inescapable part of marketing and promotion campaigns for cosmetic and skin care products, with attendant links to the ageing process. As an example, the training pamphlets for Number Seven from 1962 and 1965 asserted that dry skin was viewed as 'fine in texture . . . [and] susceptible to weather'.[108] In consequence, 'it will age quickly and lines will form round the eyes, mouth and throat', making this skin type especially vulnerable to premature ageing.[109] This mirrored scientific understandings of aged skin as dry skin: a prominent connection both within and beyond rejuvenation texts which drew on traditions established on humoral models from as early as the investigations of Bacon.[110]

In addition to the products themselves, staff working at Boots were given detailed instructions to pass on to customers about how these preparations should be applied. Although these consisted of complex massaging techniques – illustrated visually in Number Seven brochures – there was one basic overriding principle: 'the movement should always be an upward one.'[111] The idea behind this was simply that '[t]his helps lift the skin, keeping it firmer and younger looking.'[112] This represented an appeal to intuition: the loss of elasticity and structure in the skin could be mitigated by not only chemical but also physical manipulation against the undesirable natural direction of travel.

Boots was not alone in highlighting the method of application as a crucial part of the process. Organon Laboratories, a commercial organisation specialising in the production of synthetic hormones, which we encountered first in Chapter 2, entered the skin care market in the 1950s with Endocril, described as 'the first cosmetic hormone cream produced by specialists in hormones'.[113] The promotional literature noted that the cream should be applied to the face and neck 'with a circular movement, especially emphasising the upward and outward strokes'.[114] The presence of hormones in skin care products past World War Two reflected the growing interest in the potential power of such substances after various interwar breakthroughs in synthesising hormones, particularly the so-called sex hormones.[115] Product developers at Boots, led by the influential fashion writer and editor of *Women*

---

[108] 'Number Seven: Your Guide to Beauty', c.1962, 3, A30/6, Boots Archive.

[109] 'A Guide to Selling Beauty: Number Seven', c.1965, 7, A30/14, Boots Archive.

[110] Kammerer, *Rejuvenation*, 97. For more on Francis Bacon's conception of ageing as a process of cooling and drying, see: Bacon, *Historia Vitae et Mortis*, 276–77.

[111] 'A Guide to Selling Beauty: Number Seven', c.1965, 17, A30/14, Boots Archive.   [112] Ibid.

[113] 'Endocril', c.1955, n.p., EPH 625, Wellcome Library, London.   [114] Ibid.

[115] Endocril was listed in compendia of available products into the early 1960s. Scottish Wholesale Druggists' Association, *Patent Medicines*, 169.

and Beauty, Phyllis Digby Morton, who advised the company during the 1950s on the marketing and development of new products, had initially entertained the possibility of producing their own hormone cream, but this was later dismissed by the Medical Department and never taken beyond initial discussion.[116] In fact, one member of the Merchandise Committee, Dr Williams, 'felt that this should not be proceeded with on medical grounds'; this at the same time that the BMA was allegedly pondering adding hormone creams to the 'Poisons List'.[117]

As well as the use of experts such as Digby Morton, Boots also had a long heritage of surveying customers, with large-scale exercises going at least as far back as 1929 when they commissioned a study designed to assess what were the most attractive and unattractive aspects of its stores, location, pricing and products. Informal written suggestions from both staff and members of the public were given serious consideration by the Formula Committee when devising new products, updating existing lines and choosing which products should be dropped. Although the Formula Committee was composed exclusively of men, this group sought advice and input from the female 'Demonstrators', whose role largely covered in-store sales, and members of staff who attended training events. When developing the original No. 7 range, Boots hired a certain Mrs Darymple as a consultant, who was paid the not insubstantial sum of £167 for occasional work during the financial year 1934–35.[118]

Although no longer such a prominent feature of the contemporary skin care landscape, products identified as skin foods are still sold in small quantities. Indeed, although much innovation in this area came during the interwar period, skin foods were still used extensively in Britain well into the 1980s.[119]

---

[116] 'Merchandise Committee Minutes', 9 January 1953, 870; 'Own Goods Development Committee Minutes', 13 January 1953, 1182; 'Own Goods Development Committee Minutes', 31 March 1953, 1256, 'No7 Extra Rich Skin Food Product File', 843/24, Boots Archive. Digby-Morton was one of the foremost beauty editors of the period. See: 'Mrs Phyllis Digby Morton', *The Times*, 9 May 1984, 16; Tinkler, *Constructing Girlhood*, 103.

[117] 'Merchandise Committee Minutes', 17 April 1953, No7 Extra Rich Skin Food Product File, 843/24, Boots Archive.

[118] 'Statistical Record for One Year Ending March 31st 1935', 17 May 1935, 24, 461, Boots Archive.

[119] 'Beauty Care Transcends Economic Blizzard', 7 March 1978, 1, 2740/6, Boots Archive. Data gathered as part of the IPC Cosmetics and Toiletries Survey, an annual, national statistical sampling across Britain which was termed 'the "bible" of the beauty business', shows the clear ongoing popularity of skin foods through into the 1980s. As the 1979 report noted, the popularity of skin foods (which were treated as a distinct product type) remained high, with 47% of the women sampled declaring themselves to be regular users. Interestingly, despite the fact that these products were associated with ageing of the skin there was no obvious bias in age-group, with usage ranging from 43% (13–18) to 53% (19–24).' IPC Magazines, *The Cosmetics*, 90.

Nature, Gender and Beauty: Postwar Themes

Beyond their increasing prominence in justifying particular approaches to diet, vitamins also became a cornerstone of the skin care industry. Promotional literature for a wide range of beauty products developed during the interwar period emphasised the importance of a diet rich in vitamins for the upkeep of youthful skin. Vitamins C and E were particularly prominent in such discussions, with the former referenced as the complexion's 'greatest beautifier' and the latter known as 'the skin vitamin'.[120] As the *Daily Record* noted in their discussion of beauty treatments for women, 'scientists have discovered various ingredients which, when blended into skin foods or unguents, repair the ravages of the years. Vitamins, hormones, of the right kind and just the correct amount ... rejuvenate worn-out tissues.'[121] Despite this, it was far from clear that Vitamin C was absorbed through the skin, though there was strong evidence that, for example, Vitamin D was readily assimilated.[122] Similarly, the retrospective justification for the efficacy of existing skin beautifiers, such as cod livers, on the grounds that these contained vitamins was met with stubborn resistance in medical circles.[123]

Whilst the scientific mechanism of action and safety remained a matter of contention, cosmetics manufacturers, especially in Britain, could exploit an increasing number of possible means by which to persuade potential consumers. For example, Boots were able to appeal to a new and younger market for general types of skin food such as those in the Number Seven by developing more specialised products for customers with genuine signs of ageing. One example was the Vitamin Plus cream, which was explicitly designed with older skin in mind. For our purposes here this material, designed to target such audiences, highlights not only the rather different age range of women who would benefit from using rejuvenation products but also the explicit links between maintaining a youthful face and skin and one's beauty.

---

[120] 'Fresh Air Really is Greatest Beauty Treatment', *Press and Journal*, 21 July 1939, 3; '[Advertisement]', *Bristol Evening Post*, 7 September 1939, 10.

[121] 'Beauty', *Daily Record*, 21 June 1939, 20.

[122] Harry, *Modern Cosmeticology*, 63; Hume, Lucas and Smith, 'On the Absorption of Vitamin D'; Nathanial Lucas, 'The Permeability of Human Epidermis'; Lucas, 'The Production of Vitamin D'. Advertisements for foodstuffs containing Vitamin D abounded from the 1920s. See 'Vitamin D in the "Allenburys" Foods', *The Chemist and Druggist*, 25 August 1927, i.

[123] In the case of cod liver oil, for example, a number of authors attributed its beneficial action on the skin and physiologically in general to its high Vitamin A content, though this was heavily contested. Cameron, 'Cod-liver Oil'; Sandor, 'Vitamin A'. For examples of contrary publications, see: Bond, 'On Irradiated Ergosterol'; Deas, 'Vitamin A and its Variations'; Zilva, Drummond, and Graham, 'The Relation of the Vitamin A Potency'; 'The Pharmacological Value of Cod-Liver Oil'; 'Cod-Liver Oil and Vitamin A'.

As the in-house *Number Seven Magazine* produced by Boots noted, the promotional material for the Vitamin Plus cream extolled that:

> Skins no longer quite so young,
> Still can keep their youthful beauty
> If their owner makes the use
> Of *Vitamin Plus* a nightly duty.[124]

Similarly, the ageing female figure began to attain value to the extent that she was committed to combating her aged appearance and state. Advertisements for products such as Tokalon Rose Skinfood lauded the 'Beautiful Grandmother' who drew on the powers of science through ingredients such as 'Biocel – the amazing vital youth element – discovered by a famous Vienna University Professor', to maintain 'the skin and complexion of a woman of 30'.[125]

The dual properties of youth and beauty of skin became entirely intertwined; presenting a youthful face to the world also meant embodying ideas of beauty. For example, immaculate appearance as an adult was seen to recapture the lost lustre and softness of skin associated with very early childhood. The sense of duty present in marketing and press narratives about beauty was a strong feature throughout the twentieth century. The assumed ubiquity of skin care and cosmetic products led to attitudes which characterised non-users as somehow lazy or inattentive. This attitude was particularly prevalent in publications of the 1950s, when women's magazines extoled the necessity of applying products to enhance beauty and preserve youth.[126]

The most important indicators of ageing on the skin may have changed, yet certain key elements remained almost unaffected by changing trends in beauty and fashion alike. The presence of fine lines and wrinkles around the eyes was highlighted from at least as early as the 1920s as a tell-tale sign of ageing, whilst the changes in skin around the throat area gradually became more significant in terms of advertising and product development, leading to specialised 'throat creams' and instructions for protecting the neck by the early 1950s.[127] These physical changes associated with female ageing were reconfigured through the introduction of new products and techniques, and informed our understanding of what was considered beautiful. In this way, quests for younger-looking skin constituted a type of rejuvenation practice which drew

---

[124] 'A Few Verses on Number Seven…', *Number Seven Magazine* (1957) Spring, 11, Boots Archive.

[125] '[Advertisement]', *Daily Herald*, 13 October 1939, 9.

[126] 'You Are Unique', *Shopping* (March/April 1952), 30; 'A Beauty Routine', *Homes and Gardens* (May 1952), 84.

[127] 'Face Tonic at Home', *Evening Times*, 28 March 1953, Press Cuttings, Y179/4:76, Boots Archive; 'Beauty Is Now a Question of Health', *Evening Times*, 19 June 1953, Press Cuttings Y179/4:86, Boots Archive; 'When the Children are Asleep', *The Tatler*, 9 December 1953, 606.

on elements of earlier, highly medicalised approaches pioneered by Steinach and Voronoff: the presence of hormones. This was far from universal, however, and constructions of feminine beauty played a crucial role in helping to promote nourishing products such as skin food. Manufacturers made claims to scientific authority – Boots and other firms consistently highlighted the scientific purity of their products – echoing much advertising of fringe medical products during the first half of the twentieth century.[128] Women were variously castigated for failing to make maximal use of skin care regimes – cast as cheap and accessible – and encouraged to make the most of their natural looks. When it came to the use of products such as skin foods, duty and desirability were two sides of the same coin.

Belief in the indicative primacy of the skin was not a new feature of medical practice or visual aesthetic in the interwar period. Rather, it built on long-standing perceptions of the skin's status as a mediator between self and society, a theme echoed in recent scholarship on the sociocultural significance of the skin.[129] More than this, however, the late interwar period saw the scientific and commercial entrenchment of the normal ageing course for the body, which became defined by productivity, physical capacity and the visual signifiers which are now inescapably associated with ageing, such as the appearance of wrinkles.

Regulating the Rejuvenation Marketplace

The historical actors engaged in the production, promotion, use and critique of rejuvenating skin products were not, of course, acting in a neutral marketplace. Rather, they operated within marketing conventions and legal instruments which played a critical role in shaping the nature and scope of advertisement claims. Before we consider some of the key themes to emerge across different rejuvenation strategies – with skin care arguably at the intersection between these – it is worth pausing to reflect on the national differences in regulation within which manufacturers operated.

By the time that the manufacturers of hormone creams created new consumer demand (and reverence) for these preparations in the 1930s, regulation of such products in the United States still fell under the auspices of the almost thirty-year-old Pure Food and Drugs Act (1906). This legislation had been a key plank of early twentieth-century progressive reforms, and drew together a complex patchwork of inconsistent and misleading state regulations to provide a national framework for preventing adulteration of foodstuffs, demanding that manufacturers withdraw unfounded claims from their marketing. It also

---

[128] Stark, "'Recharge My Exhausted Batteries'".
[129] Benthien, *Skin*; Connor, *The Book of Skin*.

established the Bureau of Chemistry in the Department of Agriculture as the official testing body of products.[130] An increasing marketplace of invalid foodstuffs, preparations for specific diets and, of course, cosmetics containing powerful chemical and biological agents, created the context for further regulation in the 1930s, yet it was much publicised 1937 Elixir Sulfanilamide poisoning incident – in which at least ninety-three people died after taking a preparation manufactured using the highly toxic chemical diethylene glycol – which accelerated efforts to further tighten controls on the production, testing and marketing of foods, drugs and, now, cosmetics.[131]

A major consequence of the revised, expanded Food, Drug and Cosmetic Act, passed in 1938, was the power afforded to the Food and Drug Administration to remove from the market any cosmetic products which contained banned substances or were mislabelled.[132] Hormone and vitamin creams sat at the interface between medical and cosmetic products.[133] On the one hand, many of the claims made about these preparations were explicitly physiological in nature; on the other, beauty and youthfulness were the main objects of their action. According to the definition of the 1938 Act (and most subsequent pieces of legislation), cosmetics were defined as 'articles intended to be rubbed, poured, sprinkled, or sprayed on, introduced into, or otherwise applied to the human body or any part thereof for cleansing, beautifying, promoting attractiveness, or altering the appearance'.[134] This clearly captured the essence of the rejuvenating skin care products on the market in the United States.

There was no such regulation in Britain, which relied instead on the Pharmacy and Poisons Act (1933) and Dangerous Drugs Act (1920), the intention behind which was to control mainstream as well as patent medicines, and certainly not cosmetic products. As an editorial in the *British Medical Journal* noted in 1938 on the recent passage of the updated US legislation, 'Great Britain is the only large English-speaking community in which the law does nothing to protect the public against fraud in this field.'[135] Indeed, whilst the legislation designed to protect British consumers from fraudulent and potentially medical products was relatively strong, cosmetics remained unregulated, despite the acknowledged and 'important borderland

---

[130] For more on the original Pure Food and Drugs Act, see Young, *Pure Food*; Okun, *Fair Play in the Marketplace*.

[131] '"Death Drug" Hunt Covered 15 States. Wallace Reveals How Federal Agents Traced Elixir to Halt Fatalities', *New York Times*, 26 November 1937, 42.

[132] 'Act of June 25, 1938 (Federal Food, Drug, and Cosmetic Act)'.

[133] Gwen Kay has provided some important insights into the regulation of cosmetics in the context of the United States. See, for example: Kay, 'Healthy Public Relations'; Kay, *Dying to Be Beautiful*.

[134] 'Federal Food, Drug, and Cosmetic Act', 5.

[135] 'The New U.S.A. Food and Drug Act', 457.

which lies between the provinces of the dermatologist and the beauty specialist's parlour'.[136] The following year, another editorial noted two dangerous features of the cosmetic landscape in Britain. The first was the continued lack of oversight, in a marketplace 'practically unfettered by legislative regulation'; the second was that '[v]ast sections of womankind ... now devote a considerable portion of their weekly earnings to beauty culture.'[137] Cases of serious injury from cosmetic preparations were rare, but they attracted the attention of the medical press, reflecting ongoing concerns about the composition of these comparatively under-regulated products. For example, at a meeting of the Section of Dermatology of the British Medical Association in the summer of 1936, Agnes Savill (1875–1964), a London-based dermatologist and practitioner in electro-therapeutics, noted a number of 'disastrous cases of grave eye injury' and a number of cosmetic products which contained mercury or lead.[138]

Amongst those practitioners who engaged closely with the production, efficacy and safety of scientific beauty preparations was Ralph G. Harry, an analyst and consulting chemist who worked at Port Sunlight to develop a range of cosmetic products for Unilever in the 1930s. Despite his commercial affiliations, Harry provided a balanced overview of the efficacy of different cosmetic preparations, arguing that 'a sound knowledge of the dermatological principles underlying their use' was necessary, so 'that a suitable choice of raw materials may be made for the particular product in view.'[139] Amongst the many classes of skin care product which he considered – providing both evaluation and sample recipes – were skin foods, vitamin and hormone creams and lubricating creams. In his evaluation, which drew on studies carried out through the 1920s and 1930s, Harry argued that the composition of the base of skin creams had a minimal effect on whether the active ingredients were absorbed through the skin.[140] This was in marked contrast to many of the claims made by manufacturers during the 1930s about the readiness with which specific preparations were assimilated after application.

In contrast, Harry argued, '[t]he absorption of vitamins and hormones appears very definite.'[141] The use of hormones – 'not substances to be lightly trifled with' – invariably focussed on the sex hormones, which various authors had already claimed to have cancer-inducing properties following a series of

[136] 'The Science of Cosmetics', 832.   [137] 'Labels for Cosmetics'.
[138] 'British Medical Association', 258. Savill had trained at Glasgow after graduating from St. Andrew's in 1895. Savill published an authoritative treatise on conditions affecting the hair and scalp. See: Brock, British Women Surgeons, 205; Savill, The Hair and Scalp.
[139] Harry, Modern Cosmeticology, iii. This text went through a number of subsequent editions, published eventually simply as Harry's Cosmeticology in its sixth edition in 1975.
[140] Ibid., 52–55.   [141] Ibid., 55.

studies in the early 1930s.[142] It was far from clear that this supposed cancerous risk involved in the application of hormone creams played out clinically, however. Indeed, the appearance of cosmetic hormone creams and, especially, the relaxed regulatory environment prior to the Food, Drug and Cosmetic Act (1938), prompted a more rigorous interrogation of the dangers posed by these substances, which proved negative.[143] Even in the hands of 'an ordinary woman without medical supervision', Harry considered the possibility of harm arising from the use of creams containing sex hormones to be 'extremely remote'.[144] The fact that he nevertheless asserted that 'the use of therapeutic agents is rightly the domain of the medical profession' was therefore more a reflection of long-standing anxieties about the arrogation of medico-scientific expertise by the cosmetics industry, not a response to concerns over safety.[145]

Although medical practitioners were generally reluctant to engage in public discourse over products considered cosmetic, within the pages of professional journals occasional commentaries lamented the appropriation and extrapolation of scientific ideas to the realm of beauty culture. For example, as one correspondent noted in *The Lancet* in 1937, as well as the 'exploitation of up-to-date fancies, like skin-foods full of vitamins and hormones', the mobilisation of acid as 'a cause, a disease, and an almost ritual diagnosis' for the complexion, hair and constitution, was created solely to keep 'the wolf from the beauty-parlour door'.[146] According to a leading article from the following year, '"hormone face creams" enjoy an undeserved popularity'; to make matters worse, they were considered 'not without danger, for if they have an appreciable content of oestrogen and are applied continuously as recommended they may derange the menstrual cycle, if they do nothing worse.'[147] More specifically, the *Journal of the American Medical Association* actively warned its readership that overuse of the hormone cream Endocreme – 'a cosmetic with a menace' – 'may lead to dangerous consequences ... bringing about serious changes in the genital and reproductive organs of women', not to mention the possibility of carcinogenic action.[148]

As well as organised institutional safeguards and forms of regulation, more informal forms of control existed, for example through advice offered to consumers by independent sources of monitoring. In the United States, for example, organisations such as Consumer's Research Inc. issued pamphlets to consumers on a wide range of products.[149] Formed originally in 1927, Consumer's Research was the first organisation of its kind in the United

---

[142] Cook, Hewitt and Hieger, 'The Isolation of a Cancer-Producing Hydrocarbon'; Lacassagne, 'Apparition des cancers de la mamelle'; Burrows, 'Pathological Changes'.
[143] 'Royal Society of Medicine'; Cramer and Gye, 'Œstrin and Cancer', 1365.
[144] Harry, *Modern Cosmeticology*, 60.   [145] Ibid., 61.   [146] 'Grains and Scruples', 156.
[147] 'Ways of Giving Sex Hormones', 1118.   [148] 'Endocreme', 1194.
[149] Ellwood, *The Fifties Spiritual Marketplace*, 111.

States; it tested and rated products on the market, with a view to advising consumers and testing the safety and efficacy against manufacturers' claims.[150] In a book-length synthesis of some of the key early investigations by Consumer's Research, leading members Arthur Kallet and F. J. Schlink produced a comprehensive and scathing account of regulation of the food, drug and cosmetic market.[151] In this book – graphically titled *100,000,000 Guinea Pigs* – they argued that '[t]he purchaser of cosmetics has no protection whatsoever.'[152] Kallet and Schlink highlighted numerous instances where products were found to be not just ineffective but unsafe. In many cases, rather than reversing or reducing the appearance of ageing, the treatments meant that '[h]undreds, perhaps thousands, of young women ... will go through life with the withered and wrinkled cheeks or limbs of very old women, the flesh actually atrophied.'[153]

Whilst the high-profile cases discussed by Kallet and Schlink showcase some of the most sensational adverse reactions to rejuvenating products and procedures of the period, their interventions also reveal a marketplace skewed by the dominance of rejuvenation as a social discourse. Indeed, a review of a subsequent publication from Consumer's Research dismissed the details as 'more sensational than scientific', despite the acknowledgement that 'costly and sometimes dangerous cosmetics, unguents, astringents, lotions, and other aromatic chemicals that are flamboyantly, extravagantly, and often erroneously advertised as positive aids to the attainment of female pulchritude.'[154] The reviewer was James A. Tobey, a lecturer in public health law at the Massachusetts Institute of Technology and author of numerous treatises on consumer and state protections of health, including books on milk and public health legislation.[155] Tobey was just the latest in a long line of medical professionals who had watched as manufacturers exploited physicians' reluctance to engage in commercial activities.[156] As Morris Fishbein noted in his scathing 1927 critique of the modern quasi-medical fad treatments, '[r]ejuvenation pays! ... One can almost picture him [the purveyor of rejuvenating therapies] rubbing his hands in glee as he murmurs: "Rejuvenation: That's the word that gets 'em!"'[157]

---

[150] The organisation grew out of the success of a book on the topic: Chase and Schlink, *Your Money's Worth*. For a wealth of primary source material, see 'Records of Consumers' Research, Inc.' MC 3, Rutgers University, Special Collections and University Archives, 1910–1983. Systematic interrogation of the contents of patent medicines was not new, of course. For an earlier example, see 'The Composition of Certain Secret Remedies'.
[151] Kallet and Schlink, *100,000,000 Guinea Pigs*.   [152] Ibid., 78.   [153] Ibid., 89.
[154] Tobey, 'Skin Deep', 507.
[155] Tobey, *The Legal Aspects of Milk Control*; Tobey, *Public Health Law*.
[156] Stark, 'Introduction: Plurality in Patenting'; Jones, 'A Barrier to Medical Treatment?'; Gabriel, 'Pharmaceutical Patenting'.
[157] Fishbein, *The New Medical Follies*, 113 and 115.

Legacy and Conclusion

Discussions at Boots about the possible creation of a new hormone cream in the mid-1950s demonstrate that skin care products which drew on ideas originating in the endocrine system far outlasted the attention given to surgical interventions promoting rejuvenation. Indeed, whilst hormone replacement therapy (HRT) was one of the most long-lasting effect of Steinach's researches, rejuvenating skin creams were similarly inspired by the burgeoning sciences of endocrinology and nutrition in the first half of the twentieth century.

Throughout much of the advertising associated with skin care, nature was cast both as the enemy of the skin and the possible source of salvation. For example, the 1970s saw the 'natural' content of various beauty preparations trumpeted as symbols of desirability and efficacy.[158] The launch of a new Original Formula range of No7 in 1977 was accompanied by an extensive advertising campaign highlighting natural ingredients; the Moisture Plus cream was 'rich in natural oils and humectant ingredients to leave your skin soft but not sticky.'[159] On the other hand, Boots claimed that the No7 Seasonal Supplement of the late 1980s was able to 'neutralise the effects of "Seasonal Stress"' and return 'the skin to its natural, vital state', counteracting the harmful effects of the environment on the body.[160] Similarly, the rather less subtly named Anti-Wrinkle Cream was capable of 'defending against the elements which can help to accelerate skin-ageing and the development of facial lines'.[161]

Product developments came against a backdrop of increasingly detailed and sophisticated market research, which enabled manufacturers to identify tighter gaps in an ever more crowded marketplace. Whilst reducing the appearance of ageing was one of the key claims made for skin foods and related products, it was not the sole purported benefit. Alongside 'a lovely youthful glow to the skin', using the preparations appropriately to one's skin type offered 'the modern woman many wonderful ways to make her delightfully feminine'.[162] This points us straightforwardly to the target audience of such preparations in terms of gender, yet the question of age, as might be expected, is also of great significance. By the 1980s, the promotional literature for Number Seven products characterised the 'slightly older women' as 'anyone the far side of 30'.[163] Yet the impression that products associated with anti-ageing and rejuvenation have targeted increasingly younger women and girls is somewhat

---

[158] See, for a fuller discussion of the 1970s context, Binkley, *Getting Loose.*
[159] 'Advertising: Woman's Journal', 1978, Y159, Boots Archive.
[160] 'No7 Extra Care', [1986], 23, A30/9, Boots Archive.   [161] Ibid.
[162] 'Number Seven: Your Guide to Beauty', [1962], 8 and 16, A30/6. Boots Archive.
[163] '[Untitled]', *No7 Magazine* (1980) Autumn-Winter, 11, A30/7, Boots Archive.

misleading. Even during the 1950s, for example, the *Number Seven Magazine* noted that,

after thirty the natural oil supply of the skin starts to diminish. This makes it necessary to increase external applications of oil-concentrating preparations. Skin foods and nourishing creams become of first importance to maintain the suppleness and softness of the skin.[164]

More informally, advice pages in Boots publications made it clear that for these products to be maximally effective in preventing the signs of ageing from appearing, they should be used 'as soon as you start to use make-up'; in the case of one letter to *Number Seven Magazine*, this was from the age of eighteen, where the correspondent was advised that 'the few minutes that you spend each night taking care of your skin by using Number Seven Cleansing Cream, Skin Freshener and Extra-Rich Skin Food, will keep your skin young and fresh looking all your life.'[165] Another enquiry brought the response that any woman over the age of twenty-five should use skin food as an essential part of a daily beauty regime.[166] Nor was Boots alone in high-lighting the assumed importance of using products of this type earlier in life. One of Max Factor's promotional brochures from the 1960s, which featured a skin cream named 'The Cup of Youth' and dubbed '[e]ssential for every woman past her teens', warned that 'the time to start disciplined skin care is in the teens onwards.'[167]

Promotional claims surrounding skin care products from the late 1920s drew extensively on scientific understandings of the ageing process – particularly the role of hormones and vitamins – and tapped into powerful trends which emphasised to women the importance, and potential, of modern innovations. Veneration of youthfulness and modernity went hand-in-hand, resulting in a radical transformation from 'the day of the matured women' – when 'the matured woman [was] "the fashion"' – proclaimed by the *Evening Dispatch* in 1915.[168] More than this, the appropriation of hormones ensured that, long after their potential as a whole-body rejuvenation elixir had been called into question, the close link between endocrine balance and youthfulness was perpetuated. Indeed, whilst we know that the early application of endocrine research to the ageing (predominantly male) body was rooted in sexuality and

---

[164] '[Back cover]', *Number Seven Magazine* (1953) 3, 16.

[165] 'Mary Severn's Pages', *Number Seven Magazine* (1953) 4, 14–15, 14.   [166] Ibid.

[167] Also in this range and promotional literature was a 'vitamin massage cream' and 'Exuberance … a cream of unique formula, containing humectants, Vitamin A, the skin vitamin, and Vitamin D, the sun vitamin' 'Max Factor: You at Your Loveliest', [1960], 3, 3193/24, Boots Archive.

[168] 'The Charm of the Matured Woman. Forty the Popular Age To-day', *Evening Dispatch*, 23 February 1915, 2.

virility, enterprising skin care manufacturers were able to use public fascination with hormones to make new links between aesthetics, commerce and bodily chemistry, only revealed by considering a wider cross-section of the diverse rejuvenation practices of the early twentieth century.[169]

When we contextualise the case of skin care in the interwar period, two major themes emerge. The first is the incomplete yet highly significant shift in the gender dynamics of rejuvenation, with the focus of products and procedures moving from men to women. This mirrored anxieties over the fitness of the male body in the immediate aftermath of World War One and the consequent developments of a mass skin care and cosmetic market, open to and targeted towards a far broader social class.[170] Second, rejuvenation discourse, already laden with commercial imperatives in the 1920s, became increasingly subsumed within trade, not medical, literature and advertising, not editorial, columns. This was driven in a large part by the inclusion of hormones within skin care preparations, but also the normalisation of vitamins in the same way. As a result, skin care manufacturers became significant authorities on the skin, regardless of whether or not they laid claims to scientific expertise.

Many aspects of our relationship with ageing and a quest for rejuvenation were, and remain, embodied in the use of skin care products, from an increasing need to perpetuate a state of youthful appearance by correct nourishment to the desire to do so without recourse to the attentions of medical specialists. There is an important distinction, too, between the prolongation of life and the maintenance of youth; in the twentieth century, the former was bound up with medicalised ideas of public health, vaccination and battle against mortality, whilst the latter was a far broader category, encompassing not just the much-studied hormone surgeries but the use of everyday products in a domestic context. In some critical ways, too, the desirable ends of rejuvenation were little changed through the early twentieth century. As Mrs John Webster argued in her 1907 manifesto, *Beauty and Health in Old Age*, a 'natural diet' was the sure way to secure the most desirable of rejuvenatory outcomes:

An old age free from suffering, with a mind unimpaired, holding the experience of a life! A body free from the deformities which make old age ugly! The face having a beauty of its own, because its expression is not marred by a weakened brain and vacant mind – the muscles remaining well nourished [*sic*] instead of shrivelling! The skin not dried up and mummified, like the faces of the rare people who now live to be a hundred![171]

---

[169] Sengoopta, *The Most Secret Quintessence*; Hirshbein, 'The Glandular Solution'.

[170] Relevant here, too, is the changing social role of women across the interwar period. For more on this, see: Hapke, *Daughters of the Great Depression*; Sharp and Stibbe, 'Women's International Activism'; Schmid, 'The "New Woman"'; and, especially: Todd, *Young Women, Work, and Family*.

[171] Webster, *Beauty and Health in Youth and Old Age*, 60.

These ends were predicated on configurations of manufacturer–consumer relations, bodily awareness, gender, class and race; by the late interwar period, skin care products were the axis around which these themes clustered, with every advert representing a window into changing expressions of female beauty, scientific authority and the perceptions of ageing. The outward signs and aesthetics of ageing – experienced socially through inscriptions on the skin – were therefore just as critical components of rejuvenation discourse and practices as those which sought to extract maximal functionality from internal bodily machinery in the service of modern labour and social capital.

7   Conclusion

Though I look old, yet I am strong and lusty;
For in my youth I never did apply
Hot and rebellious spirits in my blood,
Nor did with unbashful forehead woo
The means of weakness and debility,
Therefore my age is as a lusty winter,
Frosty but kindly.[1]

Age aping youth is pathetic, yet a perfectly poised, suitably dressed woman can, by her serene self-confidence and her charming assurance, hold her own, even against the freshness and sparkle of youth.[2]

In 1932, Alexis Carrel performed a striking *volte-face*. Carrel, whose research on cellular immortality was critical in creating a space of intellectual credence within which the idea of rejuvenation could flourish, publicly denounced two of its chief flagbearers. Leaving open the possibility that rejuvenation might one day be achieved, Carrel nevertheless argued that '[n]o senescent organism has ever been rejuvenated by the procedures of Steinach and Voronoff ... The process of aging remains irreversible.'[3] Similarly, reflecting on the modern manifestation of rejuvenation, the tropical medicine specialist and historian of medicine Pan S. Codellas noted in his brief 1934 history of longevity in the ancient world that '[t]he very recent rerippling of the same subject had its usual fancy captivation, without any definite results. Concerning the rejuvenescence elixirs we stand just where our predecessors were thousands of years ago.'[4]

When compared with the cautious optimism of many medical practitioners in the early to mid-1920s, accompanied by more frenzied discussion in the popular periodical press, this might suggest that rejuvenation – and hormone-based rejuvenation in particular – was a short-lived craze for professionals and

---

[1] William Shakespeare, 'As you Like it', Act II, Scene 3.
[2] 'At 50! Are you Growing Old or Young?', *Northern Daily Mail*, 14 October 1930, 2.
[3] 'Medicine: No Rejuvenation'.   [4] Codellas, 'Rejuvenations and Satyricons', 520.

public alike which had largely fallen into abeyance by the advent of World War Two, perhaps even by the early 1930s. Chandak Sengoopta's characterisation of the 1920s as 'the decade of rejuvenation' certainly serves to reinforce this view.[5] However, the picture which emerges when we take into account a wider range of rejuvenatory ideas, practices and products is rather different: the 1920s was rather a decade of a particular *kind* of rejuvenation. The frenetic public enthusiasm for and fascination with rejuvenation in the immediate aftermath of World War One was gradually replaced with a less sensational, but arguably far more significant, deeply socially embedded assimilation of rejuvenatory ideas, languages and practices into everyday life. Even as late as 1939, mainstream texts on the biology of ageing approached the endocrinology of the life course with some caution. The major edited collection, *Problems of Ageing: Biological and Medical Aspects*, edited by Edmund Vincent Cowdry, Professor at Washington University, noted that 'the glamour of the gonads ... has given rise to the spectacular pseudo-science of "rejuvenation" via the route of the gonad hormones or gonad implantation.'[6] At the same time, however, A. J. Carlson, who authored the chapter on the endocrine system, argued that the evidence on the subject was 'largely fragmentary and inconclusive', even if specific glands could not be implicated in the ageing process to the extent that proponents of glandular rejuvenation therapy claimed.[7]

Arlene Weintraub has claimed that 'the new world of anti-aging medicine ... emerged in the 1990s and is promoted with a deceptively simple but incredibly appealing sales pitch: Hormones rage when we're young and then wane as we age.'[8] This is, however, at odds with the overwhelming documentary evidence of rejuvenation practices at the heart of both medical science and everyday domestic life during the early decades of the twentieth century. In a different vein, Patricia Cohen's claim that, whilst '[a]ltering the body to create an identity or fulfill [*sic*] a desire is commonplace today ... this notion took root in the twenties with rejuvenation treatments and plastic surgery' also requires some scrutiny.[9] Whilst it is clearly the case that attempts to restore lost youth underwent a fundamental transformation in this period, such changes were dependent not only on medical or cosmetic treatments and products but also on a diverse array of everyday practices inspired by such efforts.

Additionally, whilst different modes of rejuvenation practice came to prominence in the social, economic, cultural and scientific contexts of the interwar period, their resonance with human anxieties and aspirations concerning the life course was not new and continued unabated. Rejuvenation was a pivotal theme not just of a decade but of an era, and had a lasting legacy in the form of

---

[5] Sengoopta, 'Dr Steinach coming to make the old young!'   [6] Carlson, 'The Thyroid', 363.
[7] Ibid.   [8] Weintraub, *Selling the Fountain of Youth*, 3.   [9] Cohen, *In Our Prime*, 13.

an established anti-ageing marketplace, a cultural preoccupation with youth and youthfulness and a changing female aesthetic. This is the more remarkable given that the chief architects of hormone rejuvenation were accused of subverting key aspects of the established sexual lifecycle by 'nothing more than a re-erotization' of ageing individuals, predominantly men, which came with the attendant 'dangers of putting new wine into old bottles'.[10]

Taking a broader sweep of the early twentieth-century engagement with rejuvenation methods reveals that the interwar period concretised many of the features which have since persisted: an imperative for women to remain young and attractive, deep commercial drivers behind product generation and marketing, appeals to the importance of enhanced productivity and social utility in later life. The foundation of the commodification of the life course was essentially complete; since World War Two, the process has simply been amplified and translated across new media, with a continued valorisation of youthfulness in the face of ongoing demographic change. Matthew Thomson has argued that a yearning for a lost, imagined childhood was a distinctive feature of postwar British life.[11] In the first half of the twentieth century, a similar impulse – to cling to or recapture a lost youth, but with the experience afforded by adulthood – was just as pervasive. The effect of such fervour was significant and long-lasting. Such veneration of youthfulness played a central role in what Charlotte Greenhalgh has identified as the periodic marginalisation of older people throughout the twentieth century, particularly in the development and implementation of welfare policy specifically related to 'the elderly'.[12]

Although some of the methods favoured in the interwar period retained a degree of prominence beyond World War Two – exercise, diet, skin care – others, such as electrotherapy and endocrine treatments, have been reimagined in ways not as straightforwardly connected with rejuvenation. Considering five principal modes of achieving a renewed or continuing state of youthfulness has allowed us to see myriad connections which existed across these and, of course, additional approaches to combating the ageing process – for example, sleep, occupation, relaxation and recreation, and radiotherapy – have the potential to complexify things further.[13]

---

[10] Warthin, *Old Age*, 172–73.   [11] Thomson, *Lost Freedom*.

[12] Charlotte Greenhalgh sets her excellent account against the backdrop of broader social and cultural change, arguing that '[t]he meaning and experience of old age in the twentieth century have been bound up with the history of the British welfare state.' Greenhalgh, *Aging*, 10.

[13] Writing in 1928, the Georgetown pathologist and physical culture advocate Eugene R. Whitmore argued that 'all of us know how rapidly persons age, and how soon they die, upon complete retirement from all of their accustomed activities.' Whitmore, *Keeping Young after Forty*, 166.

In the interwar period, the sensational practices and claims associated with 'hard' surgical hormone rejuvenation in the professional and non-specialist press, driven by the promotion of Steinach and Voronoff, were out of all proportion with the actual results of the procedures on which they commentated. Their principal long-term effect was to embed both the desirability and feasibility of rejuvenation in a receptive social milieu. Indeed, advertisers mobilised the changing habits and practices of everyday life in the first half of the twentieth century as a reason why rejuvenation was necessary, not just for the elderly but throughout the life course. For example, Sanatogen, first viewed as a more general 'popular restorative' in the period before World War One, was gradually reframed by its manufacturers as a way of promoting 'youthful health'.[14] They claimed that '[i]t is difficult to imagine nowadays the restfulness of the world 50 years ago. Radio, motorcars, sensational newspapers and film – all these things to which we are so accustomed are nevertheless a constant strain on the nerves.'[15] On such a view, modernity put a new kind of strain on bodies, leading to premature ageing and a need to preserve and restore. Protection in earlier life was a critical element of this. Following a rigorous skin care regimen in one's forties, according to purveyors of skin foods, muscle oils and vitamin creams, was only sufficient to ward off the visual decline of older age if sensible routines had been observed since teenagerhood.

As well as scientific innovation and trustworthiness, personal endorsement was a key strategy deployed by manufacturers in an effort to persuade consumers of the efficacy of their products. Affirmation by users of significant status, such as medical practitioners, actors, singers and military personnel, was a further method designed to confer authority on devices and preparations. Promotional material for rejuvenation products and procedures relied heavily on such personal testimony, whilst newspaper reports of claimed cases of rejuvenation made continued reference to the social position of consumers. For marketeers and writers alike, the subject offered glorious opportunities. Gertrude Atherton's 1923 novel *Black Oxen* set the tone. It explored the imagined implications of youth restored in an older woman by means of hormone treatments and X-ray therapy. Instead of the anticipated glorious return to youthful beauty and happiness, however, Atherton's rejuvenated protagonist, Madame Zatianny, experienced a sense of isolation, social exclusion and, ultimately, humiliation after her secret was revealed and she was rejected by her lover.[16]

[14] Saundby, *Old Age*, 249; Genatosan Ltd., *Sanatogen*, title page.
[15] Genatosan Ltd., *Sanatogen*.   [16] Atherton, *Black Oxen*.

Atherton's exploration of the social dimensions of rejuvenation captured the moment and was far from alone.[17] Other prominent examples of rejuvenation fiction include Mabelle Burbridge's *The Road to Beauty* (1924), in which two older women embark on a radical programme of exercise and 'reducing' in order to attain an aesthetic ideal under instruction from their virtuous, rejuvenated friend, Gloria.[18] Bertram Gayton's *The Gland Stealers* (1922), in which the rejuvenated 'Gran'pa' leads an expedition to Africa to secure a supply of testicular tissue from monkeys to provide the raw material for his friends to enjoy the benefits, highlights the folly which successful rejuvenation might induce in ageing, over-sexualised men.[19] The power of hormones was also long-lasting in the public imagination. Market research carried out for Boots in 1967 revealed that '[m]ore esoteric products such as hormone creams are thought of, rather unclearly, as contributing more fundamentally to the health and growth of the skin cells.' Having started their public life as a way of explaining diverse physiological effects and sexuality, the connection between hormones and longevity, made so publicly visible by Steinach and Voronoff, had become rather less clear-cut, but just as fundamental.[20]

For women, age and overall health were now not just intimately linked with beauty; different stages of life demanded the use of different products, and the advent of World War Two only served to reinforce the message that 'beauty is duty.'[21] Rejuvenation methods spoke directly to these social concerns; the prolific beauty columnist 'Portia', writing in the *Daily Mail* in January 1933, noted with considerable approval the 'many "over forties" we see with necks without a wrinkle', lauding 'the youthful-looking grandma', attributed in no small part to '[t]he "emancipation" ... [which] has taken 20 years off the age of women'.[22] That is not to say, of course, that rejuvenation was universally regarded as a positive, or even interesting, enterprise. Dismissing some of the latest findings on the subject, a leading article from the *Daily Herald* rubbished the claim that Francesco Cavazzi had donned 'the alchemist's cloak' and discovered 'the latest elixir'; according to the paper, 'the majority of people are too busy getting the most out of life, whether at work or play, to worry about staying the hands of the clock.'[23]

---

[17] For a specific study of C. P. Snow's anonymously published second novel, *New Lives for Old*, see Oakley, 'Sexual Rejuvenation and Hegemonic Masculinity'.

[18] Burbridge, *The Road to Beauty*.   [19] Gayton, *The Gland Stealers*.

[20] J. C. P., 'Report on Qualitative Research into Skin Care and Reactions to Six New Product Concepts', September 1967, 1507, Boots Archive.

[21] The concept that '[t]he old, in order to be really alive, must act', articulated in different ways across numerous rejuvenation guides, adverts and other texts, further reflected the popular view that rejuvenation was a necessary and personal responsibility. Lacassagne, *A Green Old Age*, v.

[22] 'Portia's Weekly Topics. The Modern Woman of Fifty', *Daily Mail*, 19 January 1933, 7.

[23] 'The Latest Elixir', *Daily Herald*, 26 August 1929, 4. Cavazzi's approach nevertheless demonstrated significant staying power, with none other than the Nobel Prize–winning French

There was nevertheless a deep-seated public fascination and medical curiosity surrounding rejuvenation, predicated on new understandings of the body, its composition and its desirable features. The narrow scope of early histories, which focused on surgeries inspired by endocrinology, left uncovered the wider-reaching impact of such therapies on the everyday commercial landscape of anti-ageing more generally.[24] This both drew on and transformed long-standing perceptions of the value and utility of individuals, lauding youthfulness and suggesting that the search for a plausible manifestation of vital force was far from over, exemplified by writings such as Goizet's *Never Grow Old*, a practical guide for longer life and extended health in which the author proclaimed the circulatory system to be 'a revictualling network for the great vital current ... [constituting] *true streams of life*'.[25] This came despite prewar assertions from leading figures in British medicine and science that vitalism was dead. In his Presidential Address to the British Association for the Advancement of Science meeting in Dundee on 4 September 1912, E. A. Schäfer, Professor of Physiology at the University of Edinburgh, took as his subject the broad theme of 'The Nature, Origin, and Maintenance of Life'. Schäfer was uncompromising:

vitalism as a working hypothesis has not only had its foundations undermined, but most of the superstructure has toppled over, and if any difficulties of explanation still persist, we are justified in assuming that the cause is to be found in our imperfect knowledge of the constitution and working of living material. At the best vitalism explains nothing, and the term 'vital force' is an expression of ignorance which can bring us no further along path of knowledge. Nor is the problem in any way advanced by substituting for the term 'vitalism', 'neo-vitalism' and for 'vital force' 'biotic energy'.[26]

The retention of the language of vitalism was also accompanied by the persistence of aspects of humoural medicine in both language and ambition. Balancing or, just as commonly, remedying the electrical or hormonal composition of the body was predicated on a view of the body as a homogeneous entity, with external manifestations of the ageing process underpinned by

---

physiologist Charles Richet providing a ringing endorsement of Cavazzi's method and results, even as late as 1934. He wrote in a preface to Cavazzi's book: 'Thus Cavazzi was able, by *natural* means, to restore the organic, physical and psychical energies to men weakened by age and work, that is, to rejuvenate them. Certainly, his method is far superior to that of Voronoff and to any other method of rejuvenation, reinvigoration, restoration of energies, etc., known to this day.' 'Ainsi Cavazzi a pu, par des moyens *naturels*, redonner les énergies organiques, physiques et psychiques, aux hommes affaiblis par l'âge et par le travil, c'est-à-dire les rajeunir. Certes, sa méthode est bien supérieure à celle de Voronoff et à toute autre méthode de rajeunissement, de revigoration, de restauration des énergies, etc., connue jusqu'à ce jour.' Cavazzi, *Vie et Rajeunissement*, xi, my translation from French, original emphasis.

[24] Trimmer, *Rejuvenation*; McGrady, *The Youth Doctors*; Hamilton, *The Monkey Gland Affair*.
[25] Goizet, *Never Grow Old*, 30 and 35, original emphasis.
[26] Schäfer, 'Presidential Address', 677.

common physiological conditions. The view that particular life stages were invariably accompanied by the dominance of specific character traits – the 'sanguine youth' of Thomas Bodley Scott, who also noted that in 'old age . . . the temperature of the body is low' – served to reinforce the connection between the internal and external faces of the body.[27]

Perhaps most broadly of all, rejuvenation spoke to a pressing desire for human renewal and regeneration, made all the more urgent by the vexed question as to 'why there is so much sickness among civilized mankind'.[28] As Stefanos Geroulanos and Todd Meyers have recently argued, medical science in the early twentieth century was broadly constructed around 'a body that was both brittle and tightly integrated'.[29] However, the view of 'the body' as a singular, predominantly male, conflict-damaged entity belies the fact that bodies were also fragmented temporally, nationally and by gender, subject to natural decay as well as pathology and injury wrought by everyday manifestations of modernity. Even as the architects of an integrated physiological body constructed elaborate historical narratives to celebrate their own success, methods of intervention remained hugely contested.[30] Against this backdrop, rejuvenation in its many forms responded to and reinforced the expectation that a combination of technological innovation, modern medical science and lifestyle changes might serve to continue an indefinite increase in both average lifespan and the healthy period of life which had emerged through the latter part of the nineteenth century: Could rejuvenation be the new public health, the new germ theory of disease? This was partly because, as Chandak Sengoopta has argued, 'the concept of internal secretions pushed medical thinking in bold new directions', but also owed much to the social pressures present in the immediate aftermath of World War One and the rehabilitation and reformulation of existing understandings of the human body.[31] The American Army Medical Officer Eugene R. Whitmore, writing in his 1928 practical rejuvenation guide, *Keeping Young After Forty*, argued that

A very important cause of nervous and mental disturbances of all degrees is the stress and strain of life as lived to-day; the strain and worry connected with business care, sedentary habits, improper diet, insufficient and improper rest and recreation, misfit in employment, and attempts to make both ends meet.[32]

---

[27] Scott, *The Road to a Healthy Old Age*, 5 and 16.   [28] Mallett, *Nature's Way*, 9.
[29] Geroulanos and Meyers, *The Human Body*, x.   [30] Ibid., 291–95.
[31] Sengoopta, *The Most Secret Quintessence*, 2.
[32] Whitmore, *Keeping Young after Forty*, 164. Whitmore also developed significant new methods in vaccination and serum production. See Eugene R. Whitmore to Doctor Reagh, 2 June 1919, University of Massachusetts Medical School, http://massbiologicshistory.umassmed.edu/?attachment_id=348, accessed 18 January 2019.

Like many of British contemporaries, Whitmore lamented the state of men who submitted for service during World War One, of whom almost half had at least 'minor defects'.[33] The disturbing findings of these national exercises, assessing the physical capacity of service-age men, coupled with the much-recognised economic anxiety and demographic shock of the interwar period, contributed to a social environment in which rejuvenation became a highly desirable end. At the same time, the gender-specific claims associated with almost all forms of rejuvenation reveal a deep-seated belief in the inherent physiological, sexual, social and psychological differences between male and female bodies, whether they were thought of as fundamentally electrical or chemical in nature. We only have to look to guides which instructed that to 'retain your youthful looks and mind', women should 'preserve menstruation' for as long as possible through appropriate diet and exercise to see how extensively the change of life or climacteric was characterised as a point of decline, until 'the flame of life becomes gradually extinguished.'[34] The experience of older women was not, of course, homogeneous, but depended on numerous other social factors such as class and marital status.[35] The language of hysteria and debility – prevalent in discussions of strictly female and male maladies, respectively, during the nineteenth century – was no longer quite so dominant, yet the underlying assumptions remained. Similarly, those who promoted rejuvenation as a desirable end drew on language and imagery of the stable body, reflecting what we know from Mark Jackson's work on stress to be a view of bodies as in dynamic flux, subject to the influence of 'both biological and cultural forces rendered visible by the technology and language of biomedical science'.[36] To this, of course, we might add the importance of commercial exploitation of perceived bodily decay, whether through expensive surgical intervention, cheaper over-the-counter products or supposedly cost-neutral lifestyle management.

In keeping with this diverse range of explanatory mechanisms, the first half of the twentieth century saw a highly pluralised land-grab for scientific and moral authority over the human body, with numerous groups – women and men, specialists and non-specialists, manufacturers and professionals – exploiting, appropriating and repackaging (sometimes literally) a vast swathe of medical science to claim a new kind of bodily expertise. This can be seen in several high-profile areas of interwar medical practice, such as the treatment and management of shell shock and the rapid rise and fall of Salvarsan

---

[33] Whitmore, *Keeping Young after Forty*, 199.   [34] Baird and Cossley-Batt, *Elixir of Life*, 71.
[35] As Pat Thane and Lynn Botelho have argued, narratives of older age 'have had to overcome the notion that the lives of older people were relatively uniform'; such a point might be usefully extended to encompass rejuvenation strategies which lay claim to universality. Thane and Botelho, 'Introduction', 3.
[36] Jackson, *The Age of Stress*, 16.

606, which depended on the primacy of particular conceptualisations of bodies. By taking seriously rejuvenation – as much a social movement as a field of medical enquiry or practice – we see the persistence of a number of medical concepts which had supposedly fallen by the wayside. Advocates of electrotherapy vied with endocrinologists, and an emerging and highly visible class of experts such as dieticians, nutritionists, beauty therapists and instructors in physical culture challenged traditional medical authorities in ways which had profound long-term consequences for personal management of health, fitness and vitality, as well as the centrality of youthfulness in an ageing society.

8   Postscript

In the immediate aftermath of World War Two, the Nuffield Foundation, established in 1943 with the aim of improving social well-being through research in the sciences and social sciences and policy development, investigated 'the problems of ageing and the care of older people' in order to determine how best to manage national resources.[1] One of the foundational questions was what actually constituted 'old age', a complex term which determined the scope of the report. The Committee, chaired by the researcher and social reformer B. Seebohm Rowntree who was himself in his seventies, took a blunt and pragmatic approach, effectively treating the age of seventy as a watershed moment in human capacity. They noted that those under this age were 'still capable of leading substantially normal lives, though at a somewhat reduced tempo ... [whilst] those above that age ... tend, in most cases, to become really old, with an accelerating diminution of intellectual and physical power, and with consequently reduced ability to lead normal and independent lives.'[2] Somewhat ironically, this mirrored almost exactly Jean Frumusan's satirical mockery from twenty years earlier, in which he critiqued the simplistic concept of age which characterised seventy-year-olds as 'wrinkled old men, endowed with numerous infirmities ... miraculous that we are still alive. For we no longer live, we are merely lasting out.'[3] Frumusan's insistence that years were not an accurate measure of true age had gone unheeded.

The crude demarcation of life into periods of supposed vitality, energy and productivity, and lethargy, physical degradation and incapacity serves to highlight three important features of the debates around the process of ageing in the first half of the twentieth century. First, it hints at the power of attempts by commercial interests to break up the life course along arbitrary lines in order to target consumer groups based on age. Second, it reveals strong connections between biological and social conceptions of ageing in the period immediately following World War Two. Finally, it articulates an

---

[1] Nuffield Foundation Survey Committee on the Problems of Ageing and the Care of Old People, *Old People*.
[2] Ibid., 1.   [3] Frumusan, *Rejuvenation*, 33.

understanding of ageing which is strongly linked to utility, efficiency and both social and economic value. The goal of the Nuffield report was to provide recommendations to improve care for the elderly and suggest ways in which resources for the purpose might be better targeted. However, labouring under the impression that the elderly were a collective and growing burden on society reflected a continuation of interwar perspectives which extolled the benefits of rejuvenating ageing individuals. In many ways, the report in its entirety provides ample evidence that some of the key goals of would-be rejuvenators – maintaining youthful energy, restoring sexual potency and fertility, and ensuring the ability to act as useful citizens – had profound long-term impacts on our perception of the lifecycle, ageing and youthfulness.

By the early 1950s, even strong advocates of rejuvenation still operating in the mainstream, such as the author George Ryley Scott, had all but abandoned claims about the literal reversal of the ageing process. Scott, who published extensively on sex and contraception in the interwar period, still held the belief that 'hormonal deficiencies' were the chief cause of the degenerative process of senility, yet he also acknowledged that medical science was likely to have far more success in 'postponing or doing away with the period of senescence' than prolonging life.[4]

In some respects, Scott was echoing the earlier focus of Peter Schmidt and others who, in the early 1930s, worked to recast rejuvenation as the search for enhanced vitality and energy, as well as enhanced or protected intellectual capacity, not a source of radical life extension.[5] Scott argued that rejuvenation was concerned with remaining 'resilient, active, ever grappling with new ideas'; he sought not to rekindle enthusiasm for hormonal treatments, but rather to encourage 'the cultivation of an absorbing *interest* in life and in living, the retention of ambition, the fixing of a goal at which to aim' in older age.[6] Perhaps unsurprisingly for a writer whose work focussed on matters of sexual habits and birth control, Scott bemoaned the stigma associated with attempts to rejuvenate the human body: '[t]he idea has been mooted abroad that those seeking rejuvenation are the immoral, the debauched, the libidinistic, the lecherous members of society; that the treatment prescribed appeals to men who had led dissolute lives, and are in search of a means whereby they can continue their careers of lust and excess.'[7] This lays bare the anxiety of the interwar period that successful rejuvenation would lead to a society where immoral habits in earlier life had no long-term consequences.

---

[4] Scott, *The Quest for Youth*, 7 and 10.
[5] Schmidt, *The Conquest of Old Age*. Scott was also a prominent advocate of eugenic birth control in the interwar period. See Scott, *Birth Control*.
[6] Scott, *The Quest for Youth*, 146.   [7] Ibid., 8.

The era of rejuvenation had a lasting effect on the commercial world of products associated with the ageing process as well as social perceptions of the aged. In her seminal work on the subject, *The Coming of Age* (published in English in 1972 from the original 1970 work *La Vieillesse*), Simone de Beauvoir presented a frank and revealing consideration of the role of the elderly in society, and of the individual reality of being an old person in the modern world. Although de Beauvoir's critique of social attitudes towards age was rooted in its immediate context, her historical study made clear that the circumstances which she experienced as an ageing woman were but an extension of modes of thought concretised in the interwar period when a new and lasting value was placed on youth and youthfulness.[8]

More recently still, the necessity of the pronouncement on 19 February 2019 by the US Food and Drug Administration that '[t]aking a young person's plasma and infusing it into an older person to ward off aging ... has no proven clinical benefit' highlights the continuing appeal of rejuvenation and its challenge to professional medical bodies, regulators and policymakers.[9] The supposedly transformative power of human blood, visible in the claims of start-up companies such as Ambrosia which until the FDA pronouncement sold plasma from young donors for around $8,000 per litre, echoes long-standing beliefs in the potency of younger bodily fluids.[10] In language which could have been taken verbatim from the Australian government's assertion in the mid-1930s that public consumers should be protected from the hyperbolic marketing claims associated with the Overbeck Rejuvenator, the FDA statement noted that 'some patients are being preyed upon by unscrupulous actors touting treatments of plasma from young donors as cures and remedies.'[11] As Aldred Scott Wartin, Professor of Pathology and the University of Michigan, wrote in 1929, 'the idea of physical rejuvenation is but a myth of ancient lineage disguised in quasi-scientific garments.'[12]

Catherine Oakley has recently called for a 'critique of biomedical innovations in blood rejuvenation *in the era of medical neoliberalism*', yet we can see similar attitudes towards the economy of the body and its contents across a much longer period.[13] The youthful human body as a repository of vital force or energy has transcended socio-economic circumstances, class and gender. Such attitudes were formalised for the modern period, at least in part, by Francis Bacon's assertion in his *History of Life and Death* that '[i]f any man

---

[8] De Beauvoir, *Coming of Age*.
[9] Edney, 'Beware of Using Young People's Blood'. Many thanks to Lisa Haushofer for bringing this article to my attention.
[10] Charles, 'Young Blood'. Ambrosia's website noted that they 'ceased patient treatments' from 19 February 2019 'in compliance with the FDA announcement': Ambrosia, 'Ambrosia Health'.
[11] U.S. Food and Drug Administration, 'Statement from FDA Commissioner'.
[12] Warthin, *Old Age*, 174.   [13] Oakley, 'Towards Cultural Materialism', 5, my emphasis.

could procure that a young man's spirit could be conveyed into an old man's body, it is not unlikely but this great wheel of the spirits might turn about the lesser wheels of the parts, and so the course of nature become retrograde.'[14]

Blood, alongside other bodily fluids, may have retained its pre-anatomical significance, yet rejuvenation in the interwar period was neither a singular process nor dependent on a single substance. We can characterise at least four different end goals which advocates of rejuvenation held in view. First, human immortality, the discussion of which inspired both scientific research and speculative fictions.[15] Second, radical or significant life extension, which occupied an appreciable number of scientific figures as well as proponents of everyday health-promoting activities. Third, the restoration of youthful energy and vigour later in life, effectively postponing the period of senescence without necessarily prolonging lifespan. And fourth, a prolongation of youthful appearance, complexion and physique with a goal of maintaining outward and moral beauty and charm as well as health. The accumulation of new approaches to rejuvenation saw the centuries-long search for the elixir of life gradually displaced by pragmatic means of perpetuating a state of physical and mental youthfulness to enhance the capacity of older people. This dovetailed with wider social concerns about ageing populations, particularly in the Western world, a lack of confidence in national security and economic turbulence exemplified by the Great Depression. Such attitudes remain visible in present-day debates about social care, the complex intergenerational relationships between baby-boomers, millennials and Generation Z, and the promised dawn of transformative personalised, genomic and regenerative medical therapies.[16] When we consider the broader influence of the Financial Crisis and an environment of increasing global insecurity, it is hardly surprising that products, procedures and lifestyles which claim to exert a rejuvenating effect on the internal and external surfaces of bodies retain a place of such pre-eminence in the developed world.

---

[14] Montagu and Bacon, *The Works of Francis Bacon*, 490.

[15] For an exploration of how such kinds of rejuvenation were discussed in the context of post–World War One Russia, see Krementsov, *Revolutionary Experiments*.

[16] The connections between competing models of age, such as chronological and biological age, and broad policy issues in the 'ageing society' are explored in Tiago Moreira's superb recent book, *Science, Technology and the Ageing Society*.

Bibliography

Archive Repositories

Australian Hansard Parliamentary Papers, Australia
Bodleian Library, Oxford, UK
Bolton Council Records, Bolton, UK
Boots Company Archive, Nottingham, UK
Duke University Library, Durham, NC, US
Hansard Parliamentary Papers, London, UK
Mass Observation Archive, The Keep, Sussex, UK
National Archives, Kew, UK
National Trust, UK
Oregon State University Library, Corvallis, OR, US
Royal Society of Medicine, London, UK
Rutgers University Archives, New Brunswick, NJ, US
Smithsonian National Museum of American History, Washington, DC, US
St. John's Library, Cambridge, UK
Unilever Archives, Port Sunlight, UK
Victoria and Albert Museum, London, UK
Wellcome Library, London, UK
Worcestershire Archive and Archaeology Service, Worcester, UK

Newspapers

Aberdeen Evening Express
Aberdeen Press and Journal
Adelaide Advertiser
Age, The
Airdrie and Coatbridge Advertiser
Arbroath Herald
Bedford Record
Bedfordshire Times and Independent
Bee, The
Belfast News-letter
Belfast Telegraph
Bellshill Speaker
Berwick Advertiser

Berwickshire News
Bexhill-on-Sea Observer
Bioscope, The
Birmingham Gazette
Birmingham Mail
Border Watch
Bournemouth Graphic
Bristol Evening Post
Britannia and Eve
Buckingham Advertiser and North Bucks Free Press
Buckinghamshire Herald
Burnley Express
Bystander, The
Cairns Post
Cambridge Daily News
Cheltenham Chronicle
Cheltenham Looker-on
Chemist and Druggist
Citizen, The
Contemporary Review
Daily Herald
Daily Mail
Daily Mirror
Daily Record
Daily Telegraph
Derby Daily Telegraph
Devon and Exeter Gazette
Diss Express and Norfolk and Suffolk Journal
Dumfries and Galloway Standard
Dundee Courier
Dundee Evening Telegraph
Eastborne Gazette
English Review
Evening Dispatch
Evening News
Evening Telegraph
Everybody's Magazine
Exeter and Plymouth Gazette
Falkirk Herald
Farmer and Settler
Framlingham Weekly News
Globe
Gloucestershire Echo
Grantham Journal
Graphic, The
Hampshire Advertiser
Harper's Bazaar

Hartlepool Northern Daily Mail
Health Saver
Hereford Times
Homes and Gardens
Illustrated London News
Jarrow Express
Jedbugh Gazette
Jewish Daily Bulletin
Johnstone Advocate
Kent and Sussex Courier
Lancashire Evening Post
Leamington Spa Courier
Leeds Mercury
Lincolnshire Echo
Lincolnshire Free Press
Liverpool Evening Express
London Gazette
Manchester Evening News
Manchester Guardian
Merchandise Bulletin
Milngavie and Bearsden Herald
Motherwell Times
Nature
New York Times
News, The
Northern Whig
Nottingham Evening Post
Observer, The
Pall Mall Gazette
Penny Illustrated, The
People, The
Petit Parisien, Le
Pittsburgh Press
Portadown Times
Portsmouth Evening News
Press and Journal
Punch
Reporter, The
Retail Chemist
Rugby Advertiser
Scotsman, The
Sheffield Daily Telegraph
Sheffield Evening Telegraph
Sheffield Independent
Shopping
Shrewsbury Chronicle
Sketch, The

Sphere, The
Sporting Times
St. Andrew's Citizen
Staffordshire Advertiser
Stage, The
Straits Times
Sunday Post, The
Tamworth Herald
Tatler, The
Time
Times, The
Tit-Bits
Todmorden and District News
Townsville Daily Bulletin
Warwick Daily News
Washington Post
Weekly Welcome, The
Wellington Journal
Wells Journal
West London Observer
West Sussex County Times and Standard
Western Daily Press
Western Gazette
Western Morning News
Worthing Gazette
Yorkshire Evening Post
Yorkshire Post

Primary

A. Abplanalp, 'Exercising Apparatus for Use in a Lying Position', US Patent
    1,144,085, 22 June 1915
    In Perfect Shape All Your Life. London: Health for All, c.1947
    *Slimness and Health: For Both Sexes and All Ages: The Hygienic, Aesthetic and
    Practical Value of Scientifically Devised and Graduated Exercise*. London:
    Simpkin and Marshall, c.1931
    'The Hygienic Value of Muscular Exercise', *The Sketch*, 11 November 1925, 42
O. Abramowski, *Fruitarian Diet and Physical Rejuvenation*. London: The Order of the
    Golden Age, 1916
'Act of June 25, 1938 (Federal Food, Drug, and Cosmetic Act)', Public Law 75-717,
    52 STAT 1040, https://catalog.archives.gov/id/299847, accessed 24 January
    2018
G. Mercer Adam ed., *Sandow on Physical Training*. New York: J. Selwyn Tait & Sons,
    1894
'Alfred Eichholz C.B.E., M.D. Former Chief Medical Inspector, Board of Education',
    British Medical Journal, 18 February 1933, 294–95
Alfred Eichholz Clinic & Institute of Massage and Physiotherapy. London, 1934

E. Allen, 'Female Reproductive System' in E. V. Cowdry ed., *Problems of Ageing: Biological and Medical Aspects*. London: Balliere, Tindall and Cox, 1939, 398–433

Ambrosia, 'Ambrosia Health', www.ambrosiaplasma.com, accessed 20 February 2019

H. Amos, *The Humane Diet Leaflets: 15. Medical and Scientific Testimony*. London: London Vegetarian Society, c.1925

'Arthur Abplanalp', *The Swiss Observer*, 8 November 1968, 53138, http://doi.org/10.5169/seals-696070, accessed 8 March 2019

G. Atherton, *Black Oxen*. New York: A. L. Burt, 1923

F. Bacon, *Historia Vitae et Mortis*. Leiden: J. Maire, 1636

I. Baird and J. Cossley-Batt, *Elixir of Life*. London: Python Publishing Co., 1933

H. Bailey, 'Testicular Grafting', *The Lancet*, 5 February 1927, 284

A. Balfour, 'Problems of Acclimatisation', *The Lancet*, 14 July 1923, 84–8

W. Bayliss and E. Starling, 'The Mechanism of Pancreatic Secretion', *Journal of Physiology* 28:5 (1902), 325–53

S. Beard, *A Comprehensive Guide-Book to Natural, Hygienic and Humane Diet*. London: The Order of the Golden Age, c. 1921

   Is Flesh-Eating Morally Defensible? 11th ed. London: The Order of the Golden Age, 1923

W. Beaufort, *Diathermy: Short-Wave Therapy, Inductothermy, Epithermy, Long-Wave Therapy*. London: H. K. Lewis, 1951

Z. Beckley, 'There is no Eternal Youth, but We Can Curb Old Age, Woman Researcher Says', *Brooklyn Daily Eagle*, 19 January 1928, 5

G. Beddoes, *Habit and Health: A Book of Golden Hints for Middle Age, with Especial Reference to Ailments Besetting Professional and Business Men at the Present Day*. London: Swan Sonnenschein, 1890

M. Beddow Bayly, 'The Menace of Dr Voronoff', *The Graphic*, 27 April 1929, 147

   Dr Sergius Voronoff and Rejuvenation by means of Grafting Monkey-Glands. London: The Animal Defence and Anti-Vivisection Society, 1928

   The Gland-Grafting Operations of Dr. Voronoff, reprinted from *Medical World*, 20 July 1928

W. Belfield, 'Some Phases of Rejuvenation', *The Journal of the American Medical Association* 82:16 (1924) 1237–42

S. Belfrage, *What's Best to Eat?* London: William Heinemann (Medical Books) Ltd., 1926

F. Benedict, W. Miles, P. Roth and H. Smith, *Human Vitality and Efficiency under Prolonged Restricted Diet*. Washington, DC: Carnegie Institute of Washington, 1919

S. Bennett, *Exercising in Bed: The Simplest and Most Effective System of Exercise Ever Devised*. San Francisco: Edward Hilton, 1907

   Old Age: Its Cause and Prevention: The Story of an Old Body and Face Made Young. New York: The Physical Culture Publishing Co., 1912

The Bioglan Laboratories Hertford, *Bioglan Hormone Compounds: Compositions and Indications for Use* 4th ed. Hertford: Bioglan Laboratories, 1938

E. Björkstén, *Principles of Gymnastics for Women and Girls* trans. A. Dawson, 2 vols. London: J. & A. Churchill, 1932 and 1934

J. Boeke, 'The Histological Basis of Health. I. The Tissues in Youth and Old Age', *The Lancet*, 25 January 1930, 218–21, 220

C. Bond, 'On Irradiated Ergosterol as a Dressing for Wounds', *British Medical Journal*, 3 March 1928, 339–40

'Causes of Racial Decay. Distribution of Natural Capacity. The Need for a National Stocktaking. The Galton Lecture, 1928', *The Eugenics Review* 20 (April 1928), 5–19

B. Booth, *The Advantages of Vegetarian Diet*. London: The Order of the Golden Age, c.1925

W. Brady, *The 7 Keys to Vite*. Beverly Hills, CA: Dr William Brady, c.1932

'Your Health', *Milwaukee Sentinel*, 20 April 1939, 5

'Brine Baths Closed for Good', *Droitwich Spa Advertiser*, 29 September 2009, www.droitwichadvertiser.co.uk/news/4654871.brine-baths-closed-for-good/, accessed 5 October 2018

'British Electro-Therapeutic Society', *The Lancet*, 22 February 1902, 519–20

British Glandular Products Ltd., *The Essence of Life: An Illustration of a Natural Method of Rejuvenation of the Human System by Gland Substances*, 11th edn. London: British Glandular Products Ltd., c.1933

'British Medical Association. Meeting at Oxford', *The Lancet*, 1 August 1936, 253–62

P. Brock, *Charlatan: The Fraudulent Life of John Brinkley*. London: Weidenfeld & Nicolson, 2008

H. Brown, *Sleep and Sleeplessness*. London: Hutchinson, 1910

Vitality and Diet. London; New York: Andrew Melrose Ltd., 1924

L. Brown, *Scientific Living for Prolonging the Term of Human Life. The New Domestic Science, Cooking to Simplify Living and Retain the Life Elements in Food*. Passaic, NJ: Health Culture Co., 1909

C. Brown-Séquard, 'The Effects Produced on Man by Subcutaneous Injection of a Liquid Obtained from the Testicles of Animals', *The Lancet*, 20 July 1889, 105–07

H. Ellen Browning, *Beauty Culture*. London: Hutchinson, 1898

M. Burbridge, *The Road to Beauty: An Adventure in Rejuvenation*. New York: Greenberg, 1924

H. Burrows, 'Pathological Changes Induced in the Mamma by Œstrogenic Compounds', *British Journal of Surgery* 23:89 (1935), 191–213

'The By-Effects of Salvarsan', *British Medical Journal*, 4 July 1914, 4

A. Cameron, 'Cod-Liver Oil in External Eye Affections', *British Medical Journal*, 17 October 1936, 785

'Can Old Age Be Deferred?', *Scientific American*, October 1925, 226–27

'A Canine Rejuvenation Experiment', *The Lancet*, 29 April 1922, 857

A. Cantor, *Dr Cantor's Longevity Diet: How to Slow Down Aging and Prolong Youth and Vigor*. West Nyack, NY: Parker Pub. Co., 1967

A. Carlson, 'The Thyroid, Pancreatic Islets, Parathyroids, Adrenals, Thymus and Pituitary', in E. V. Cowdry ed., *Problems of Ageing: Biological and Medical Aspects*. London: Baillière, Tindall & Cox, 1939, 361–97

A. Carrel, 'On the Permanent Life of Tissues Outside of the Organism', *Journal of Experimental Medicine* 15:5 (1912), 516–28

'The Immortality of Animal Tissues and Its Significance', in *Proceedings of the Third Race Betterment Conference, January 2–6, 1928*. Battle Creek, MI: The Race Betterment Foundation, 1928

F. Cavazzi, *Vie et Rajeunissement: Une Nouvelle Méthode Générale de Traitment et mes Expériences de Rajeunissement de Bologne et de Paris*. Paris: Gaston Doin & Cie, 1934

S. Charles, '"Young Blood" Company Ambrosia Halts Patient Treatments after FDA Warning', 19 February 2019, www.nbcnews.com/health/aging/young-blood-company-ambrosia-halts-patient-treatments-after-fda-warning-n973266, accessed 20 February 2019

S. Chase and F. Schlink, *Your Money's Worth*. New York: The MacMillan Company, 1927

C. Child, *Senescence and Rejuvenescence*. Chicago: University of Chicago Press, 1915

J. Clark, *The Business of Beauty: Gender and the Body in Modern London*. London: Bloomsbury, 2020.

J. Clement, *Human Power*, 6th edn. London: Mills & Boon, 1934

I. Cobb, *The Glands of Destiny: A Study of the Personality*. London: William Heinemann (Medical Books) Ltd, 1928

'Cod-Liver Oil and Vitamin A', *British Medical Journal*, 30 September 1922, 610

'Commons Sitting of Thursday, 17th March, 1927', Hansard Parliamentary Papers, Series 5, Volume 203, page columns 2167–2316, 2181–2182, parlipapers.proquest.com/parlipapers/docview/t71.d76.cds5cv0203p0-0014?accountid=14664, accessed 15 January 2019

'Comparative Physiology of the Iris', *The Lancet*, 22 November 1890, 1112

'The Composition of Certain Secret Remedies, Nerve Tonics, Etc.' *British Medical Journal*, 7 January 1911, 26–28

R. Conniff, 'The Hunger Gains: Extreme Calorie-Restriction Diet Shows Anti-Aging Results', *Scientific American*, 16 February 2017, www.scientificamerican.com/article/the-hunger-gains-extreme-calorie-restriction-diet-shows-anti-aging-results/, accessed 17 June 2017

J. Cook, C. Hewitt and I. Hieger, 'The Isolation of a Cancer-Producing Hydrocarbon from Coal Tar. Parts I, II, and III', *Journal of the Chemical Society* (1933), 395–405

G. Corners, *Rejuvenation: How Steinach Makes People Young*. New York: Thomas Seltzer, 1923

G. Cruden, *The British Institute of Physical Training*. Aberdeen: Rosemount Press, 1925

W. Cramer and W. Gye, 'Œstrin and Cancer', *The Lancet*, 5 December 1936, 1365

'The Cure of Obesity. By Dr Jean Frumusan', *Journal of the American Medical Association* 84:9 (1925), 701

H. Dale, 'Otto Loewi. 1873–1961', *Biographical Memoirs of Fellows of the Royal Society* 8 (1962), 67–89

A. Davies, 'The Hunterian Oration on Organo-Therapy', *The Lancet*, 19 April 1902, 1089–96

N. Davies, *Foods for the Fat: A Treatise on Corpulency, with Dietary for Its Cure*. London: Chatto and Windus, 1889

B. Dawson, 'Physical Education in England. Symposium on Physical Medicine', *Medical Record*, 2 June 1937, 455–56

S. de Beauvoir, *The Coming of Age*. New York: G. P. Putman, 1972

J. Deas, 'Vitamin A and Its Variations in Cod Liver Oil', *Canadian Medical Association Journal* 14:10 (1924), 959–61

Development Commission. Nineteenth Report of the Development Commissioners for the Year Ended the 31st March, 1929. London: HMSO, 1929

W. Douglass, *The Elements of Medical High Frequency and Diathermy: For Assistants and Nurses.* London: J. K. Lewis & Co. Ltd., 1930

'Dr Bernard Hollander', *British Medical Journal,* 17 February 1934, 316

'Dr Hollander on Localisation of Mental Faculty', *The Phrenologist* 42 (1907), 402–03

L. Dundas Irvine, 'Foreword', in Abplanalp, *Slimness and Health,* 11–17
  'Rejuvenation: A Reply to Dr Voronoff', *English Review* 40 (1925), 167–71

N. Eberhart, *A Working Manual of High Frequency Currents.* Chicago: New Medicine Publishing Co., 1911

A. Edney, 'Beware of Using Young People's Blood to Halt Aging, FDA Says' *Bloomberg,* 19 February 2019, www.bloomberg.com/news/articles/2019-02-19/beware-of-buying-young-people-s-blood-to-prevent-aging-fda-says, accessed 20 February 2019

The Elizabeth Arden Exercises for Health and Beauty. London: Elizabeth Arden, 1924

M. Ellison [Mary H. Youde]. *The Key to Rejuvenation,* 1948

'Endocreme – A Cosmetic with a Menace', *Journal of the American Medical Association,* 9 April 1938, 1194–96

J. English, *A Treatise on the Renewal and Rejuvenation of the Physical Body, with Affirmations for Use in the Work.* San Diego, CA: George P. Sikes, 1919

J. L. Faure, *Congrès Français de Chirurgie.* Paris: F. Alcan, 1919

'Federal Food, Drug, and Cosmetic Act', 13 March 2013, 21 U.S.C. 321, (i), http://legcounsel.house.gov/Comps/FDA_CMD.pdf, accessed 24 January 2018

D. Ferrier, *The Functions of the Brain.* London: Smith, Elder, 1876

'Fighting Father Time: A Beauty Parlour Peep', 27 July 1922, www.britishpathe.com/video/fighting-father-time-a-beauty-parlour-peep/query/ageing, accessed 12 May 2016

M. Fishbein, *The Medical Follies.* New York: Boni & Liveright, 1925
  The New Medical Follies. New York: Boni and Liveright, 1927

E. Fisher, 'Experiments on the Bactericidal Action of the Violet Ray', *California State Journal of Medicine* 21:5 (1924), 218–19

Foreign Prescriptions: Hormone Therapy. London: Anchor Press, c.1930

'The Function of the Prostate', *British Medical Journal,* 5 June 1909, 1382–83

J. Frumusan, Rejuvenation: The Duty, the Possibility, and the Means of Regaining Youth, trans. Elaine C. Wood. London: John Bale, Sons & Danielsson, 1923

W. Gallichan, *The Conflict of Owen Prytherch.* London: Watts & Co, 1905
  Modern Woman and How to Manage Her. London: T. Werner Laurie Ltd, 1909
  A Soul From The Pit. London: David Nutt, 1907
  The Art of Courtship and Marriage; or, How to Love. London: Health Promotion, Ltd., 1915
  The Great Unmarried. London: T. Werner Laurie Ltd., 1916
  The Critical Age of Woman. London: Health Promotion, Ltd., 1920
  Youth and Maidenhood. London: Health Promotion, Ltd., 1920
  The Sterilization of the Unfit. London: T. Werner Laurie Ltd., 1929
  Youthful Old Age: How to Keep Young. London: T. Werner Laurie Ltd., 1929

W. Gantt, 'A Medical Review of Soviet Russia. V. – The Medical Profession, Soviet Science, and Soviet Sanitation', *British Medical Journal*, 19 February 1927, 338–40

J. Gardner, *Longevity: The Means of Prolonging Life after Middle Age*, 3rd edn. Boston: William F. Gill and Co., 1875

B. Gayton, *The Gland Stealers*. Philadelphia; London: J. B. Lippincott Co., 1922

D. L. George, 'Foreword', in E. Samson, *Old Age in the New World*. London: The Pilot Press, 1944, 5

Genatosan Ltd., *The Good Life*. Loughborough: Genatosan Ltd., c.1944
    Sanatogen for Youthful Health and New Vitality. Loughborough: Genatosan, c.1930

J. Gloag, *Winter's Youth*. London: George Allen and Unwin, 1934

L. Goizet, *La Vie Prolongée au Moyen de la Méthode Brown-Séquard: Force et Santé*. Paris: E. Flammarion, c.1891
    Never Grow Old: How to Live for More Than One Hundred Years. New York; London: G. P. Putnam's Sons, 1920

'Grains and Scruples', *The Lancet*, 17 July 1937, 156–57

J. Gravener, 'How to Keep Your Health. Special Exercise Hints for Ladies', *The News*, 23 May 1930, 19

A. Gray, 'People Who Want to Look Young and Beautiful', *The American Magazine* 94 (1922), 32–33

H. Gubbins, *The Elixir of Life or 2905 A.D.: A Novel of the Far Future*. London: Henry J. Drane, 1914

N. Haire, *Rejuvenation: The Work of Steinach, Voronoff, and Others*. London: George Allen and Unwin, 1924

G. S. Hall, *Senescence: The Last Half of Life*. New York; London: D. Appleton and Company, 1922

Hancock & Co., *Foreign Prescriptions: Hormone Therapy*. London: Anchor Press, c.1930

B. Harrow, *One Family: Vitamins, Enzymes, Hormones*. Minneapolis: Burgess, 1950

R. Harry, *Modern Cosmeticology: The Principles and Practice of Modern Cosmetics*. London: Chapman and Hall, 1941

G. Hauser, 'Prolong Youth . . . but without the Surgery', *New Health* 14:4 (April 1939), 8–10
    Look Younger, Live Longer. London: Faber & Faber, 1955

L. Hayflick and P. Moorhead, 'The Serial Cultivation of Human Diploid Cell Strains', *Experimental Cell Research* 25 (1961), 585–612

'Health and Beauty on Parade!', 1933, British Pathe Historical Collections, Film ID 707.10, www.britishpathe.com/video/health-and-beauty-on-parade, accessed 25 September 2018

L. Heilbronn and E. Ravussin, 'Calorie Restriction and Aging: Review of the Literature and Implications for Studies in Humans', *American Journal of Clinical Nutrition* 78:3 (2003), 361–69

Heudebert Laboratories, *The Diet in Diseases of the Digestive Tract. Part I – Diseases of the Stomach*. Alperton: Heudebert Laboratories, c.1924
    The Diet in Diseases of the Digestive Tract. Part 2 – Diseases of the Intestine. Alperton: Heudebert Laboratories, c.1925

A. Hill, 'Enemies of Knowledge', *The Lancet*, 29 June 1929, 1385–88

G. Hinsdale, 'Memorial: John Madison Taylor', *Transactions of the American Clinical and Climatological Association* 48 (1932), 41

B. Hirst, 'Secretin and the Exposition of Hormonal Control', *Journal of Physiology* 560:2 (2004), 339

F. Hoffman, *Some Problems of Longevity*. Chicago; New York: Spectator, 1928

B. Hollander, *Scientific Phrenology: Being a Practical Mental Science and Guide to Human Character; An Illustrated Textbook*. London: Grant Richards, 1902

   The Mental Symptoms of Brain Disease: An Aid to the Surgical Treatment of Insanity, Due to Injury, Haemorrhage, Tumours, and Other Circumscribed Lesions of the Brain. London: Rebman, 1910

   In Search of the Soul: The Mechanism of Thought, Emotion and Conduct, Vol 2. London: Kegan Paul, 1920

   Old Age Deferred: The Prevention of the Disabilities and Diseases of Old Age. London: Watts & Co., 1933

H. Hopkinson, 'Exercise for the Elderly', *New Health* (November 1936), 26–27

C. Horn, 'Ultra-Violet-Ray Electrode', US Patent 761,183, 21 June 1904

N. Hosali, *The Humane Diet Leaflets: 16. The Vegetarian Diet for Busy People*. London: Vegetarian Society, c.1925

'House of Representatives', 14th Parliament, 1st Session, 29 November 1934, https://historichansard.net/hofreps/1934/19341129_reps_14_145/#subdebate-25-1-s3, accessed 14 February 2019

'House of Representatives', 14th Parliament, 1st Session, 12 December 1934, https://historichansard.net/hofreps/1934/19341212_reps_14_145/#subdebate-11-0-s2, accessed 14 February 2019

R. Hovarth, 'The Key to Rejuvenation', *Health Saver* 3:2 (1960), 36–39

E. Hume, Nathanial Lucas and Hannah Smith, 'On the Absorption of Vitamin D from the Skin', *Biochemical Journal* 21:2 (1927), 362–67

F. Humphris, *Artificial Sunlight and Its Therapeutic Uses*. Oxford: Oxford University Press, 1929

F. Humphris and L. Williams, *Emanotherapy*. London: Bailliere, Tindall and Cox, 1937

A. Huxley, *After Many a Summer*. London: Chatto and Windus, 1939

Ideal Home Electrical Appliances, *Health, Healing & Recovery by Means of Rogers Vitalator High Frequency Treatment*. London: Ideal Home Electrical Appliances, c.1935

'The Internal Secretion of the Reproductive Glands', *The Lancet*, 3 November 1917, 687

IPC Magazines, *The Cosmetics and Toiletries Survey, 1979*, London: IPC Magazines, 1980

B. Jancke, 'Violet-Ray Generator', US Patent 1,506,344, 26 August 1924

A. Kallet and F. Schlink, *100,000,000 Guinea Pigs: Dangers in Everyday Foods, Drugs, and Cosmetics*. New York: The Vanguard Press, 1933

P. Kammerer, *Rejuvenation and the Prolongation of Human Efficiency: Experiences with the Steinach-Operation on Man and Animals*. London: Methuen & Co., 1924

B. Katz, 'Archibald Vivian Hill. 26 September 1886–3 June 1977', *Biographical Memoirs of Fellows of the Royal Society* 24 (1978), 71–149

J. Kellogg, *Autointoxication or Intestinal Toxemia*. Battle Creek, MI: Modern Medicine Publishing Company, 1919

The Natural Diet of Man. Battle Creek, MI: Modern Medicine Publishing Company, 1923

G. Knight, *Sex and Rejuvenation*. London: New World Publishing, 1933

E. Kromayer, *The Cosmetic Treatment of Skin Complaints*. Oxford: Oxford University Press, 1930

'Labels for Cosmetics', *British Medical Journal*, 21 October 1939, 815

A. Lacassagne, 'Apparition des cancers de la mamelle chez la souris mâle soumise à des injections de folliculine', *Comptes rendus de l'Académie des sciences* 195 (1932), 630–32

A Green Old Age. London: John Bale, Sons & Danielsson Ltd., 1923

W. Lane, 'Chronic Intestinal Stasis', *British Medical Journal*, 12 June 1909, 1408–11

Le Brasseur Surgical Manufacturing Co. Ltd., *Le Brasseur's Revised List of Medical Goods 1925: Catalogue "C"*. Birmingham, AL: Le Brasseur Surgical Manufacturing Co., 1925

'League of Health and Beauty Perform in Hyde Park', 1930, British Pathe Historical Collections, Film ID VLVAF47HQHFF8BELNYGQG8DFF2G50

Lloyd George's Message: Looking Forward: Substance of a Speech Delivered by the Prime Minister at Manchester, September 12, 1918. London: National War Aims Committee, c.1918

O. Loewi, 'Über humorale Übertragbarkeit der Herznervenwirkung', *Pflügers Archiv für die Gesamte Physiologie des Menschen und der Tiere* 204 (1924), 629–40

A. Lorand, *Health and Longevity through Rational Diet: Practical Hints in Regard to Food and the Usefulness or Harmful Effects of the Various Articles of Diet*. Philadelphia: F. A. Davies Co., 1913

Old Age Deferred: The Causes of Old Age and Its Postponement by Hygienic and Therapeutic Measures. Philadelphia: F. A. Davis, 1913

Life Shortening Habits and Rejuvenation. Montreal: Canadian Medical Book Co., 1922

'Steinach's Rejuvenation Operation', *Journal of Nervous and Mental Disease* 58:5 (1923), 470

N. Lucas, 'The Permeability of Human Epidermis to Ultra-Violet Irradiation', *Biochemical Journal* 25:1 (1931), 57–70

'The Production of Vitamin D by Irradiation of Ergosterol through the Epidermis of a Rat', *Biochemical Journal* 27:1 (1933), 132–35

B. Macfadden, *Strength from Eating: How and What to Eat and Drink to Develop the Highest Degree of Health and Strength*. New York: Physical Culture Publishing Co., 1901

Eating for Health and Strength. New York: Physical Culture Corporation, 1921

Physical Culture Cook Book. New York: Macfadden Book Company, 1932

G. MacKeen, 'The High Frequency Spark in the Treatment of Premature Alopecia', *New York Medical Journal*, 28 July 1906, 180–84

R. Mallett, *The Gospel of Feeding, from Childhood to Old Age*. London: Watts & Co., 1925

Nature's Way: A Means of Health without Medicine. Melbourne: E. W. Cole, c.1930

F. Marshall and F. Crew, 'Super-sheep', *The Times*, 21 November 1927, 21

F. Marshall, F. Crew, A. Walton and W. Miller, *Report on Dr Serge Voronoff's Experiments on the Improvement of Livestock*. London: HMSO, 1928

G. Massey, *Practical Electrotherapeutics and Diathermy*. London: J. & A. Churchill, 1924

W. Masters, 'Sex Steroid Influences on the Aging Process', *American Journal of Obstetrics and Gynecology* 74:4 (1957), 733–46

W. Masters and V. Johnson, 'Sex and the Aging Process', *Journal of the American Geriatrics Society* 29:9 (1981), 385–90

J. Mattison, R. Colman, T. Beasley et al., 'Caloric Restriction Improves Health and Survival of Rhesus Monkeys', *Nature Communications* 8 (2017) doi:10.1038/ncomms14063

J. Mattison, G. Roth, T. Beasley et al., 'Impact of Caloric Restriction on Health and Survival in Rhesus Monkeys: The NIA Study', *Nature* 489:7415 (2012) doi:10.1038/nature11432

E. McCollum, *The Newer Knowledge of Nutrition: The Use of Food for the Preservation of Vitality and Health*. New York: The Macmillan Co., 1919

E. McCollum and C. Kennedy, 'The Dietary Factors Operating in the Production of Polyneuritis', *Journal of Biological Chemistry* 24: 493 (1916), 491–502

E. McCollum and W. Pitz, 'The "Vitamine" Hypothesis and Deficiency Diseases', *Journal of Biological Chemistry* 31:1 (1917), 229–53

L. McCormick, *Family Record and Biography*. Chicago: 1896

W. McGovern, *To Lhasa in Disguise: A Secret Expedition through Mysterious Tibet*. London; New York: The Century Co., 1924

'The Medical and Surgical Uses of Diathermy', *British Medical Journal*, 31 January 1931, 181–82

Medical Research Committee, *Report on the Present State of Knowledge Concerning Accessory Food Factors (Vitamines)*. London: HMSO, 1919

Medical Research Council, *Vitamins: A Survey of Present Knowledge, Compiled by a Committee Appointed Jointly by the Lister Institute and Medical Research Council*. London: HMSO, 1932

'Medical Societies. Royal Society of Medicine. Section of Therapeutics and Pharmacology', *The Lancet*, 20 January 1923, 130–32

Medical Supply Association, *New Electro-Medical Apparatus for A.C. Mains, Diathermy and Short Wave Apparatus*. London: Medical Supply Association, 1934

'Medicine: No Rejuvenation', *Time*, 4 January 1932, http://content.time.com/time/subscriber/article/0,33009,742813,00.html, accessed 26 June 2017

F. Meier, *The Artistry of Mixing Drinks*. Paris: Fryam Press, 1936

M. Melendy, *Perfect Womanhood for Maidens-Wives-Mothers: A Book Giving Full Information on All the Mysterious and Complex Matters Pertaining to Women*. Chicago: Monarch Book Co., 1903

L. Mervyn, *The B Vitamins: Their Major Role in Maintaining Your Health*. Wellingborough: Thorsons, 1981

Vitamin C: The Enemy of the Common Cold. Wellingborough: Thorsons, 1981

Vitamins A, D, K: All You Need to Know to Ensure a Balanced Intake. Wellingborough: Thorsons, 1984

E. Metchnikoff, *The Prolongation of Life: Optimistic Studies*, trans. P. Chalmers Mitchell. New York; London: G. P. Putnam's Sons, 1908

Middlesex Laboratory of Glandular Research Ltd., *The Fires of Life Replenished: The Influence of the New Sex-Hormones in the Twilight of the Ductless Glands*. London: Middlesex Laboratory of Glandular Research Ltd., c.1929

The Treatment of Impotence. London: Middlesex Laboratory of Glandular Research, Ltd., c.1930

A. Milinowski Jr, 'Electrotherapy', GB Patent 554,848, 18 March 1942

D. Mills, *Phoenix*. London: Hutchinson, 1926

F. Mitchell, *A Key to Health and Long Life*. London: C. W. Daniel, 1914

A Key to Health and Long Life (The Secret of Healthy Nutrition), 2nd edn. London: C. W. Daniel, 1922

B. Montagu and F. Bacon, *The Works of Francis Bacon, Lord Chancellor of England, with a Life of the Author*, vol. 3. Philadelphia: M. Murphy, 1876

G. Morrell, 'Youth Regained by Thyroid?', *The Graphic*, 11 December 1920, 22

I. Morus, *Nikola Tesla and the Electrical Future*. London: Icon Books, 2019

J. Muller, *My System: Fifteen Minutes' Work a Day for Health's Sake*, trans. G. Fox-Davies. Copenhagen: Tillge's Boghandel, 1905

My System for Ladies. London: Ewart Seymour and Co., 1911

My System for Children. London: Ewart Seymour and Co., 1912

My System: 15 Minutes' Exercise a Day for Health's Sake. London: Athletic Publications, c.1925

T. Muller and T. Lorenze, 'Holder for Terminals of Violet-Ray Apparatus', US Patent 1,524,876, 3 February 1925

National Health Service, 'TENS (transcutaneous electrical nerve stimulation)', 10 August 2018, www.nhs.uk/conditions/transcutaneous-electrical-nerve-stimulation-tens/, accessed 28 February 2019

'The New U.S.A. Food and Drug Act', *British Medical Journal*, 27 August 1938, 457–58

A. Nicholls, 'Youthful Old Age', *Canadian Medical Association Journal* 21:2 (1929), 252

J. Nixon, 'The Long Fox Memorial Lecture: The Influence of Food on the Production and Prevention of Disease', *Bristol Medico-Chirurgical Journal*, 47:178 (1930), 255–86

H. Norman, 'In Search of the Soul', *Journal of Neurology and Psychopathology* 2:5 (1921), 95–97

'Notices of Books', *British Journal of Tuberculosis* 25:4 (1931), 192–97

Nuffield Foundation Survey Committee on the Problems of Ageing and the Care of Old People, *Old People: Report of a Survey Committee on the Problems of Ageing and the Care of Old People, under the Chairmanship of B. Seebohm Rowntree*. Oxford: Oxford University Press, 1947

'Nutrition and Longevity', *Nature* 104 (1920), 527–28

J. Oliver, 'Food and the Natural Limited of Man's Life', *The Medical Press*, 14 October 1931, 293–97

'On Rejuvenation', *Nature* 119 (1927), 396–97

G. Orwell, *Nineteen Eighty-Four*. London: Penguin, 2000

The Art of Donald McGill. Adelaide: The University of Adelaide, 2014, https://ebooks.adelaide.edu.au/o/orwell/george/art-of-donald-mcgill/, accessed 15 March 2019

Overbeck's New Electronic Theory of Life and Rejuvenation. Lincoln, NE:
   J. W. Ruddock & Sons, 1925

O. Overbeck, *A New Electronic Theory of Life.* Lincoln: Chantry House, 1926
   A New Electronic Theory of Life, 4th edn. Lincoln, NE: Chantry House, 1932
   The New Light. London: Metchim & Son, 1936

Overbeck's Rejuvenator Ltd., *Overbeck's Rejuvenator: Supreme Model: Directions for
   Use.* Grimsby: Overbeck's Rejuvenator Ltd., 1938

T. Parsons, *Brain Culture through Scientific Body Building.* Chicago: The American
   School of Mental and Physical Development, 1912

L. Pauling, *How to Live Longer and Feel Better.* New York: Freeman, 1986

'The Pharmacological Value of Cod-Liver Oil', *British Medical Journal*, 13 August
   1921, 245–46

'Physiology', *British Medical Journal*, 3 October 1914, 586–87

J. Pilates and W. Miller, *Return to Life through Contrology.* Boston: Christopher
   Publishing House, 1960

A. Pitcairn-Knowles, *The History and Development of the Schroth Cure: With and
   Explanation of Many Important Details of the Treatment.* Hastings: Knowledge
   Health Hydro, c.1929
   The Schroth Regeneration Cure. Letchworth: Garden City Press, 1929

W. Pitkin, *Life Begins at Forty.* New York; London: McGraw-Hill Book Company,
   1932

Prunella, 'Seeking Beauty. Long Faces to Be Seen in Beauty Parlour', *The News*,
   23 May 1930, 19

J. Pulvermacher, *J. L. Pulvermacher's Patent Portable Hydro-Electric Voltaic Chains.*
   New York: William Fillmer & Co., 1853

'Quest for Youth', directed by C. Roeder, Tees-Side Cine Club, 1935, http://player
   .bfi.org.uk/film/watch-quest-for-youth-1935/, accessed 31 August 2016

C. Ramus, *Outwitting Middle Age.* London: George Allen & Unwin, 1926

M. Ravenel, 'Why Not Grow Young? Or Living for Longevity', *American Journal of
   Public Health* 19:7 (1929), 840

C. Reinhardt, *Diet and the Maximum Duration of Life.* London: London Publicity Co.,
   c.1910

Riposo Recipes, *Two Completely Meatless Meals.* Hastings: Riposo Nature Cure
   Resort, c.1925

M. Roth, *Movements or Exercises, According to Ling's System for the Due
   Development and Strengthening of the Human Body, in Childhood and in Youth.*
   London: Groombridge & Sons, 1852

Royal Commission on Congestion in Ireland, *Appendices to the First Report: Minutes
   of Evidence (Taken in Dublin, 7th September to 5th October, 1906).* Dublin:
   HMSO, 1906

'Royal Society of Medicine', *The Lancet*, 28 November 1936, 1269–73

H. Rubinstein, *My Life for Beauty: Helena Rubinstein.* London: Bodley Head, 1965

E. Ruddock, *Vitalogy: An Encyclopedia of Health and Home.* Chicago: Vitalogy
   Association, 1929

C. Saberton, *Diathermy in Medical and Surgical Practice.* London; New York: Cassell
   and Company Limited, 1920

C. Saleeby, *The Eugenic Prospect: National and Racial.* New York: Dodd, Mead, 1921

A. Salter and W. Barwick, *Be Rejuvenated*. Sydney: W. M. Nash, 1925

S. Sandor, 'Vitamin A in the Local Treatment of Wounds', *The Lancet*, 26 September 1936, 738–40

E. Sandow, *Strength and How to Obtain It: With Anatomical Chart Illustrating the Exercises for Physical Development*. London: Gale and Polden, 1897

R. Saundby, *Old Age: Its Care and Treatment in Health and Disease*. London: Edward Arnold, 1915

A. Savill, *The Hair and Scalp: A Clinical Study with a Chapter on Hirsuties*. London: Edward Arnold & Co., 1935

E. Schäfer, 'Presidential Address on the Nature, Origin, and Maintenance of Life', *The Lancet*, 7 September 1912, 675–85

E. Schliephake, *Short Wave Therapy: The Medical Uses of Electrical High Frequency*, trans. R. King Brown. London: The Actinic Press, 1935

A. Schneider, 'Some Suggestions on Reactivation and Rejuvenation Experiments', *American Medicine* 23 (1928), 722–36

'The So-Called Rejuvenation Treatment. Its Present Status and Indicated Social and Economic Significance', *Medical Review of Reviews* 34 (1928), 49–74

P. Schmidt, *The Theory and Practice of the Steinach Operation: A Report on One Hundred Cases*. London: William Heinemann (Medical Books) Ltd., 1924

Das überwundene Alter: Wege zu Verjüngung und Leistungssteigerung. Leipzig: Paul List Verlag, 1928

The Conquest of Old Age: Methods to Effect Rejuvenation and to Increase Functional Activity, trans. E. and C. Paul. London: George Routldge & Sons, Ltd., 1931

G. Scott, *Birth Control: A Practical Guide for Working Women*. London: T. W. Laurie, 1933

The Quest for Youth: A Study of All Available Methods of Rejuvenation and of Retaining Physical and Mental Vigour in Old Age. London: Torchstream, 1953

T. Scott, *The Road to a Healthy Old Age: Essays Lay and Medical*. London: H. K. Lewis, 1914

Scottish Wholesale Druggists' Association, *Patent Medicines and Proprietary Articles Catalogue, 1959–1960*. Edinburgh, 1959

'Science: Rejuvenation', *Time*, 23 April 1928, http://content.time.com/time/subscriber/article/0,33009,787185,00.html, accessed 26 June 2017

'The Science of Cosmetics', *British Medical Journal*, 14 December 1940, 832–33

E. Scripture, 'An Unsuccessful Steinach Operation', *The Lancet*, 2 December 1922, 1206

Seventeenth Report of the Board of Agriculture for Scotland Being for the Year Ended 31st December 1928. London: HMSO, 1929

E. Sharpey-Schafer, 'Endocrine Physiology', *Irish Journal of Medical Science* 69 (1931), 483–505

L. Simpson, *The Handbook of Dining or How to Dine Theoretically, Philosophically and Historically Considered*. London: Longman and Co., 1859

'Sir Arthur Balfour', *British Medical Journal*, 7 February 1931, 245–46

Sixteenth Report of the Board of Agriculture for Scotland Being for the Year Ended 31st December 1927. London: HMSO, 1928

T. Smith, *The Glorious Pool*. New York: Doubleday, 1934

C. Snow, *New Lives for Old*. London: Gollancz, 1933

T. Standwell, *Do You Desire Health? If you do you are in need of the advice contained in this book*. [London], [1945]

E. Starling, 'The Croonian Lectures on The Chemical Correlation of the Functions of the Body, Lecture I', *The Lancet*, 5 August 1905, 339–41

E. H. S[tarling]., 'Hormones', *Nature* 111 (1923), 694–96

'The Wisdom of the Body: The Harveian Oration', *British Medical Journal*, 20 October 1923, 685–90

E. Steinach, 'Untersuchungen zur vergleichenden Physiologie der männlichen Geschlechtsorgane insbesondere der accessorischen Geschlechtsdrüsen', *Pflügers Archiv* 56 (1894), 304–38

'Geschlechtstrieb und echt sekundäre Geschlechtsmerkmale als Folge der innersekretorischen Funktion der Keimdrüsen', *Zentralblatt für Physiologie* 24 (1910), 551–66

Verjüngung durch experimentelle Neubelubung der alternden Pubertätsdrüse. Berlin: Verlag Von Julius Springer, 1920

'The Steinach Operation', *The Lancet*, 4 October 1924, 702

'Steinach's Operation', *British Medical Journal*, 4 April 1925, 662–63

'Steinach's Operation', *The Lancet*, 24 February 1923, 393

G. Stoney, 'Of the "Electron" or Atom of Electricity', *Philosophical Magazine* 5:38 (1894), 418–20

G. Stuart, *Gland Treatment for Renewal or Rejuvenation of the Body through Applied New Thought*. London: L. N. Fowler, 1925

'The Sun-Burnt Face', *The Lancet*, 20 August 1910, 574

Sylvania, 'Madame and the Monkey Gland' *The Sphere*, 27 October 1922, iv

J. Taylor, *The Old, Old, Very Old Man*. London, 1635

N. Tesla, 'High Frequency Oscillators for Electro-Therapeutic and Other Purposes', *The Electrical Engineer* 26:550 (1898), 477–81

Théiron School of Life. *The Théiron Method: A Correspondence Course in Youth, Personality, Achievement & Rejuvenation*. London: The Théiron School of Life, 1931

F. Tisdall, 'The Etiology of Rickets', *Canadian Medical Association Journal* 11:12 (1921), 934–43

'A Note on the Kramer-Tisdall Method for the Determination of Calcium in Small Amounts of Serum', *The Journal of Biological Chemistry* 56 (1923), 439–41

J. Tobey, *Public Health Law: A Manual of Law for Sanitarians*. Baltimore: Williams and Wilkins, 1926

'Skin Deep: The Truth about Beauty Aids – Safe and Harmful', *American Journal of Public Health and the Nation's Health* 25:4 (1935), 507

The Legal Aspects of Milk Control. Chicago: International Association of Milk Dealers, 1936

'Transplantation of the Sex Glands', *British Medical Journal*, 12 March 1921, 42

'Treatment of Industrial Rheumatism in Germany', *British Medical Journal*, 17 September 1927, 502–04

W. Troup, 'Individual Overdose of Ultra-Violet Rays', *British Medical Journal*, 20 February 1926, 349

'An Unsuccessful Steinach Operation', *The Lancet*, 25 November 1922, 1154

U.S. Food and Drug Administration, 'Statement from FDA Commissioner Scott Gottlieb, M.D., and Director of FDA's Center for Biologics Evaluation and Research Peter Marks, M.D., Ph.D., cautioning consumers against receiving young donor plasma infusions that are promoted as unproven treatment for varying conditions', 19 February 2019, www.fda.gov/NewsEvents/Newsroom/PressAnnouncements/ucm631568.htm, accessed 20 February 2019

'Vienna (from our own Correspondent)', *The Lancet*, 26 February 1921, 454

'Vienna (from our own Correspondent)', *The Lancet*, 28 March 1925, 683

'Vienna: Some Recent Medical Work', *British Medical Journal*, 18 November 1922, 988–89

S. Vincent, 'The Endocrine Functions of the Female Reproductive Organs', *The Lancet*, 11 February 1922, 303–06

'The Violet Ray', *Journal of the National Medical Association* 9:3 (1917), 153

A. Vischer, *Old Age: Its Compensations and Rewards*. London: George Allen, 1947

S. Voronoff, *Life: A Study of the Mean of Restoring Vital Energy and Prolonging Life*, trans. E. Voronoff. New York: E. P. Dutton and Co., 1920

Vivre: Étude des Moyens de Relever L'énergie Vitale et de Prolonger la Vie. Paris: B. Grasset, 1920

Rejuvenation by Grafting, trans. F. Imianitoff. London: George Allen and Unwin, 1925

The Study of Old Age and my Method of Rejuvenation, trans. F. Imianitoff. London: Gill, 1926

The Conquest of Life, trans. G. Rambaud. London: Williams and Norgate, 1933

'Voronoff's Method of Rejuvenation', *The Lancet*, 26 February 1927, 446–47

K. Walker and J. Cook, 'Steinach's Rejuvenation Operation', *The Lancet*, 2 February 1924, 223–26

A. Warthin, *Old Age: The Major Involution. The Physiology and Pathology of the Aging Process*. London: Constable & Co., 1929

'Ways of Giving Sex Hormones', *The Lancet*, 14 May 1938, 1117–18

H. Weber, *On Longevity and Means for the Prolongation of Life*, ed. F. Parkes Weber. London: Macmillan, 1919

H. Weber and F. Weber, *Climatotherapy and Balneotherapy*. London: Smith, Elder & Co., 1907

J. Webster, *Beauty and Health in Youth and Old Age: An Appeal to Men and Women of All Ages*. London: Swan Sonnenschein & Co., 1907

F. Weidman, 'Ageing of the Skin', in E. Cowdry ed., *Problems of Ageing: Biological and Medical Aspects*. London: Balliere, Tindall and Cox, 1939, 339–60

M. Weinbren, 'The Public, the Doctor, and the Masseuse', *British Medical Journal*, 8 January 1917, 80–81

A. Weismann, *The Germ-Plasm: A Theory of Heredity*. New York: Charles Scribner's Sons, 1893

E. Whitmore, *Keeping Young after Forty*. New York; London: D. Appleton and Company, 1928

T. Whittaker, 'Alcoholic Beverages and Longevity', *Contemporary Review* 85, March 1904, 413–29

C. Willi, 'Appareil pour la Réduction du Double Menton et des Hanches', French Patent No. 441537, 20 March 1912

Facial Rejuvenation: How to Idealise the Features and the Skin of the Face by the Latest Scientific Methods. London: Cecil Palmer, 1926

Secret of Looking Young, with the Aid of the Hystogen-derma-process: Based on 10,000 Successful Cases & Twenty-five Years' Experience. London: Cecil Palmer, 1932

The Face, and Its Improvement by Aesthetic Plastic Surgery. Birkenhead: Melville Press, 1949

The Face, and Its Improvement by Aesthetic Plastic Surgery, 3rd edn. London: Macdonald and Evans, 1955

C. Williams, *High-Frequency Currents in the Treatment of Some Diseases*. New York: Rebman Company, 1903

L. Williams, 'Chronic Intestinal Stasis', *The Lancet*, 19 October 1918, 538

'Fasting', *The Lancet*, 10 December 1921, 1245

'The Interstitial Gland', *British Medical Journal*, 27 May 1922, 833–35

'Endocrines, Vitamins, and Subtleties', *British Medical Journal*, 16 June 1923, 1010–13

'The Present Position of Organotherapy', *The Lancet* 201:5188 (1923), 255–56

'Testicular Grafts', *British Medical Journal*, 20 January 1923, 130

The Science and Art of Living. London: Hodder and Stoughton, 1924

Obesity. Oxford: Oxford University Press, 1926

, 'Senescence and Senility', *The Lancet*, 4 June 1927, 1179–81

Growing Old Gracefully: Health Laws & Lessons Meanwhile. London: Jarrolds, 1929

L. Williams and H. Lyon-Smith, 'Chronic Intestinal Stasis', *The Lancet*, 5 October 1918, 472

C. Williamson, 'Turn Back the Clock!', *Pall Mall Magazine*, December 1922, 234–46

C. Wilson, 'Calorie Restriction Diet Extends Life of Monkeys by Years', *New Scientist*, 17 January 2017, www.newscientist.com/article/2118224-calorie-restriction-diet-extends-life-of-monkeys-by-years/, accessed 17 June 2017

E. Wilson ed., *Hufeland's Art of Prolonging Life*. London: John Churchill, 1849

'Written Answers (Commons) of Monday, 17th May, 1926', Hansard Parliamentary Papers, Series 5, Volume 196, page column 13-14, https://parlipapers.proquest.com/parlipapers/docview/t71.d76.cas5cv0196p0-0001?accountid=14664, accessed 15 January 2019

Zenobé, *The New 'Bioserm' (Trade mark) Way to Beauty: Serum Treatment without Injections for the Rejuvenation of the Skin*. Dermo-Serum Co., Ltd., c.1939

S. Zilva, J. Drummond and M. Graham, 'The Relation of the Vitamin A Potency of the Liver Oil to the Sexual Condition and Age of the Cod', *Biochemical Journal* 18:1 (1924), 178–81

Secondary

J. Adams, *Healing with Water: English Spas and the Water Cure, 1840–1960*. Manchester: Manchester University Press, 2015

M. Adams, *Mr America: How Muscular Millionaire Bernarr Macfadden Transformed the Nation Through Sex, Salad, and the Ultimate Starvation Diet*. New York: HarperCollins, 2009

L. Alexander, 'BFI Screenonline: Lion Has Wings, The (1939)', 2014,
    www.screenonline.org.uk/film/id/479863/index.html, accessed 9 October 2018

M. Anderson, 'The Emergence of the Modern Life Cycle in Britain', *Social History*
    10:1 (1985), 69–87

R. Apple, *Vitamania: Vitamins in American Culture*. New Brunswick, NJ: Rutgers
    University Press, 1996

D. Armstrong, *Political Anatomy of the Body: Medical Knowledge in Britain in the
    Twentieth Century*. Cambridge: Cambridge University Press, 1983

T. Armstrong, *Modernism, Technology, and the Body: A Cultural Study*. Cambridge:
    Cambridge University Press, 1998

M. Ash, *Gestalt Psychology in German Culture, 1890–1967: Holism and the Quest for
    Objectivity*. Cambridge: Cambridge University Press, 1995

F. Augier, E. Salf and J. Nottet, 'Le Docteur Samuel Serge Voronoff (1866–1951) ou
    "la quête de l'éternelle jeunesse"', *Histoire des Sciences Médicales* 30 (1996),
    163–71

I. Barkan, 'Industry Invites Regulation: The Passage of the Pure Food and Drug Act of
    1906', *American Journal of Public Health* 75:1 (1985), 18–26

A. Bates, *Anti-Vivisection and the Medical Profession in Britain*. Basingstoke: Palgrave
    Macmillan, 2017

N. Bauch, *A Geography of Digestion: Biotechnology and the Kellogg Cereal
    Enterprise*. Berkeley: University of California Press, 2016

J. Bennett, 'Rubinstein and the Rejuvenationists', 17 December 2017,
    www.cosmeticsandskin.com/fgf/rejuvenation.php, accessed 18 March 2019

C. Benthien, *Skin: On the Cultural Border between Self and the World*, trans.
    T. Dunlap. New York: Columbia University Press, 2002

A. Bingham, *Gender, Modernity and the Popular Press in Interwar Britain*. Oxford:
    Oxford University Press, 2004

S. Binkley, *Getting Loose: Lifestyle Consumption in the 1970s*. Durham, NC: Duke
    University Press, 2007

R. Bivins, H. Marland and N. Tomes, 'Histories of Medicine in the Household:
    Recovering Practice and "Reception"', *Social History of Medicine* 29:4 (2016),
    669–75

E. Bleiler and R. Bleiler, *Science Fiction: The Early Years*. Kent, OH; London: Kent
    State University Press, 1990

L. Boia, *Forever Young: A Cultural History of Longevity*. London: Reaktion, 2003

M. Borell, 'Brown-Séquard's Organotherapy and Its Appearance in America at the End
    of the Nineteenth Century', *Bulletin of the History of Medicine* 50 (1976), 309–20

L. Botelho and P. Thane, 'Introduction', in L. Botelho and P. Thane eds, *Women and
    Ageing in British Society since 1500*. Harlow: Pearson Education, 2001, 1–12

P. Bowler, *Charles Darwin: The Man and His Influence*. Cambridge: Cambridge
    University Press, 1996

    Evolution: The History of an Idea, 3rd edn. Berkeley: University of California Press,
    2003

R. Brandon, *Ugly Beauty: Helena Rubinstein, L'Oreal, and the Blemished History of
    Looking Good*. New York: Harper, 2011

C. Breathnach, *The Congested Districts Board of Ireland, 1891–1923: Poverty and
    Development in the West of Ireland*. Dublin; Portland, OR: Four Courts, 2005

C. Brock, *British Women Surgeons and Their Patients, 1860–1918*. Cambridge: Cambridge University Press, 2017

W. Brock, *Justus Von Liebig: The Chemical Gatekeeper*. Cambridge: Cambridge University Press, 2002

P. Brown, 'Nineteenth-Century American Health Reformers and the Early Nature Cure Movement in Britain', *Medical History* 32 (1988), 174–94

R. Campenot, *Animal Electricity: How We Learned That the Body and Brain Are Electric Machines*. Cambridge, MA; London: Harvard University Press, 2016

A. Carden-Coyne, *Reconstructing the Body: Classicism, Modernism, and the First World War*. Oxford: Oxford University Press, 2009

K. Carpenter, *The History of Scurvy and Vitamin C*. Cambridge: Cambridge University Press, 1986

G. Casadesus, G. Perry, J. Joseph and M. Smith, 'Eat Less, Eat Better, and Live Longer: Does It Work and Is It Worth It? The Role of Diet in Aging and Disease', in S. Post and R. Binstock eds, *The Fountain of Youth: Cultural, Scientific, and Ethical Perspectives on a Biomedical Goal*. Oxford; New York: Oxford University Press, 2004, 201–27

S. Cayleff, *Nature's Path: A History of Naturopathic Healing in America*. Baltimore, MD: Johns Hopkins University Press, 2016

L.-C. Celestin, *Charles-Edouard Brown-Séquard: The Biography of a Tormented Genius*. Heidelberg; New York; London: Springer, 2014

D. Chapman, *Sandow the Magnificent: Eugen Sandow and the Beginnings of Bodybuilding*. Chicago: University of Chicago Press, 1994

B. Chow, 'A Professional Body: Remembering, Repeating and Working Out Masculinities in fin-de-siécle Physical Culture', *Performance Research* 20:5 (2015), 30–41

A. Christen and J. Christen, 'Horace Fletcher (1849–1919): "The Great Masticator"', *Journal of the History of Dentistry* 45:3 (1997), 95–100

J. Clark, '"Beauty on Bond Street": Gender, Enterprise, and the Establishment of an English Beauty Industry, 1850-1910'. Unpublished PhD dissertation, Johns Hopkins University, 2012

'Pomeroy v. Pomeroy: Beauty, Modernity, and the Female Entrepreneur in fin-de-siècle London', *Women's History Review* 22:6 (2013), 877–903

'"Clever Ministrations": Regenerative Beauty at the fin de siècle' *Palgrave Communications* 3 (2017), doi.org/10.1057/s41599-017-0029-9

G. Cocks, *The State of Health: Illness in Nazi Germany*. Oxford: Oxford University Press, 2012

H. Cocks, *Classified: The Secret History of the Personal Column*. London: Random House, 2009

P. Codellas, 'Rejuvenations and Satyricons of Yesterday', *Annals of Medical History* 6 (1934), 510–20

P. Cohen, *In Our Prime: The Invention of Middle Age*. New York; London: Scribner, 2012

T. Cole, *The Journey of Life: A Cultural History of Aging in America*. Cambridge: Cambridge University Press, 1997

T. Cole, D. van Tassel and R. Kastenbaum eds., *Handbook of the Humanities and Aging*. New York: Springer, 1992

S. Connor, *The Book of Skin*, Ithaca, NY: Cornell University Press, 2004

S. Constantine, *Social Conditions in Britain 1918–1939*. London: Routledge, 2006

D. Cooper and R. Lanza, *Xeno: The Promise of Transplanting Animal Organs into Humans*. Oxford: Oxford University Press, 2000

R. Cooter ed., *Studies in the History of Alternative Medicine*. Basingstoke: MacMillan, 1988

I. Crozier, 'Becoming a Sexologist: Norman Haire, the 1929 London World League for Sexual Reform Congress, and Organizing Medical Knowledge about Sex in Interwar England', *History of Science* 39:3 (2001), 299–329

C. Culotta, 'Arsonval, Arsène D', in C. Gillispie ed., *Dictionary of Scientific Biography*. New York: Charles Scribner's Sons, 1971, 302–05

E. Cuperschmid and T. de Campos, 'Dr Voronoff's Curious Glandular Xenoimplants', *História, Ciências, Saúde – Manguinhos* 14:3 (2007), 1–24

S. Currell, 'Depression and Recovery: Self-Help and America in the 1930s', in D. Bell and J. Hollows eds, *Historicizing Lifestyle: Mediating Taste, Consumption and Identity from the 1900s to 1970s*. Aldershot: Ashgate, 2006, 131–44

J. Day, 'The Ideological Development of Physical Activity as Medicine in Britain, 1870-1939'. Unpublished MSc thesis: University of Chester, 2013

A. Digby, *Making a Medical Living: Doctors and Patients in the English Market for Medicine, 1720–1911. Cambridge: Cambridge University Press*, 1994

R. Dowbiggin, *The Sterilization Movement and Global Fertility in the Twentieth Century*. Oxford: Oxford University Press, 2008

E. Dyck, *Facing Eugenics: Reproduction, Sterilization, and the Politics of Choice*. Toronto: University of Toronto Press, 2013

P. Elliott, '"More Subtle than the Electric Aura": Georgian Medical Electricity, the Spirit of Animation and the Development of Erasmus Darwin's Psychophysiology', *Medical History* 52 (2008), 195–220

R. Ellwood, *The Fifties Spiritual Marketplace: American Religion in a Decade of Conflict*. New Brunswick, NJ: Rutgers University Press, 1997

K. Endres, 'The Feminism of Bernarr Macfadden: *Physical Culture* Magazine and the Empowerment of Women', *Media History Monographs* 13:2 (2011), 2–14

R. Ernst, *Weakness Is a Crime: The Life of Bernarr Macfadden*. Syracuse, NY: Syracuse University Press, 1991

L. Evans, 'The Problem of Death: Dr Maurice Ernest and his Longevity Library', *Electronic British Library Journal* (2013), 1–24

M. Fairclough, '*Frankenstein* and the "Spark of Being": Electricity, Animation, and Adaptation', *European Romantic Review* 29:3 (2018), 399–407

W. Feldberg, 'Henry Hallett Dale. 1875–1968', *Biographical Memoirs of Fellows of the Royal Society* 16 (1970), 77–174

G. Fendley, 'McCoy, Sir Frederick (1817–1899)', in D. Pike, B. Nairn, G. Serle and R. Ward eds., *Australian Dictionary of Biography*, vol. 5. Melbourne: Melbourne University Press, 1974, 134–36

M. Finlay, 'Early Marketing of the Theory of Nutrition: The Science and Culture of Liebig's Extract of Meat', in H. Kamminga and A. Cunningham eds., *The Science and Culture of Nutrition, 1840-1940*. Amsterdam: Rodopi, 1995, 48–74

M. Finn, 'The West Riding Lunatic Asylum and the Making of Modern Brain Sciences in the Nineteenth Century'. Unpublished PhD thesis: University of Leeds, 2012

M. Fitoussi, *Helena Rubinstein: The Woman Who Invented Beauty*, trans. K. Bignold
and L. Ramaskishnan Iyer. London: Gallic, 2013

R. Foster, *W. B. Yeats: A Life II: The Arch-Poet, 1915–1939*. Oxford: Oxford
University Press, 2003

M. Foucault, *The Birth of the Clinic: An Archaeology of Medical Perception*. New
York: Pantheon Books, 1973

L. Foxcroft, *Calories and Corsets: A History of Dieting over Two Thousand Years*.
London: Profile Books, 2012

R. French, *Antivivisection and Medical Science in Victorian Society*. Princeton, NJ:
Princeton University Press, 1975

J. Gabriel, 'Pharmaceutical Patenting and the Transformation of American Medical
Ethics', *British Journal for the History of Science* 49:4 (2016), 577–600

L. Gälmark, 'Women Antivivisectionists: The Story of Lizzy Lind af Hageby and Leisa
Schartau', *Animal Issues* 4:2 (2000), 1–32

G. Geison, *Michael Foster and the Cambridge School of Physiology: The Scientific
Enterprise in Late Victorian Society*. Princeton, NJ: Princeton University Press,
1978

S. Geroulanos and T. Meyers, *The Human Body in the Age of Catastrophe: Brittleness,
Integration, Science, and the Great War*. Chicago: University of Chicago Press,
2018

J. Gilheany, *Familiar Strangers: The Church and the Vegetarian Movement in Britain
(1809–2009)*. Cardiff: Ascendant Press, 2010

S. Gilman, 'Fat as Disability: The Case of the Jews', in J. Metzl and S. Poirier eds,
Difference and Identity: A Special Issue of Literature and Medicine. Baltimore,
MD: Johns Hopkins University Press, 2005, 46–60
   Fat: A Cultural History. Cambridge; Malden, MA: Polity Press, 2008
   'Thoughts on the Jewish Body, Baseball and the Problem of Integration', in
   E. Mendelsohn ed., *Jews and the Sporting Life*. Oxford; New York: Oxford
   University Press, 2008, 5–16

G. Gooday, *Domesticating Electricity: Technology, Uncertainty, and Gender,
1880–1914*. London: Pickering and Chatto, 2008

G. Gooday and S. Arapostathis, *Patently Contestable: Electrical Technologies and
Inventor Identities on Trial in Britain*. Cambridge, MA; London: MIT Press,
2013

S. Grant, *Physical Culture and Sport in Soviet Society: Propaganda, Acculturation, and
Transformation in the 1920s and 1930s*. London: Routledge, 2013
   'Bolsheviks, Revolution and Physical Culture', *International Journal of the History
   of Sport* 31:7 (2014), 724–34

A. Gray, 'People Who Want to Look Young and Beautiful', *The American Magazine*
94 (1922), 32–33

S. Greenblatt, 'Huglings Jackson's First Encounter with the Work of Paul Broca: The
Physiological and Philosophical Background', *Bulletin of the History of Medicine*
44:6 (1970), 555–70

C. Greenhalgh, *Aging in Twentieth Century Britain*. Oakland: University of California
Press, 2018

A. de Grey, *Ending Aging: The Rejuvenation Breakthroughs That Could Reverse
Human Aging in Our Lifetime*. New York: St. Martin's Press, 2007

R. Griffith, 'Apostles of Abstinence: Fasting and Masculinity in the Progressive Era', *American Quarterly* 52:4 (2000), 599–638

M. Gullette, *Safe at Last in the Middle Years: The Invention of the Midlife Progress Novel: Saul Bellow, Margaret Drabble, Anne Tyler, and John Updike*. Berkeley: University of California Press, 1988

Declining to Decline: Cultural Combat and the Politics of the Midlife. Charlottesville; London: University Press of Virginia, 1997

Aged by Culture. Chicago: University of Chicago Press, 2004

E. Haiken, *Venus Envy: A History of Cosmetic Surgery*. Baltimore, MD: Johns Hopkins University Press, 1997

D. Hamilton, *The Monkey Gland Affair*. London: Chatto & Windus, 1986

J. Hand, 'Marketing Health Education: Advertising Margarine and Visualising Health in Britain from 1964–c.2000', *Contemporary British History* 31:4 (2017), 477–500

L. Hapke, *Daughters of the Great Depression: Women, Work, and Fiction in the American 1930s*. Athens: University of Georgia Press, 1995

A. Harrington, *Medicine, Mind, and the Double Brain: A Study in Nineteenth Century Thought*. Princeton, NJ: Princeton University Press, 1987

Reenchanted Science: Holism in German Culture from Wilhelm II to Hitler. Princeton, NJ: Princeton University Press, 1996

M. Harrison, 'Cantlie, Sir James (1851–1926)' in *Oxford Dictionary of National Biography*. Oxford University Press, 2004; online edn, Oct 2008, www.oxforddnb.com.wam.leeds.ac.uk/view/article/50530, accessed 15 May 2017

M. Hau, *The Cult of Health and Beauty in Germany: A Social History, 1890–1930*. Chicago: University of Chicago Press, 2003

L. Haushofer, 'Between Food and Medicine: Artificial Digestion, Sickness, and the Case of Benger's Food', *Journal of the History of Medicine and Allied Sciences* 73:2 (2018), 168–87

D. Haycock, *Mortal Coil: A Short History of Living Longer*. New Haven, CT: Yale University Press, 2008

R. Hayward, *The Transformation of the Psyche in British Primary Care, 1870–1970*. London: Bloomsbury, 2014

K. Heath, *Aging by the Book: The Emergence of Midlife in Victorian Britain*. Albany: State University of New York Press, 2009

L. Hirshbein, 'The Glandular Solution: Sex, Masculinity, and Aging in the 1920s', *Journal of the History of Sexuality* 9:3 (2000), 277–304

K. Hooper, 'Hartley, Catherine Gasquoine (1866/7–1928)' in *Oxford Dictionary of National Biography*. Oxford: Oxford University Press, 2011, www.oxforddnb.com/view/article/101278, accessed 13 October 2017

R. Hornsey, '"The Modern Way to Loveliness": middle-class cosmetics and chain-store beauty culture in mid-twentieth-century Britain', *Women's History Review* 28:1 (2018), 111–38

U. Houe, 'Frankenstein without Electricity: Contextualizing Shelley's Novel', *Studies in Romanticism* 55:1 (2016), 95–118

B. Hurwitz, 'Narrative Constructs in Modern Clinical Case Reporting', *Studies in History and Philosophy of Science* 62 (2017), 65–73

M. Jackson, *The Age of Stress: Science and the Search for Stability*. Oxford: Oxford University Press, 2013

J. Jahiel, 'Rejuvenation Research and the American Medical Association in the Early
    Twentieth Century: Paradigms in Conflict'. Unpublished PhD thesis: Boston
    University, 1992
A. Jamieson, 'More Than Meets the Eye: Revealing the Therapeutic Potential of
    "Light", 1896–1910', *Social History of Medicine* 26:4 (2013), 715–37
E. Jensen, *Body by Weimar: Athletes, Gender, and German Modernity*. Oxford: Oxford
    University Press, 2010
T. Jensen, 'The Importance of Age Perceptions and Nutritional Science to Early
    Twentieth-century Institutional Diets', *Social History of Medicine* 30:1 (2017),
    158–74
R. Jobs, *Riding the New Wave: Youth and the Rejuvenation of France after the Second
    World War*. Stanford, CA: Stanford University Press, 2007
P. Johnson and P. Thane eds., *Old Age from Antiquity to Post-Modernity*. London:
    Routledge, 1998
C. Jones, *The Medical Trade Catalogue in Britain, 1870–1914*. London: Pickering and
    Chatto, 2013
    'A Barrier to Medical Treatment? British Medical Practitioners, Medical Appliances
    and the Patent Controversy, 1870–1920', *British Journal for the History of Science*
    49:4 (2016), 601–25
G. Jones, *Beauty Imagined: A History of the Global Beauty Industry*. Oxford; New
    York: Oxford University Press, 2010
G. Kay, *Dying to Be Beautiful: The Fight for Safe Cosmetics*. Columbus: Ohio State
    University Press, 2005
    'Healthy Public Relations: The FDA's 1930s Legislative Campaign', *Bulletin of the
    History of Medicine* 75:3 (2001), 446–87
H. Kean, 'The "Smooth Cool Men of Science": The Feminist and Socialist Response to
    Vivisection', *History Workshop Journal* 40 (1995), 16–38
    Animal Rights: Political and Social Change in Britain since 1800. London: Reaktion
    Books, 1998
D. Kirk, 'Foucault and the Limits of Corporeal Regulation: The Emergence,
    Consolidation and Decline of School Medical Inspection and Physical Training in
    Australia, 1909-30', *International Journal of the History of Sport* 13:2 (1996),
    114–31
P. Kirkham and J. Thumim eds, *You Tarzan: Masculinity, Movies and Men*. London:
    Lawrence & Wishart, 1993
G. Koureas, *Memory, Masculinity and National Identity in British Visual Culture,
    1914–1930: A Study of 'Unconquerable Manhood'*. London; New York:
    Routledge, 2016
N. Krementsov, *Revolutionary Experiments: The Quest for Immortality in Bolshevik
    Science and Fiction*. Oxford: Oxford University Press, 2014
C. Lansbury, *The Old Brown Dog: Women, Workers, and Vivisection in Edwardian
    England*. Madison: University of Wisconsin Press, 1985
Y. Laporte, 'Charles-Édouard Brown-Séquard. Une vie mouvementée et une
    contribution importante à l'étude du système nerveux', *Comptes Rendus Biologies*
    329 (2006), 363–68
H. Levenstein, *Revolution at the Table: The Transformation of the American Diet*.
    Berkeley: University of California Press, 1988

L. Loeb, 'Consumerism and Commercial Electrotherapy: The Medical Battery Company in Nineteenth-Century London', *Journal of Victorian Culture* 4 (1999), 252–75

C. Logan, *Hormones, Heredity and Race: Spectacular Failure in Interwar Vienna*. New Brunswick, NJ: Rutgers University Press, 2013

V. Long and H. Marland, 'From Danger and Motherhood to Health and Beauty: Health Advice for the Factory Girl in Early Twentieth-Century Britain', *Twentieth Century British History* 20:4 (2009), 454–81

D. Loriaux, *A Biographical History of Endocrinology*. Ames, IA; Chichester: John Wiley & Sons Ltd., 2016

L. Ludovici, *Cosmetic Scalpel: The Life of Charles Willi, Beauty-Surgeon*. Bradford-on-Avon: Moonraker Press, 1981

C. Macdonald, 'Body and Self: Learning to be Modern in 1920s–1930s Britain', *Women's History Review* 22:2 (2013), 267–79

P. Mackowiak, 'Recycling Metchnikoff: Probiotics, the Intestinal Microbiome and the Quest for Long Life', *Frontiers in Public Health* 1:52 (2013), doi:10.3389/fpubh.2013.00052

E. Macrae, *Exercise in the Female Lifecycle in Britain, 1930–1970*. Basingstoke: Palgrave Macmillan, 2016

J. Mangan and J. Walvin eds, *Manliness and Morality: Middle-class Masculinity in Britain and America, 1800–1940*. Manchester: Manchester University Press, 1991

M. Marsh, *Compacts and Cosmetics*. Barnsley: Pen and Sword, 2009

B. Marshall and S. Katz, 'From Androgyny to Androgens: Resexing the Aging Body', in T. Calasanti and K. Slevin eds, *Age Matters: Realigning Feminist Thinking*. New York; London: Routledge, 2006, 75–98

J. Martschukat, '"The Necessity for Better Bodies to Perpetuate Our Institutions, Insure a Higher Development of the Individual, and Advance the Conditions of the Race." Physical Culture and the Formation of the Self in the Late Nineteenth and Early Twentieth Century USA', *Journal of Historical Sociology* 24:4 (2009), 472–93

M. Mason, 'The Impact of World War II on Women's Fashion in the United States and Britain'. Unpublished MA Dissertation: University of Nevada, Las Vegas, 2011

L. McFarland, 'From Yaks to Yogurt: The History, Development, and Current Use of Probiotics', *Clinical Infectious Diseases* 60:2 (2015), 85–90

P. McGrady, Jr, *The Youth Doctors*. London: Barker, 1969

S. McKenzie, *Getting Physical: The Rise of Physical Culture in America*. Lawrence: University of Kansas Press, 2013

A. McLaren, *Reproduction by Design: Sex, Robots, Trees, and Test-Tube Babies in Interwar Britain*. Chicago: University of Chicago Press, 2012

P. McDevitt, *May the Best Man Win: Sport, Masculinity, and Nationalism in Great Britain and the Empire, 1880–1935*. New York: Palgrave Macmillan, 2004

A. Medeiros and E. Watkins, 'Live Longer Better: The Historical Roots of Human Growth Hormone as Anti-Aging Medicine', *Journal of the History of Medicine and Allied Sciences* 73:3 (2018), 333–59

I. Miller, *A Modern History of the Stomach: Gastric Illness, Medicine and British Society, 1800–1950*. London: Pickering & Chatto, 2011

S. Mintz, *The Prime of Life: A History of Modern Adulthood*. Cambridge, MA: Harvard University Press, 2015

W. Mitchinson, *Body Failure: Medical Views of Women, 1900–1950*. Toronto; London: University of Toronto Press, 2013

D. Monger, *Patriotism and Propaganda in First World War Britain: The National War Aims Committee and Civilian Morale*. Liverpool: Liverpool University Press, 2012

T. Moreira, *Science, Technology and the Ageing Society*. London; New York: Routledge, 2017

I. Morus, *Shocking Bodies: Life, Death and Electricity in Victorian England*. Stroud: The History Press, 2011

O. Mouristen, *Seaweeds: Edible, Available and Sustainable*. Chicago: University of Chicago Press, 2013

R. Nye, 'The Rise and Fall of the Eugenics Empire: Recent Perspectives on the Impact of Bio-Medical Thought in Modern Society', *Historical Journal* 36 (1993), 687–700

P. O'Higgins, *Madame: An Intimate Biography of Helena Rubinstein*. New York: Viking Press, 1971

C. Oakley, 'Sexual Rejuvenation and Hegemonic Masculinity in C. P. Snow's suppressed novel *New Lives for Old* (1933)', *Palgrave Communications* 4:93 (2018), doi:10.1057/s41599-018-0142-4

'Vital Forms: Bodily Energy in Medicine and Culture, 1870–1925'. Unpublished PhD thesis: University of York, 2016

D. Oddy, *From Plain Fare to Fusion Food: British Diet from the 1890s to the 1990s*. Woodbridge: Boydell, 2003

D. Oddy, P. Atkins and V. Amilien eds, *The Rise of Obesity in Europe: A Twentieth Century Food History*. Farnham: Ashgate, 2009

M. Okun, *Fair Play in the Marketplace: The First Battle for Pure Food and Drugs*. Dekalb: University of Illinois Press, 1986

S. Olsen, *Juvenile Nation: Youth, Emotions and the Making of the Modern British Citizen, 1880–1914*. New York: Bloomsbury Academic, 2014

D. Omodei and L. Fontana, 'Calorie Restriction And Prevention Of Age-Associated Chronic Disease', *FEBS Letters* 585:11 (2011), 1537–42

J. Oppenheim, *'Shattered Nerves': Doctors, Patients and Depression in Victorian England*. London: Oxford University Press, 1991

N. Oudshoorn, *Beyond the Natural Body: An Archaeology of Sex Hormones*. London; New York: Routledge, 1994

R. Overy, *The Morbid Age: Britain between the Wars*. London: Allen Lane, 2009

Oxford English Dictionary Online, Oxford University Press, 2017, www.oed.com

H. Park, *Old Age, New Science: Gerontologists and Their Biosocial Visions, 1900–1960*. Pittsburgh, PA: University of Pittsburgh Press, 2016

D. Paul, 'Darwin, Social Darwinism and Eugenics' in J. Hodge and G. Radick eds, *The Cambridge Companion to Darwin*. Cambridge: Cambridge University Press, 2003, 214–39

S. Peitzman, *Dropsy, Dialysis, Transplant: A Short History of Failing Kidneys*. Baltimore, MD: Johns Hopkins University Press, 2007

C. de la Peña, *The Body Electric: How Strange Machines Built the Modern American*. New York: New York University Press, 2003

M. Petitt, 'Becoming Glandular: Endocrinology, Mass Culture, and Experimental Lives in the Interwar Age', *American Historical Review* 118:4 (2013), 1052–76

J. Phillips and M. French, 'Adulteration and Food Law, 1899–1939', *Twentieth Century British History* 9:3 (1998), 350–69

W. Pickren and A. Rutherford, *A History of Modern Psychology in Context*. London: Wiley, 2010

R. Porter, *Blood and Guts: A Short History of Medicine*. London: Allen Lane, 2002

A. Rabinbach, *The Human Motor: Energy, Fatigue, and the Origins of Modernity*. Berkeley: University of California Press, 1992

J. Real, *Voronoff*. Paris: Stock, 2001

J. Rechter, '"The Glands of Destiny": A History of Popular, Medical and Scientific Views of the Sex Hormones in 1920s America'. Unpublished PhD thesis: University of California, Berkeley, 1997

F. Reid, *Broken Men: Shell Shock, Treatment and Recovery in Modern Britain*. London: Bloomsbury, 2011

D. Rhees, 'Electricity – "The Greatest of All Doctors". An Introduction to "High Frequency Oscillators for Electro-Therapeutic and Other Purposes"', *Proceedings of the IEEE* 87:7 (1999), 1277–81

R. Romani, *National Character and Public Spirit in Britain and France, 1750–1914*. Cambridge: Cambridge University Press, 2002

C. Ross, *Naked Germany: Health, Race and the Nation*. Oxford; New York: Berg, 2005

Royal College of Surgeons of England, 'Crile, George Washington (1864–1943)', 20 June 2013, https://livesonline.rcseng.ac.uk/client/en_GB/search/asset/338623/0, accessed 22 January 2019

J. Savage, *Teenage: The Creation of Youth, 1875–1945*. London: Pimlico, 2008

C. Schmid, 'The "New Woman", Gender Roles and Urban Modernism in Interwar Berlin and Shanghai', *Journal of International Women's Studies* 51:1 (2014), 1–16

W. Schneider, *Quality and Quantity: The Quest for Biological Regeneration in Twentieth-Century France*. Cambridge: Cambridge University Press, 1990

P. Scott, 'Body-Building and Empire-Building: George Douglas Brown, The South African War, and *Sandow's Magazine of Physical Culture*', *Victorian Periodicals Review* 41:1 (2008), 78–94

G. Scrinis, *Nutritionism: The Science and Politics of Dietary Advice*. New York: Columbia University Press, 2013

C. Searing and H. Zeilig, '*Fine Lines*: Cosmetic Advertising and the Perception of Ageing Female Beauty', *International Journal of Ageing and Later Life* 11:1 (2017), 7–36

K. Segrave, *Baldness: A Social History*. Jefferson, NC; London: McFarland & Company Inc., 1996

C. Sengoopta, 'Rejuvenation and the Prolongation of Life: Science or Quackery?', *Perspectives in Biology and Medicine* 37:1 (1993), 55–66

'Glandular Politics. Experimental Biology, Clinical Medicine, and Homosexual Emancipation in fin-de-siècle Central Europe', *Isis* 89:3 (1998), 445–73

'Transforming the Testicle: Science, Medicine and Masculinity, 1800–1951', *Medicina nei Secoli* 13 (2001), 637–55

'"Dr Steinach Coming to Make Old Young": Sex Glands, Vasectomy and the Quest for Rejuvenation in the Roaring Twenties', *Endeavour* 27 (2003), 122–26

The Most Secret Quintessence of Life: Sex, Glands, and Hormones, 1850–1950. Chicago: University of Chicago Press, 2006

J. Senior, 'Rationalising Electrotherapy in Neurology, 1860-1920'. Unpublished PhD thesis: Oxford University, 1994

I. Sharp and M. Stibbe, 'Women's International Activism during the Interwar Period, 1919–1939', *Women's History Review* 26 (2017), 163–72

H. Small, *The Longer Life*. Oxford: Oxford University Press, 2007

V. Smith, *Clean: A History of Personal Hygiene and Purity*. Oxford: Oxford University Press, 2007

P. Södersten, D. Crews, C. Logan and R. Soukup, 'Eugen Steinach: The First Neuroendocrinologist', *Endocrinology* 155:3 (2014), 688–95

S. Spindler, 'Biological Effects of Caloric Restriction: Implications for Modification of Human Aging' in G. Fahy, M. West, L. Coles and S. Harris eds., *The Future of Aging: Pathways to Human Life Extension*. Dordrecht; London: Springer 2010, 367–438

J. Stark, '"Recharge my Exhausted Batteries": Overbeck's Rejuvenator, patenting, and public medical consumers, 1924–1937', *Medical History* 58:4 (2014), 498–518

'Introduction: Plurality in Patenting: Medical Technology and Cultures of Protection', *British Journal for the History of Science* 49:4 (2016), 533–40

'"Replace Them by Salads and Vegetables": Dietary Innovation, Youthfulness, and Authority, 1900–1939', *Global Food History* 4:2 (2018), 130–51

P. Steans, *Old Age in European Society: The Case of France*. London: Croome Helm, 1977

P. Stearns, *Fat History: Bodies and Beauty in the Modern West*. New York; London: New York University Press, 1997

E. Stoilova, 'The Bulgarianization of Yoghurt: Connecting Home, Taste, and Authenticity', *Food and Foodways* 23:1–2 (2015), 14–35

F. Sypher ed., *Frederick L. Hoffman: His Life and Works*. Philadelphia: Xlibris, 2002

A. Tauber and L. Chernyak, *Metchnikoff and the Origins of Immunology: From Metaphor to Theory*. New York; Oxford: Oxford University Press, 1991

M. Tausk, *Organon: de Geschiedenis van een Bijzondere Nederlandse Onderneming*. Nikmegen: Dekker en Van de Vegt, 1978

C. Tebbutt, 'Popular and Medical Understandings of Sex Change in 1930s Britain'. Unpublished PhD thesis: University of Manchester, 2014

M. Thomson, *Psychological Subjects: Identity, Culture, and Health in Twentieth Century Britain*. Oxford: Oxford University Press, 2006

Lost Freedom: The Landscape of the Child and the British Post-War Settlement. Oxford: Oxford University Press, 2013

I. Thompson, 'The Acceptance of a National Policy for Physical Education in Scotland, 1872–1908'. Unpublished PhD dissertation: University of Stirling, 1976

C. Timmermann, 'Constitutional Medicine, Neoromanticism, and the Politics of Antimechanism in Interwar Germany', *Bulletin of the History of Medicine* 75:4 (2001), 717–39

'Rationalizing "Folk Medicine" in Interwar Germany: Faith, Business, and Science at "Dr. Madaus & Co."', *Social History of Medicine* 14:3 (2001), 459–82

P. Tinkler, *Constructing Girlhood: Popular Magazines for Girls Growing Up in England, 1920-1950*. Abingdon: Taylor & Francis, 1995

S. Todd, *Young Women, Work, and Family in England, 1918–1950*. Oxford: Oxford University Press, 2005

N. Tomes, *Remaking the American Patient: How Madison Avenue and Modern Medicine Turned Patients into Consumers*. Chapel Hill: University of North Carolina Press, 2016

E. Trimmer, *Live Long and Stay Young: An Essay on Positive Health and Rejuvenation*. London: George Allen & Unwin Ltd, 1965

Rejuvenation: The History of an Idea. London: Hale, 1967

J. Tumblety, *Remaking the Male Body: Masculinity and the Uses of Physical Culture in Interwar and Vichy France*. Oxford: Oxford University Press, 2012

M. Turda, *Modernism and Eugenics*. Basingstoke: Palgrave MacMillan, 2010

T. Ueyama, 'Capital, Profession and Medical Technology: The Electro-Therapeutics Institutes and the Royal College of Physicians, 1888–1922', *Medical History* 41 (1997), 150–81

Health in the Marketplace: Professionalism, Therapeutic Desires, and Medical Commodification in Late-Victorian London. Palo Alto, CA: The Society for the Promotion of Science and Scholarship, 2010

C. Usborne, *The Politics of the Body in Weimar Germany: Women's Reproductive Rights and Duties*. Basingstoke: Palgrave Macmillan, 1992

M. Verbrugge, *Active Bodies: A History of Women's Physical Education in Twentieth-Century America*. Oxford: Oxford University Press, 2012

P. Vertinsky, 'The Social Construction of the Gendered Body: Exercise and the Exercise of Power', *International Journal of the History of Sport* 11:2 (1994), 147–71

'"Building the Body Beautiful" in The Women's League of Health and Beauty: Yoga and Female Agency in 1930s Britain', *Rethinking History* 16:4 (2012), 517–42

Victoria and Albert Museum, 'Andrew Pitcairn-Knowles – Victoria and Albert Museum', 2016, www.vam.ac.uk/content/articles/t/andrew-pitcairn-knowles/, accessed 2 August 2018

S. Walch, *Triebe, Reize und Signale. Eugen Steinachs Physiologie der Sexualhormone. Vom biologischen Konzept zum Pharmapräparat, 1894–1938*. Wien: Böhlau, 2016

E. Watkins, *The Estrogen Elixir: A History of Hormone Replacement Therapy in America*. Baltimore, MD: Johns Hopkins University Press, 2007

C. Watt, 'Cultural Exchange, Appropriation and Physical Culture: Strongman Eugen Sandow in Colonial India, 1904–1905', *The International Journal of the History of Sport* 33:16 (2017), 1921–42

A. Weintraub, *Selling the Fountain of Youth: How the Anti-Aging Industry Made a Disease out of Getting Old and Made Billions*. New York: Basic Books, 2010

A. Wexler, 'The Medical Battery in the United States (1870–1920): Electrotherapy at Home and in the Clinic', *Journal of the History of Medicine and Allied Sciences* 72:2 (2017), 166–92

'Recurrent Themes in the History of the Home use of Electrical Stimulation: Transcranial Direct Current Stimulation (tDCS) and the Medical Battery (1870–1920)', *Brain Stimulation* 10 (2017), 187–95

J. Whorton, *Inner Hygiene: Constipation and the Pursuit of Health in Modern Society*. New York: Oxford University Press, 2000

Nature Cures: The History of Alternative Medicine in America. Oxford: Oxford University Press, 2002

C. Wolff, *Magnus Hirschfeld: A Portrait of a Pioneer in Sexology*. London: Quartet Books, 1986

T. Woloshyn, *Soaking up the Rays: Light Therapy and Visual Culture in Britain, c.1890–1940*. Manchester: Manchester University Press, 2017

L. Woodhead, *War Paint: Elizabeth Arden and Helena Rubinstein*. London: Virago, 2012

World Health Organisation, 'What Is Active Ageing?', 2019, www.who.int/ageing/active_ageing/en/, accessed 23 January 2019

D. Wyndham, 'Versemaking and Lovemaking – W. B. Yeats' "Strange Second Puberty": Norman Haire and the Steinach Rejuvenation Operation', *Journal of the History of Behavioral Sciences* 39:1 (2003), 25–50

Norman Haire and the Study of Sex. Sydney: Sydney University Press, 2012

J. Young, *Pure Food: Securing the Federal Food and Drugs Act of 1906*. Princeton, NJ: Princeton University Press, 1989

I. Zweiniger-Bargielowska, 'The Culture of the Abdomen: Obesity and Reducing in Britain, ca. 1900–1939', *Journal of British Studies* 44:2 (2005), 239–73

'Building a British Superman: Physical Culture in Interwar Britain', *Journal of Contemporary History* 41:4 (2006), 595–610

Managing the Body: Beauty, Health, and Fitness in Britain, 1880–1939. Oxford: Oxford University Press, 2010

Index

A New Electronic Theory of Life, 115, 136
Abplanalp, Arthur, 146
Abramowski, Otto, 68, 82–83, 91
adolescence, 7, 139
Adulteration of Food and Drugs Acts, 95
aesthetics, 3, 5, 13, 15, 69, 106, 120, 122, 129,
　　133, 146, 158, 171, 174, 176, 183, 196,
　　207, 209
af Hageby, Lizzy Lind, 49
ageing
　biological, 7, 22, 206
　premature, 25–26, 42, 60, 63, 66, 80, 98,
　　139, 155, 167–68
　signs of, 1, 20, 22, 104, 119, 130, 132–33,
　　136–37, 159, 161, 170, 191, 194, 202
alcohol, 19, 85, 104, 157
Alfred Eichholz Clinic, 128
alimentary canal. *See* intestine
Allbutt, Sir Clifford, 11
animal foods. *See* meat
anti-vivisectionism, 49–50, 68, 74
anxiety, 2, 5–6, 8, 11, 13, 16, 20, 38–39, 48,
　　50, 62–63, 66, 74, 79, 81, 94, 99, 103,
　　117, 122, 140, 149, 158, 168, 178, 199,
　　203, 206, 212
appetite, 34, 38, 59, 70–73, 81–82, 100, 104,
　　135
Apple, Rima D., 88
Arden, Elizabeth, 13, 16, 107, 129, 166, 173,
　　177, 185–86
arthritis, 134, 162
Atherton, Gertrude, 17, 42, 208
atomic structure, 111, 136
attractiveness, 2, 175, 197
Australia, 24, 39, 51, 55, 91, 113, 117, 186,
　　216

Back, Ivor, 30
Bacon, Francis, 22, 192, 216
Bagot Stack, Mary, 151–52
Bagot Stack, Prunella, 151
Baird, Irvin, 90–91, 212

baldness, 41, 89, 120, 133, 158
bathroom, 16, 165
Bayliss, William, 24
Beaton, Cecil, 64
beauty, 3, 11, 13–14, 17, 20, 22, 59, 62, 88, 91,
　　93, 107, 113, 119, 124–25, 127, 129,
　　132–34, 149, 151, 153, 158–59, 161–62,
　　164–65, 168, 170, 172, 175, 177, 179–80,
　　182, 185–87, 190, 194, 197–98, 201–3,
　　208, 213, 217
beauty culture, 158, 160, 162, 165, 170, 172,
　　177, 179–80, 185, 198–99
Beddow Bayly, Maurice, 49–50
Belfield, William, 31
Benjamin, Harry, 37
Bennett, Sanford, 80, 82–83, 109, 141, 144,
　　167, 180
beri-beri, 87, 92
Bioglan Laboratories Limited, 62
Bioserm, 62
birth control, 39, 215
Björkstén, Kristina Elisabeth, 149
Black Oxen, 17, 42, 208
Blackpool illuminations, 2
blood, 24, 28–29, 42, 75, 78–79, 83, 94–95,
　　97–98, 100, 102, 113, 124, 134, 136, 162,
　　166, 175–76, 205, 216
bodies
　as chemical, 24, 136
　exposed, 125
　faded by time, 134
　function of, 67
　limits of, 22, 66
　male and female, 3, 13, 19, 38, 144, 212
　management of, 24
　normal versus pathological, 109
　potential of, 20
Bond Street, 88, 126, 172, 185–86
Boots, 16, 21, 65, 107, 159, 162, 165, 177,
　　182, 186–87, 189–90, 192–94, 196,
　　201–2, 209
bowels, 75

Brady, William, 170
Briant, Frank, 48
Brinkley, John R., 5
British Electrotherapeutic Society, 108
British Glandular Products Ltd., 58–60
British Medical Association, 5, 115, 193, 198
Brittain, Sir Harry, 47, 123
Broca, Paul, 108
Brown, Haydn, 92
Brown-Séquard, Charles, 9, 28, 58, 110
Buffon, Comte de, 73

caloric restriction, 6, 102
Campenot, Robert B., 135
Cantlie, James, 138, 140, 145
carbohydrate, 78, 87
Carrel, Alexis, 5, 7, 12, 27, 88, 179, 205
Carslbad Spa, 80
case histories, 41, 54, 71
Cavazzi, Francesco, 58, 209–10
celebrity, 19, 149
Centenarian Club, 49
Chamberlain, Neville, 122
charm, 17, 26, 161, 173, 187, 205
Chartered Society of Massage and Medical
    Gymnastics, 123
Chartered Society of Physiotherapy, 128
childbirth, 135
childhood, 1, 7, 75, 144, 195, 207
Clark, Jessica P., 159, 172
climacteric. *See* menopause
Cocks, Geoffrey, 3
cod liver oil, 103, 194
Cole, Thomas R., 8, 11
commerce, 5, 16, 203
complexion, 13, 53, 90, 132, 140, 162, 172–73,
    176, 178, 182, 185, 194–95, 199, 217
constipation, 95, 145
consumers, 7, 15, 17, 20, 95, 98, 103, 106, 113,
    115, 119, 123–24, 136, 165, 169, 171,
    174, 176, 185, 190, 194, 197, 199, 208,
    216
cooking, 84, 86, 91
cosmetic surgery, 174
cosmetics, 1, 13, 17, 62, 95, 162, 173, 177–79,
    182, 185, 187, 193–94, 197, 199–200
Cossley-Batt, Jill, 90–91, 212
Crichton Browne, James, 68
crows feet, 95
Cruden, George, 139, 156
Curie, Marie, 134

d'Arsonval, Jacques Arsene, 119
Darwin, Charles, 40, 51, 118
de Beauvoir, Simone, 216

deafness, 38, 41
decline, 6–8, 22, 67, 72, 83, 140, 148–49, 169,
    208, 212
degeneration, 6, 20, 50, 68, 74, 81, 101, 104,
    168, 181
demographic change, 8
diathermy, 37, 56, 105, 107, 113, 118, 123–24,
    126–29, 135, 174
diet, 3, 5, 10, 12–13, 17–20, 22, 40–41, 48,
    53, 67–70, 73–75, 77–81, 83–85, 87–88,
    90, 92–95, 97, 101–3, 106, 108, 110,
    139, 141–42, 145, 154, 159, 194, 203,
    207, 211
dietetics, 68, 75, 77, 89
Digby-Morton, Phyllis, 193
digestive tract, 78, 94, 103
disability, 2
Duchess of Hamilton, The, 49
Dundas Irvine, L. C., 31, 148

Earle, Phyllis, 159, 172
economic productivity, 8, 10–11, 141
efficiency, 3, 40, 66, 126, 149
electric belts, 106, 108
electric combs, 133
electric hair brush, 118
electricity, 2, 10, 12–13, 18–20, 24, 32, 56, 98,
    105–7, 109–12, 115, 118, 124, 128–29,
    131–32, 134–36, 139, 162, 210
electro-convulsive therapy, 107
electrotherapy, 5, 9, 12–13, 16, 20, 42,
    105–7, 109, 111, 113–14, 119–20, 122,
    126–27, 132, 135, 149, 157, 176, 207,
    213
emanotherapy, 41, 132
Endocril, 65, 192
endocrinology, 5, 7, 10–13, 18, 24–25,
    27–28, 30–31, 35, 39, 41, 54, 58, 61,
    63, 65, 72–73, 79, 93, 101, 103, 111,
    113–14, 179–80, 183, 186, 201–2,
    206–7, 210
English, Jessie Millard, 52
enhancement, 21
entrepreneurs, 12, 14, 21, 82, 114, 135, 146
Ernest, Maurice, 90
eugenics, 10, 14, 26, 31, 66, 111, 140, 144,
    150, 155, 215
exercise, 1, 5–6, 10–11, 13, 17–20, 34, 40, 42,
    53, 60–61, 70, 75–76, 80–81, 89–90, 103,
    106–7, 131, 134, 136, 138–39, 141,
    144–45, 148, 150–54, 156–58, 161–62,
    164, 166, 168, 185, 207, 209, 212

facial massage, 159–61, 164, 192
faddism, 71, 94, 110, 200

family, 8, 10, 57, 75
faradism, 127, 162
fasting, 6, 19, 69, 73–74, 76–77, 79–80, 82,
    103–4
fat, 41, 63, 71, 76, 80, 87, 103, 131, 161, 175
feminine beauty, 196
femininity, 148, 152, 167
Ferrier, David, 108, 111
fertility, 8, 10, 14, 16–17, 22, 30, 34, 48, 215
fiction, 2, 17, 42, 57, 133, 209
fifty, 33, 41, 58, 65, 72–73, 100, 110, 138, 154,
    157, 161, 164
film, 2, 17, 42, 141, 152, 154, 208
Financial Crash, 9
fine lines, 20, 22, 161, 195
Finsen, Nils, 132
Fishbein, Morris, 25, 168, 176–77, 200
fitness, 8, 11, 14, 20, 42, 66, 79, 99, 140, 146,
    149, 154, 156, 167, 203, 213
food
    bread, 77–78, 87, 89
    dietetic foods, 77
    extracts, 69, 71, 101
    fruit, 19, 82–83, 87, 91, 97
    nutritional content of, 81, 93
    raw, 19, 79, 85, 98, 102, 104
    rich foods, 53, 71, 170
    supplements, 71
    vegetables, 19, 80, 83, 87, 90–91
    yoghurt, 85, 104
Food and Drugs Act (1938), 95
Food, Drug and Cosmetic Act (1938), 197,
    199
Formula Committee of Boots, 186–87, 189–90,
    193
forty, 99–100, 208–9
Foucault, Michel, 139
Frankenstein, 133
fresh air, 40, 75, 162, 167
Frumusan, Jean, 37, 39, 75–76, 140, 214

Galen, 69
Gallichan, Walter M., 144–45
galvanism, 106, 127–28, 133
Gayton, Bertram, 17, 45, 209
gender, 2–3, 5, 13, 16–17, 21, 23, 65, 106, 120,
    139, 175, 201, 203–4, 211
geriatrics, 8
Germany, 3–4, 6, 37, 81, 151, 153, 169, 183
gerontology, 8
Gilman, Sander, 76
glands
    extracts, 63, 100, 181
    feeding the, 89
    grafting, 16, 29, 31–32, 36, 48, 50, 53, 115

secretions of, 180–81
sex, 28–29, 33–34, 37, 40–41
testicles, 9, 28–30, 33, 36, 41, 48, 56, 59, 74,
    209
thyroid, 24, 39, 54–55, 59, 176, 206
Goizet, Louis Henri, 110, 210
gonads, 25, 41, 59, 206
gout, 51
Great Depression, 9, 91, 159, 203, 217
grey hair, 20, 22, 90, 125, 133, 159
Gubbins, Herbert, 133–34
Gullette, Margaret, 6
gymnastics, 128, 149–50

Haire, Norman, 27, 39, 41, 57, 72, 178
Hancock & Co., 61, 99
Hau, Michael, 3
Hauser, Benjamin Gayelord, 89, 93
Hayflick, Leonard, 7
Heath, Kay, 6
Heudebert Foods, 77
high-frequency treatment. *See* violet ray
Hill, A. V., 117
Hirshbein, Laura, 28, 73, 203
Hoffman, Frederick L., 79, 86, 157
holism, 4
Hollander, Bernard, 22, 111–12
Hopkins, Frederick Gowland, 87, 92
Hormone Twin Youthifiers, 180–81
hormones, 9, 11–13, 15–16, 18, 23–25,
    28–29, 35–36, 38, 40–42, 51, 53–54,
    57–60, 62–65, 67, 69–70, 74, 79, 88,
    101, 104, 107, 109, 111, 130, 136, 146,
    149, 169–71, 176–77, 179, 181, 183,
    186, 191, 193, 196, 198–99, 201–3, 205,
    207–10, 215
hospitals, 12, 49, 100, 109, 127–28, 135
Hovarth, Roland Evin, 166
Hughes, William "Billy", 118
Hurwitz, Brian, 72
Huxley, Julian, 17, 40, 45, 54
hysteria, 38, 124, 212
Hystogen Institute, 175

imbalance, 16, 56, 60, 126
impotence, 60
Innoxa, 186
intestinal stasis, 145, 166
intestine, 73, 77, 85–86

Juvigold Tonic Life Elixir, 181

Kammerer, Paul, 33, 38, 66, 71, 192
Knight, George E. O., 63
Kromayer, Ernst, 132

Lane, William Arbuthnot, 58, 85, 146
later life, 7–8, 92, 144, 148, 207
laws of nature, 79
Leichner, Ludwig, 59
libido, 17, 38
Lichtenstern, Robert, 33, 72
Life Begins at Forty, 6, 10, 186
life extension, 15, 54, 103, 217
lifecourse, 2, 6, 8, 13, 21–22, 79, 92, 101, 139,
    146, 148, 171, 206, 208, 214
Lloyd George, David, 1, 138, 140
Loeb, Jacques, 5
Lorand, Arnold, 68, 74, 80, 99, 132
lost youth, 8, 25, 67, 134, 206

Macfadden, Bernarr, 5, 81, 84, 141, 144, 157,
    167
Macrae, Eilidh, 139
Mallett, Reddie, 75, 211
manufacturers, 8–9, 13, 17, 59, 61–62, 67,
    71, 77, 97–99, 106, 122–23, 127,
    162, 165, 169, 171, 177, 181, 183,
    187, 190, 194, 196, 198, 200, 203,
    208, 212
marketplace, 12, 14, 41, 63, 69–70, 94–95,
    100, 103, 107, 114, 132, 135, 159,
    170, 176–77, 180, 191, 196, 198,
    200–1, 207
marriage, 1, 14, 63, 139
mass exercise, 139, 150
mass observation, 140, 154, 167
massage, 72, 76, 107, 111, 124, 128, 132, 140,
    158–59, 161–62, 164–65, 167, 175, 183,
    202
Massey, G. Betton, 113
Max Factor, 171
McCollum, E. V., 86–87
McLaren, Angus, 10, 29
meat, 19, 78, 85, 87
Medical Research Council, 87, 92
Mellanby, Edward, 92
menopause, 25, 73, 212
menstruation, 199, 212
mental capacity, 6
metabolism, 42, 69
Metchnikoff, Elié, 9, 61, 68, 74, 85, 103, 145,
    166
Methuselah, 53
middle-age, 6, 14, 69, 93, 144–45, 148, 161
middle-class, 2, 8, 13, 16, 146, 151
Middlesex Laboratory of Glandular Research,
    60, 181
military, 2, 5, 138, 140, 150, 152, 155, 208
milk, 54, 77, 84, 104, 200
Milk and Dairies Act (1914), 95

minerals, 19, 87, 89, 91, 98, 103
Mitchell, F. W. D., 45, 83–84
moderation, 11, 22, 40, 70, 74, 102, 104, 149
modernisation, 10
modernity, 77, 135, 148, 175, 202
monkey glands, 36, 39, 42, 45, 50–51, 57, 67,
    79, 156, 179
moral duty, 22, 83
moral ideals, 50
moral law, 8
moral panic, 8
mortality, 5, 7, 179, 203
Morus, Iwan Rhys, 14, 24, 106, 108, 135
motherhood', 139
Mr Sparks of St. Helen's, 124
Müller, Jørgen Peter, 122, 141–42, 144, 153,
    166, 168
Müsham, Richard, 30

Nacktkultur, 4
national security, 140, 167, 217
Nature, 32, 40, 75, 78, 80, 86, 98–99, 194, 210
nervous disorders, 16, 97, 157
nervous exhaustion, 13
neuralgia, 78, 117
neurasthenia, 20, 60, 120
neuritis, 124
New Thought, 51, 113
Nobel Prize, 12, 27, 92, 109, 117
non-naturals, 11, 21, 69, 76, 140
Nuglandin Cream, 182
Number Seven, 65, 162, 165, 186, 189–90,
    192–94, 201–2

obesity, 41, 69, 76–77, 79, 81, 120
old age, 6–7, 9, 20, 22, 30, 36, 39–40, 47, 54,
    57, 63, 74–75, 80, 83, 107, 112, 144, 160,
    164, 203, 211, 214
older men, 17, 34, 66, 146, 158
Order of the Golden Age, 68, 82–83
Organon Laboratories, 65, 192
organotherapy, 9, 28, 31, 35, 59, 111
orgasm, 41
Orwell, George, 1–2, 138
ovaries, 25, 29, 41, 59, 129
Overbeck, Otto, 110, 113–15, 122, 126, 136,
    176, 216
Overones, 59
Overy, Richard, 13, 140
Oystrax, 98

Paris, 9, 27, 29–30, 45, 48, 64, 77, 110, 134,
    160, 179
Pariser, Carl, 30
Park, Hyung Wook, 7, 141

Parr, Thomas, 21
Parsons, Mrs Theodore, 5
patents, 114–15, 122, 126, 146, 176
patient experience, 126–27, 130
Pauling, Linus, 88, 102
pellagra, 87, 92
pensions, 8, 47, 57
perpetual youth, 53, 57
Phyllosan, 100–1
physical culture, 3, 5, 20, 80–81, 136, 139,
    141–42, 145, 149, 151–52, 154, 156–58,
    165, 167–68, 207, 213
physical education, 6, 11, 139, 167
physical jerks, 138, 145, 148, 153, 156, 158,
    170
physiology, 7, 9, 13, 15, 17, 19, 24, 29–32,
    35, 38–39, 42, 54, 58–59, 65, 69–70,
    73–74, 83, 87, 90, 102, 107, 109, 111,
    118, 158, 169, 174–77, 181, 187, 197,
    209, 211
pills, 13, 19, 59–60, 94–95, 98
Pitcairn-Knowles, Andrew, 77–78, 93, 99
Pitkin, Walter, 6
Pomeroy, 159, 172, 178, 187
Ponds, 16
popular culture, 11
pregnancy, 49, 139
primates, 27, 29, 66, 102
privacy, 106, 125, 149, 166
Pulvermacher Battery Belt, 106
Pure Food and Drugs Act (1906), 196

race, 8, 13, 34, 49, 62, 76, 140, 155, 204
radiation, 16, 132
radiotherapy, 18, 26, 207
radium, 18, 134
Ramus, Carl, 11
reducing, 69, 76–77, 79, 100, 136, 146, 176,
    200–1, 209
regeneration, 8, 36, 59, 100, 140, 211
rejuvenation
    as biological process, 15, 22, 90, 174
    of livestock, 47–48
    of the nation, 87
    as panacea, 66
    as prolongation of life, 5, 7, 57, 70, 104, 203
    as prolongation of youth, 15, 38, 54, 104
    relationship with longevity, 15, 26, 94, 144
    societal, 4, 13–14, 200
    surgical, 19, 25–26, 36, 62, 171, 201
retirement, 8, 14, 18, 76, 128, 207
rheumatism, 20, 31, 78, 95, 100, 120, 127, 134
rickets, 92, 120
Riposo Resort, 78

Rogers Vitalator, 124
Royal College of Physicians, 31, 40, 70, 84,
    149
Royal College of Surgeons, 30, 119
Royal Society of Medicine, 29, 35, 109, 128,
    199
Rubinstein, Helena, 107, 130, 160, 166, 171,
    177, 179, 181, 183, 185–86
Rutherford, Ernest, 51, 113, 136

Saleeby, Caleb, 84–85
Salvarsan, 2, 37, 212
Sanatogen, 101, 208
Sand, Knud, 34, 72
Sandow, Eugen, 5, 81–82, 141, 144, 146, 157,
    168
Schmidt, Peter, 36, 41, 71–73, 215
Schroth Regeneration Cure, 78
Schroth, Johann and Emanuel, 78
scientific authority, 16, 20, 22, 59, 83, 89, 115,
    175, 177, 181, 196, 204
scientific feeding, 68
Scott, George Ryley, 215
Sea-Vitoid tablets, 97
seaweed, 99
Seaweena, 99
secularisation, 8
self-help literature, 9–10, 93, 102, 154, 165
senescence, 5, 8, 25, 68, 73, 75, 102, 105, 205,
    215, 217
Sengoopta, Chandak, 7, 9, 16, 18, 28, 33–34,
    64, 73, 203, 206, 211
senility, 72, 215
Senior, John, 24, 107
seventy, 71, 79, 115, 156–57, 214
sexual desire, 38
sexual intercourse, 41
sexual potency, 10, 13, 17, 62, 73, 97, 215
sexuality, 10–11, 33–34, 67, 73, 202
sheep, 47–48
skin, 2, 11, 13, 15–16, 19–20, 23, 28, 41, 59,
    62, 65, 70, 78, 89, 95, 120, 123, 129–30,
    132, 142, 155, 158, 161–62, 165, 169–70,
    172, 174, 176–78, 180–81, 183, 186–87,
    189–91, 193–94, 196–98, 201–3, 207,
    209
skin care, 2, 5, 12–13, 17–20, 23, 95, 129, 131,
    155, 158–59, 162, 165, 170, 174, 177–78,
    181, 186–87, 190–91, 193, 195–98,
    201–3, 207
skin food, 16, 21, 65, 175, 177, 182, 186–87,
    189–90, 193–94, 196, 198, 201–2, 208
sleep, 11, 18, 70, 76, 141, 149, 207
Small, Helen, 10–11

soap, 164–65, 175
soldiers, 6, 118, 129, 150, 161
spermatic economy, 36, 67
Stanley Cox Ltd, 124, 127
Stanley Hall, G., 75
Starling, Ernest, 24, 31, 117
Steinach, Eugen, 7, 9, 15–16, 18–19, 25–27,
    29–30, 32–33, 35–38, 41–42, 47, 51,
    53, 55, 57–58, 61, 64–66, 70–71, 74,
    79, 111, 129, 179, 196, 201, 205,
    208–9
sterility, 60
stomach, 74, 77, 124
Stuart, Grace, 113
sunlight, 39, 131
surgery, 2, 15, 17–18, 25, 29, 31–32, 36, 38,
    40, 59, 62–63, 66, 71–72, 74, 111, 164,
    170–71, 174, 176, 179, 183, 201, 206,
    208, 212

tablets. See pills
Tarzan, 51
tennis, 154
Tesla, Nikola, 119
testimonials, 20, 101, 114, 156, 176
Testrones, 59
The Gland Stealers, 17, 45, 209
The Monkey Gland (cocktail), 45, 210
Théiron School of Life, 88–90, 93
thirty, 1, 79, 117, 124, 150, 195–96, 202
Thompson, J. J., 136
throat, 160–61, 164, 192, 195
Tomes, Nancy, 16, 171
toxins, 75, 85, 166
tuberculosis, 20, 120

ultraviolet rays, 123
United States, 3, 5, 9–10, 16, 26, 28, 51,
    54, 64, 72, 81, 88, 94, 103, 107, 139,
    141, 148, 150, 171, 179, 196–97,
    199
University College London, 117
upper-class, 13, 16
UV lamps, 39

vasectomy, 33, 72
vasoligature, 35, 71–73
vegetables, 94
vegetarianism, 9, 19, 68–69, 76–80, 82–83,
    86–87, 89, 104
Vienna, 9, 32–33, 35, 38–39, 53–55, 58, 72,
    111, 126, 129, 179, 195
Vienna Youth Mask, 126, 129
Viereck, George Sylvester, 26

vigour, 9–10, 19, 25, 29, 37, 59, 61, 63, 81, 88,
    98, 110, 148, 172, 175, 217
Vikelp, 98
Vincent, Swale, 35, 206
violet ray, 105, 107, 114, 118, 120, 122, 124,
    126, 128, 135, 159
virility, 8, 17, 34, 38, 59, 203
vital energy. See vital force
vital force, 19, 100, 142, 210, 216
vitality, 13–14, 18, 20, 22, 26, 34, 56, 58,
    61–63, 74, 76, 81, 88–90, 92, 97–99, 103,
    139, 146, 148, 151, 161, 168, 170, 181,
    183, 213–15
Vitalogy, 148, 157
Vitamin A, 86, 97, 194, 202
Vitamin C, 19, 101–2, 194
Vitamin D, 104, 194, 202
Vitamin E, 19, 98, 194
Vitamina, 98
vitamines. See vitamins
vitamins, 7, 11, 16, 19, 65, 67, 70, 73, 81,
    83–84, 86, 88–91, 93, 95, 97–98, 101–4,
    107, 169–70, 177, 194, 197–98, 202–3,
    208
Vivarium, The, 33, 39
Vi-vims, 62–63
Voronoff, Serge, 9, 15–16, 18–19, 24, 26–27,
    29–32, 34–36, 38–42, 45, 47–48, 50,
    53–54, 56–58, 61, 64–65, 67, 70–71,
    73, 77, 79, 111, 179, 196, 205,
    208–10

Watson & Sons Ltd., 109, 123–24
Weber, Hermann, 11, 70, 75, 84–85, 89, 102,
    104
weight gain, 33, 42, 70–73, 104
weight loss, 29, 70–72, 74
Weimar Republic, 3–4
Weismann, August, 5
Wexler, Anna, 107
Willaims, Leonard, 59
Willi, Charles E., 5, 11, 174, 176–77
Williams, Chisholm, 119
Williams, Leonard, 30, 40, 58, 66, 73, 77, 132
Women's League of Health and Beauty, 17,
    140, 151–52, 154, 167
working-class, 1, 13
World Health Organisation, 5
World War One, 8, 14, 16, 20, 22, 30,
    57, 67, 69, 75, 80, 85, 94, 108, 120,
    140, 150, 157, 168, 174, 209, 211,
    217
World War Two, 82, 93, 98–99, 101, 139, 154,
    157, 167, 207, 209

wrinkles, 10, 13, 20, 22, 38, 91, 95, 132, 158, 161, 170, 172, 175, 182, 187, 191, 195–96, 200

X-rays, 25, 37, 39, 56, 208

yeast, 88, 94–95, 102, 154
youth movement, the, 167

youthful appearance, 1–2, 14–15, 21, 53, 93, 174, 176, 203, 217

Zander Electropathic Institute, 108
Zeissl, Maximilian von, 37
Zweiniger-Bargielowska, Ina, 8, 70, 77, 154, 167, 170